Living Yoga

PSYCHIC STUDIES

Editor: Stanley Krippner, U.S.A.
Managing Editor: Irene Hall, U.S.A.

Advisory Board: V. G. Adamenko (U.S.S.R.), Duncan Blewet (Canada),
Francoise Gauquelin (France), Ruth Miller (U.S.A.),
Don Parker (U.S.A.), Alberto Villoldo (Puerto Rico),
Joseph Wolf (Czechoslovakia)

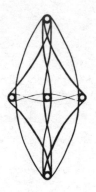

WAKING DREAMS Mary M. Watkins
SUGGESTOLOGY AND OUTLINES OF
SUGGESTOPEDY Georgi Lozanov
LIVING YOGA Swami Satchidananda

Other volumes in preparation

Living Yoga

The value of Yoga in today's life

Swami Satchidananda

and

Sant Keshavadas
Swami Nirmalananda Giri
Rabbi Joseph Gelberman
Rabbi Shlomo Carlebach
Ram Dass
Br. David Steindl-Rast, O.S.B.

AN INTERfACE BOOK

An INTERFACE book, published by Gordon and Breach Science Publishers, Inc., New York

Copyright © 1977 by
Gordon and Breach Science Publishers, Inc.
One Park Avenue
New York, NY10016

Editorial Offices for the United Kingdom
Gordon and Breach Science Publishers Ltd.
42 William IV Street
London WC2N 4DF

Editorial Offices for France
Gordon & Breach
7-9 rue Emile Dubois
Paris 75014

Library of Congress Cataloging in Publication Data

Satchidananda, Swami.
  Living Yoga.

  (Psychic studies)
  "An interface book."
  1. Yoga—Addresses, essays, lectures. 2. Conduct of
life—Addresses, essays, lectures. I. Title.
B132.Y6S375   181'.45   76–53664
ISBN 0–677–05230–8

Introduction to the Series

American history is basically a saga of people concerned with external voyages. At first the exploration, exploitation, and settlement of a new continent occupied their attention. This was followed by the development of industrial empires at home and the assertion of diplomatic power overseas. Then came the most distant venture of all – the probes into outer space.

In recent years, a small but growing number of Americans has placed a high priority on internal events and inner growth. Some individuals view this in terms of a spiritual quest while others consider it a voyage of self-discovery or a search for personal fulfillment.

The roads taken to attain these goals vary. Of current appeal are the quick and hazardous openings offered by LSD, the explosive encounters found in sensitivity training, the deep probes provided in Jungian psychotherapy, and the creative routes implicit in development of artistic and scientific creativity. Awareness of Eastern wisdom has helped facilitate the process of many seekers. Yoga, Zen, and the Oriental disciplines are all alternatives to consider, either in their original form or in the synthesis offered by many contemporary scholars.

A synthesis with the external world is offered by research workers in psychoenergetics, psychotronics, and parapsychology who seek to explain the relationships among consciousness, energy, and matter.

A Reformation of Consciousness may well evolve as, for the first time in its history, the entire gamut of human hopes, aspirations, and teachings are available for us to grasp and to incorporate. Our series is a part of this reformation and should shed light upon the road taken by many curious travelers.

Stanley Krippner

Humanistic Psychology Institute
San Francisco, California

Hari Om Tat Sat Brahmaarpanamastu
I offer this unto OM, that Truth which is Universal.

Lokaa Samastaa Sukino Bhavantu
May the entire universe find peace and joy.

Preface

Dear friends, I am really happy to see this beautiful book, *Living Yoga*, coming out. I sincerely hope that it will help people all over the world to see what is being done in this country in the name of Yoga. We hear a lot about unity and the oneness of all the religions and about finding peace, but in these ecumenical Yoga retreats, we are actually seeing and experiencing this living oneness. For ten full days, hundreds of people come together and live together in silence, in harmony and in joy.

There is a joy in being together, in living together, in thinking together. And this is the need of the hour. We have faced, we are facing, the terrible consequences of having lived apart, of having talked in terms of differences, and of having divided man and man, in all possible ways. We have divided in the name of caste, creed, color, race, religion, sex, country, language. By such division, where are we now? We are facing a great crisis.

We have been sent into this world to live together, to enjoy the world, to make use of the great potentiality of nature. But because of these differences we are making use of this very nature for our own destruction. And the whole world has understood the danger of it. That is why we are coming together. Everyone knows there is no other way to find peace and harmony except raising above all these man-made differences, realizing the oneness of the spirit, realizing our own true nature.

This is not the first time the world is facing such a crisis. Many a time in the past it has faced such situations. Always at such times, somehow, through something or somebody, nature itself provides us with a proper lesson. And Yoga today has taken up that place. In the name of Yoga, people are coming together from all over the world, to realize that oneness of the spirit.

This is the aim of Yoga. And this is the entire purpose of all the religions, philosophies, institutions, whatever name they use: to help us realize our true nature, that peace within. If you cannot have peace in you, you can never change things outside. So let us realize our own selves, and thus see the same Self in everybody. We'll be able to love everybody equally then. We'll be able to raise above these physical and mental differences. We'll be able to bring peace and harmony into the world.

And this is the purpose of this book also. This book is a record of a retreat in which hundreds of persons of all backgrounds came together in harmony and in which many teachers from different spiritual backgrounds testified to the oneness of the spirit. I want to thank those who made this possible: the retreatants themselves, who took part so beautifully; the staff of the Integral Yoga Institutes who conducted the retreat in the true spirit of selfless service; and our teachers for those ten days, who gave of their time, energy and wisdom. We owe a debt of gratitude to them all.

I hope that this book will inspire many more people to join the thousands of others across the country and all over the world in living the truths of their own faiths and of the sacred science of Yoga. We are seeing this happen. We are seeing people all over the world beginning to lead such yogic lives. And so we are really seeing the dawn of such an era. This is my sincere belief and prayer.

Swami Satchidanand

Contents

Preface vii

Introduction 1

FIRST DAY

Getting Yourself Together 8
Swami Satchidananda

SECOND DAY

The Divine Name 18
Sant Keshavadas

Stick to One Thing 27
Swami Satchidananda

Questions and Answers on Different Spiritual Paths . . 36
Swami Satchidananda

THIRD DAY

The Three Mirrors 44
Sant Keshavadas

The Secret Behind All Religions 51
Swami Satchidananda

Questions and Answers on Attachment 60
Swami Satchidananda

FOURTH DAY

Let Go of the Cat's Tail 70
Swami Nirmalananda

Undoism 88
Swami Satchidananda

Questions and Answers on Self-discipline and Meditation . . 98
Swami Satchidananda

ix

FIFTH DAY

There Is Only One Light 108
Swami Nirmalananda

The Tenth Man 121
Swami Satchidananda

Questions and Answers on the Philosophy of Yoga . . . 131
Swami Satchidananda

SIXTH DAY

Wholeness and Holiness 138
Rabbi Joseph Gelberman

Internal Cleansing 147
Swami Satchidananda

Questions and Answers on Health and Diet 150
Swami Satchidananda

SEVENTH DAY

Practical Advice on Meditation 166
Swami Nirmalananda

Questions and Answers on Meditation 175
Swami Nirmalananda

The Mother and Her Children 180
Swami Satchidananda

Questions and Answers on Women, Family Life and Monkhood 193
Swami Satchidananda

EIGHTH DAY

A Great Morning 206
Rabbi Shlomo Carlebach

Satsang with Swami Satchidananda's Devotees . . . 217

NINTH DAY

Honoring Siva 240
Ram Dass

The Three Gunas and the Three Types of People . . . 257
Swami Satchidananda

Questions and Answers on Parents and Children . . . 270
Swami Satchidananda

TENTH DAY

Staying Together 278
Brother David Steindl-Rast, O.S.B.

Questions and Answers on Yoga and Christianity . . . 287
Brother David Steindl-Rast, O.S.B.

Closing Comments by Retreatants 298

Concluding Comments 311
Swami Satchidananda

Glossary 317

Photographic Illustrations . . . *between pages 164 and 165*
Rim Ritscher
Sri Ram Austin
Shanthi Zupan

Introduction

The world is now one world. There is one humanity. In recent years we have seen this reality taking shape more and more clearly. There are no longer any countries or cultures which live in isolation. In this country, we live with images of events around the world. In the 1960's, awareness of a small nation on the continent of Asia, halfway around the globe, was brought into every home every evening by the television news. With the manned landings on the moon, the unity of the earth became both visible and imperative.

This growing unity is not limited to the physical or geographical level. As cultures come into contact with one another, they affect each other profoundly. Each absorbs from the other what it needs most. And once the superficial differences have become familiar, both become increasingly aware of values that they share in common.

This process, while it is now taking place on the popular level, has been going on for a long time. In the past centuries, with the colonization of Africa and Asia by the European nations, this influence was primarily in the direction of the transmission of European culture — literature, technology, forms of government ideals — to the non-European peoples. More recently, the converse has become more and more apparent. Even in the 19th century, the influence of Eastern thought upon America was great, through the writings and teachings of Emerson and Thoreau. But this influence was indirect. On the popular level, the traditions and teachings of Eastern culture remained exotic and distant.

This is the case with Yoga. One of the first representatives of the Yoga tradition to come to the West was Swami Vivekananda, who came to America in 1896, to attend the World Parliament of Religions in Chicago. At this convocation there were representatives of most of the great faiths of mankind, and the theme of the Parliament was the underlying unity of these religions. Swami Vivekananda was the most eloquent spokesman for this theme, electrifying the audience not only with his words but with his very presence. Young and vigorous (he was then only 30 years old), Vivekananda made several sojourns to America and Europe in the next few years, establishing centers and teaching students, sowing the seeds for future developments.

Until quite recently, however, the word Yoga remained relatively un-

1

known in this country. It was generally identified with India and Hinduism, so that it was often assumed to be some form of religion or cult,
limited to persons of that culture or faith. At the same time, the images
associated with Yoga were usually a little exotic: someone sitting in a
trance in a Himalayan cave, or standing on their head. The idea seemed
to be either one of withdrawal from the world or the adoption of
difficult and dubious postures.

During this time there were a few books available in stores and
libraries for those who were interested, but very few teaching centers and
even fewer genuine representatives of the tradition. In addition, some of
the books, and some of the instruction, were misleading. Most of what
was presented was simply Hatha Yoga, which is only one branch of
Yoga, the one which is concerned with the physical practices. When this
aspect was taken to represent the whole of Yoga, the result was often a
distortion, even a reversal, of its true significance. What was originally
meant to be a physical means (among other means) for transcending both
the body and mind and for realizing spiritual truth, was transformed into
a kind of body cult, whose aim now was to be youthful or attractive.

In the past decade, however, this partial understanding began to be
replaced by a more complete understanding. This change began with a
great upsurge of interest, primarily on the part of young people, not only
in Yoga but in all things spiritual (especially if a little exotic). In conjunc-
tion with this interest, teachers began to arrive in this country who could
speak authentically about their tradition, not merely because they knew
about it but because they themselves were living examples of it.

It was these teachers who began to clarify the real significance of the
Eastern teachings, by translating them into terms which made it clear that
these teachings were not something essentially foreign and strange, but on
the contrary were universal. In doing so, it became more and more obvious that these teachings were merely using another language to say
things that had always been said – though perhaps largely forgotten – in
the Western traditions. In this way, these teachers, by presenting the full
spiritual significance of a tradition such as Yoga, also helped to restore the
full significance of the Western traditions as well.

This, in turn, helped to broaden the significance of a very important
process that had already been taking place for some time in the West: the
ecumenical movement. This was (and is) a movement within the Christian world to reunite a badly divided Christianity, to restore a greater
degree of understanding, cooperation and unity among the different
Christian churches.

But by the present decade, with the increasing and inevitable rapprochement between East and West, the idea of ecumenism has taken on a broader meaning, in addition to the original one. Ecumenism can now be said to be a process whereby all the great faiths of mankind can come to a greater understanding and acceptance of each other: not a merging, but a realization of a common essential ground, upon which all their differences rest.

It is here that teachers of a tradition such as Yoga can serve well. For Yoga is not itself a religion and therefore does not in any sense compete with the different faiths (secular as well as religious). Instead, it is a practical and scientific system whereby a man or woman can experience for himself or herself the fundamental spiritual truths and experiences that are talked about in all of the faiths. And so you find men and women of all faiths (or of no particular religious commitment) incorporating Yoga into their lives.

One of the teachers who presented the teachings of Yoga in its fullest sense was Swami Satchidananda. Before coming to America in 1966, Swamiji (as he is known to his students) was head of a Yoga ashram, or spiritual compound, in Ceylon. Born in South India in 1914, Swamiji had followed various careers, primarily in the technical industries, until the age of twenty-eight. At that time, he began his full-time spiritual quest. He had read and been influenced by Swami Vivekananda, whose work in restoring India to her own spiritual heritage was as great as his work in transmitting it to the West. As a spiritual seeker, Swamiji studied and lived with many of the great spiritual teachers of modern India, including Sri Aurobindo and Ramana Maharshi. Finally, Swamiji met his Master, the renowned Sri Swami Sivananda, in the foothills of the Himalayas, and in 1949 entered the Order of Sannyas (monkhood). Swami Sivananda was a world spiritual teacher, whose teachings always emphasized the universality of spiritual truth, who saw no difference between people of different faiths, and many of whose disciples have traveled and taught around the world.

In 1966, a young American seeker came to Ceylon and met Sri Swamiji. Impressed by the wisdom and simplicity of Swamiji's teaching, he persuaded him to make a short visit to the West, including a two-day visit to New York. But when Swamiji came to this country, he was surrounded by hundreds of eager students and the intended two-day visit stretched into months. This was a time when there was an explosion among many young people in this country, an explosion in drugs, politics, music, religions, and life styles. Those who flocked to hear Swamiji and to learn from him were mostly young, and mostly those who had been experimenting with drugs. There was a genuine seeking on their part for something more real, more satisfying, than what they had grown up to understand. Many of them had dropped away from their schools, their faiths, and their families. Those who became involved with Swamiji felt that before this they had not found what they were seeking – that drugs were not an answer. They did not really know what they were looking for until they met him, and saw in him something they wanted to be themselves.

Because of this interest in him, Swamiji, after returning to Ceylon for a while, came back to America, and in 1967 became a permanent resident of this country. He became the director of the Integral Yoga Institutes (IYIs) and centers began to open up in cities across the country. These were teaching centers, offering a great many classes in Yoga to the general public; but they were also living centers, where boys and girls who wanted to follow the teachings of Swamiji and to help each other in this practice stayed. Many who lived in these centers were fairly young, and for many it was a new kind of home, one they could accept more easily than their own and where they could grow up. They were dedicated and hard-working, but at first not very disciplined. Often they had rejected their own religious background. But slowly they began to absorb the disciplines of Yoga and the spiritual teachings of Swamiji, and to live them. In doing so, many came to a new appreciation of their own tradition, to come back to it in a new way.

During these years, Swamiji spoke and traveled widely. While he was based primarily at the New York IYI, and for periods of many months would give talks every Friday evening at the Universalist Church in New York City, he also traveled around the country and made two world tours. He spoke at schools, prisons, drug rehabilitation centers, religious institutions and to various groups of spiritual seekers. In 1970, he opened the Woodstock Music and Peace Festival.

That year saw the beginning of something new. By this time there were many people who had heard the message of Yoga through Swamiji. There were many people who had begun some kind of Yoga practice, either on their own or by coming to the classes at the IYIs. Many of these people were interested in exploring Yoga in more depth, in experiencing what it had to offer in an environment totally given over to the practices. They were interested in the kind of experience one would have in living at a Yoga ashram or center, but they were not ready or able to commit themselves to such a complete change in the outward form of their lives. It was at this time that the first Yoga retreat was held.

The idea of a retreat is to remove yourself for a limited period of time from your day-to-day life; to go to an environment that is conducive, and there to follow the various Yoga practices with others who wish to do so, under the guidance of a teacher. The retreat may last anywhere from a weekend to ten days, and during this time complete silence is observed, in order to deepen the inwardness and to maximize the benefit of the practices. Each day's activities are scheduled, from early morning meditation to the evening *satsang*, or get-together, in which Swamiji or some other teacher talks and answers any questions that have been written out for them. Throughout the day all the other practices are given: the physical practices of *Hatha Yoga*; periods of meditative work, or *Karma Yoga*; chanting, which is one of the main practices of *Bhakti Yoga*, or the Yoga of love and devotion; and lectures, which could be said to represent *Jnana Yoga*, or the Yoga of knowledge. So each day is a blending of all the different Yoga paths, an integral whole in which there is something for persons of every temperament, and which taken together constitute an integral way of life.

The first of these retreats took place in the summer of 1970. It was held at Annhurst College, located in northeastern Connecticut. And, as many of the subsequent retreats have been, it was ecumenical in its nature, being conducted not only by Swami Satchidananda, but receiving assistance from teachers of other faiths as well: from Brother David, a Benedictine monk; from Rabbi Gelberman of the Little Synagogue in New York City; and from Father George Maloney, A Jesuit priest from Fordham University.

In the next few years, many other retreats were given. And then, in June of 1973, a very special event took place. It was also a 10-day retreat, but by far the largest to be held: largest in terms of the number of people attending, in terms of the number and variety of spiritual teachers taking part, and even in terms of physical locale. The retreat was held in Monticello, New York, on 1500 acres of wooded property belonging to the Dominican Order of the Catholic Church. There is a beautiful lake on this property, and on one side is a boys' camp, on the other a girls'. These camps provided the many cabins and the dining space for the men and women retreatants. In addition, overlooking the lake was a large wooden structure, a meeting hall, where everyone would gather for the morning talks and for the evening satsangs.

More than 600 people, of all ages and backgrounds, and from all parts of the country, came to this retreat. It seemed to signal something: that the interest in Yoga had now become a widespread phenomenon in American life and that this interest was now on a serious level. People seemed to be looking for more than postures or a few techniques; they seemed to be looking for something that would have meaning for their lives as a whole. Each day they would crowd together in friendly silence in the satsang hall, to listen to the different speakers.

The arrangement of the retreat was that each day a guest speaker would give a morning talk, and that each evening Swami Satchidananda would talk and answer questions. There were a number of topics that several of the speakers developed: topics such as the different spiritual paths that one could follow, depending upon one's temperament; the topic of meditation and the use of a *mantram* or sacred sound vibration; and the question of different ways of life, that of married life and that of monastic. But as the days went by, it became clear that each speaker, in his own way and from his own tradition, was contributing to a common theme. This was the theme of a living spiritual unity.

As developed at the retreat, this theme brought the idea of unity or ecumenism to its fullest possible significance. In a world brought to a state of crisis by division everywhere – divisions between the races and the nations, between the sexes and the generations, divisions based on religious, political, economic and cultural differences – each of the speakers pointed the way to mutual acceptance and to an underlying unity.

They did so not by encouraging acceptance for its own sake or by advocating a merely external form of unity. Instead, they said that external ecumenism, or coming together, must be based on what could be called internal ecumenism – coming together within oneself. It is in integrating spiritual truth into one's own life that one is able to be of service to others. Ultimately, the basis of true world unity lies in the individuals realizing their own inner Self, that Self which is the same in all.

This was the message of the retreat. And the experience of the retreat was one of living these yogic truths in a practical way, day by day, under the guidance of masters in whom this ancient science of Yoga is a living tool. In making these talks available, we hope to be able to share both this spirit of inner unity and this practical approach to realizing it in our own lives. May the whole world be blessed with this peace and joy.

First Day

Getting Yourself Together

Swami Satchidananda

On the first evening of the retreat, after everyone has registered and put their belongings away, there is a light fruit supper. Then everyone gathers in the satsang hall. Swamiji comes and sits at the front of the hall, on a small stage that has been prepared, so that everyone can see him. He gives a short orientation talk, telling the retreatants about the basic purpose of Yoga and of coming to a retreat, as well as some particular points about what they would be experiencing in the coming days. It is a beautifully concise talk, bringing home the theme of living a yogic life.

Every time I see people coming to such retreats I am overwhelmed with joy just to think that there is hope for the world. People seem to be talking a lot about the future of the world. Many seem to be losing hope. Can we survive with all the troubles that are arising today? There seems to be turmoil everywhere, in every area, and yet at the same time there is a flash of hope. However large the darkness is and however long it has been there, the moment a small candle is there the whole room is lit. The darkness does not go little by little. It is gone in an instant. That is the power of light.

Each one of you is a candle lit by the light of Yoga. That is what makes me so happy in seeing such a large gathering. You have come a long way, leaving the world behind for these days. There is a spirit of renunciation certainly, to come here and spend ten days under all the disciplines and restrictions. This is not a comfortable holiday, but we seem to be ready to pay the price to find that light within. To have that light within and to share it with everyone we will have to work.

This night being an orientation night, we won't go too deeply into the philosophy and practices; instead, a few hints on how to make the most of this retreat would probably be helpful.

First, let us understand that a retreat is a place to "be treated," not to have treats. This is going to be a "concentration camp," or in a more yogic word, a meditation camp. Nobody will force your minds to concentrate; instead, you yourself have come forward to practice this.

The English word "retreat" has more or less the same meaning as the

8

Sanskrit "Antar Yoga." "Antar" means inner; "Yoga" yo
"getting it together" in your own terms. Inner Yoga me:
yourself together. Together means to gather. You have gotten
and have come here to gather everything and put it in its place.
are together.

Our life is not centralized. It is scattered all around. We are on the cir-
cumference of a spinning wheel. The farther away from the center you
are, the harder it is to balance. If you want to enjoy peace on the wheel,
where must you go? To the very center. So, those who have become
tired of spinning and imbalance want to come to the center and find
peace. That is what is called being together, or concentration.

The mind must find its proper place. It must be one-pointed. Then
whatever you do will be a success and will also be Yoga. That is the purpose of Yoga.

That is the main purpose of this retreat. In the coming days, always be
in your center, even while you are doing many things, mentally and
physically. Whatever you do, keep an awareness of your center. That is
what is meant by Antar Yoga. You are doing many things; at the same
time, your mind is centered, you are doing one thing. By observing what
you are doing, you are almost a double personality. Really we are all
double personalities. Ordinarily, it has a different connotation, doesn't it?
If you look at somebody and say, "You seem to be a double personality,"
he gets a little disturbed. But the fact is that every one of us is a double
person: the doer and the observer.

It's something like an actor on a stage. He is observing his own actions.
He plays different parts without forgetting himself, his true nature, who
he is. But on the stage he is totally different, his name is different, his
form is different, his make-up is different, his action is different. A man
who may not even have a dollar in his pocket can come out as a king on
the stage. Even while he plays the part of the king he knows he is a
pauper. One is the true Self, the knower of everything. So, whatever you
do, keep an eye on it. "What am I doing? Why am I doing this? Who is
it that is doing? Am I the observer or the doer? I cannot be both at the
same time." With this attitude you slowly go into your center, the very
core of the person.

Here I would like to use a term which is not really used in the proper
sense. I want you all to be self-centered. But not self-centered meaning a
totally selfish man; not with a little "s" but a big "S." That kind of action is not selfishness, but self-fulness. That is what I would like to remind
you of. Whatever you do, whatever be the emotions, whatever be the
feelings, whatever be the thoughts, what's behind it? Then you are really

doing something as an Antar Yogi. And once you become the witness, you will see your own mind, your own body, doing many things, and as a witness you can pinpoint the motive of the mind, what it is doing, what it should do, what it should not do, till gradually you are able to exercise your mastery over the mind. The main purpose of Yoga is to keep control over the mind; to have a good control over the modifications of the mind, not to allow the mind to go as it wants but to control it to go as you want.

That is why these disciplines. In the normal life we don't seem to do this. You should do it in everyday life wherever you are. But somehow, you seem to have lost control over the mind. It's spoiled. Imagine a person buys a beautiful puppy and he pets it too much and it grows and grows, but wild. Because of his affection for his pet he just allows it to go anywhere and do anything. No manners, not house-broken, it goes and breaks the house, it does anything it wants. All of a sudden one day the master says, "What is this? This is not a nice thing any longer. It is always disturbing. At the same time, it's a lovely dog, I don't want to lose it. I paid so much. When it plays, it plays wonderfully. I enjoy it. But when it does terrible things, I don't even like to keep it here. What am I to do?"

Then one of your friends might say, "I know a good trainer. Why don't you take him there and put him in school? He will train your dog and bring it back to you. Then when you say 'Sit' it will sit, 'Walk' it will walk, 'Roll' it will roll."

"Oh, that seems to be a good idea. Where is the training place?"

"Oh, there in Monticello. Within 10 days they train it."

"But can I be there to watch?"

"Oh yes, you can be there. You leave it in their hands but you can be there. You will see how they are trained."

That's what happens here. Our mind is like a restless monkey. Even a dog is better. All the great saints, sages, thinkers say it is a restless monkey, restless as an insane monkey. Not only insane, insane and drunk. Not only insane and drunk, but bitten by a scorpion, too. An ordinary monkey itself will not keep quiet, and when it becomes a little insane you can imagine. And when it gets drunk, still worse. If at the same time it is bitten by a scorpion, no one can control it. That's what they say about the mind. That is what brings all these calamities, not only within the individual, but within the community, within the family, within the country, within the whole world; and probably we are not going to spare even the other planets. We are going to "train" them also, as we got trained here.

That is the purpose here: to train your mind. Training means discipline. Without discipline, there's no training. The very first training, the first rule, is to train the mind. It is rather difficult to handle the mind directly, though, so you have to control the instruments through which the mind functions – the senses. Sense control is indirect mind control, as the mind cannot function without the senses. The tongue, the ears, the nose, the eyes, and the touch – those are the five important senses. And of these five, the most important, the most turbulent sense is the tongue. It is just a piece of flesh; but my goodness, so many troubles are brought by this tongue.

The tongue is the most important sense because it does double function – tasting and talking. That is why they gave it the name tongue, also "t". Tastes, talks, tongue: "t," "t," "t." So the first discipline has to be with the tongue. That's why silence is to be observed all through the ten days. Try to maintain the silence. You won't lose anything. You'll gain a lot. People lose much of their energy by talking. So by observing *mouna*, silence, you will save a lot of energy. Of course, you will see all these new faces and sometimes your old, old friends whom you have not seen for several years. "How can I see their face and just keep quiet without even saying, Hi!" If you keep saying "Hi" to everybody, they will go "high" and you will stay *low*! After the tenth day you can say anything you want.

Think that you are just an individual here. You don't know anybody else. You have come for a purpose. You are doing that. Even if a couple have come here they should not treat themselves as a couple, they are individuals. Otherwise your mind cannot be indrawn always. So always do things in a meditative way, watching your own feelings, your own thoughts. If you are going to do that constantly you won't even have time to look outside and talk to somebody. It's something worth trying. We have been talking all these years, so that's why we say, seriously, "follow this!" That doesn't mean you must always be tense. No. Relax! No harm. Just a smiling face, but don't look at a particular face and smile. Just keep a smiling face always. Like a rose smiles always. It doesn't smile at you or at her. It smiles. That's all. So all the faces must be like roses, smiling. But don't smile at a particular individual. Let the smile come from within. Feel relaxed. That will help you a lot.

So the first point is that silence is to be maintained at all times. The other point also has to do with the tongue. Not talking and simple tasting. I saw the menu for the retreat a couple of days ago. It really seems to be a good menu. Then I thought, later on, that you might have been having much more delicious things outside, so to you this is rather rough. You will notice that very soon, if you are really interested in delicacies or your tongue is too long, maybe in a day or two you will go. So eat for the sake of the stomach, not for the sake of the tongue. Don't worry about the taste. Suppose you are really terribly hungry, and somebody gives you an old piece of bread. If you're really hungry, you won't even worry about the taste. So if you can relish the food, and if you can keep the tongue without talking, you have acquired a little mastery over your tongue.

So you are putting yourself into all kinds of tests. In the scriptures we read that in old days men who wanted to conquer themselves, conquer their mind, gained the mastery by doing a lot of penance, quite a lot of *tapasya*. They used to meditate for hours and hours without any movement, having a fire around them. They used to fast, just live only on water. We need not do that kind of tapasya or penance. But in the retreat, you will undergo certain hardships. Take it as tapasya. I don't know. I am only preparing you for these things. Probably after a couple of days you may say, "What's all this, we seem to be enjoying everything." I really want you to enjoy. If you accept it, you enjoy it. If you don't accept, even a palace will not bring you happiness. Remember the purpose. We are here to train the mind, to gain the mastery. That's why these restrictions are given. That's why it is a kind of "concentration camp". Not for anyone else's sake but for your sake. Don't think that you are following the schedule because somebody said to. If you don't get up at five o'clock, I'm not going to suffer. So try it. If you want, you can do it. Let nothing stop you.

Is there anything more I should say? (One of the staff says, "Karma Yoga.") Karma Yoga, I see. Well, there is a part which is called Karma Yoga. To get a sample of that they give a Karma Yoga period, a work project, here. This period is more or less like going to the office or going to the shop. At eight or nine o'clock you go to wherever you work. Instead of that, you will be going and doing some work which will be the Karma Yoga. But in a way, everything is Karma Yoga. Selfless action is Karma Yoga. Even when the hand takes the food and puts it in the mouth, the hand is doing Karma Yoga because the hand is not going to taste anything. Does the hand say, "I am not going to taste anything, so why should I work?" And the tongue — it just tastes, it is not going to keep it so, in a way, every minute we are doing selfless service, all for the sake of the life within. But, in the normal sense, when we go out and work to do something, as Karma Yoga, we do it as a selfless service to others. We are doing it for the benefit of others, not for our own sake with a selfish motive. It is a way of life which you should be able to do when you go back. Otherwise it is just a mere philosophy which you cannot use in daily life. That's why Yoga never ignores anything. The very life is Yoga.

So this retreat is a kind of baby life, which you will use later on the outside. So, when you go home, when you go to the office, say, "This is the Karma Yoga period now. I am going to the hospital, I am a doctor, I am a nurse. I am a businessman." Just as you are doing the Karma Yoga not for your own sake, neither are you going to the office for your sake, but for the sake of the humanity. That's what we learn from doing Karma Yoga, to treat every activity outside as Karma Yoga.

It's in the attitude, that's all. You don't need to change anything. Just change the attitude. See that you have a proper attitude behind every action, proper motive, a selfless motive always for the benefit of others. So when you get a project, don't think you are being made to do some work, so that some work can be gotten from you. Your mind can comment, "Oh that's a nice way of getting things done, huh. We come here and we pay and we have to work for them. I could work myself, in my home. Why should I come all the way here, giving them money and then doing all this work, huh? This is a nice way of doing things, and you call it retreat?"

The mind will bring all these pictures. At least, I had such pictures when I was like you, sitting there, and I heard the teacher saying this. Even as he was talking, I thought, "Oh, this is all kind of flowery, I don't know. He must have something behind it." So remember, constantly your mind will bring all these feelings. It will try to discourage you, because it knows you are trying to train it. So know that your mind is playing a trick on you. Don't allow your mind to play any tricks. As I said, you couldn't train your pet, so you have brought it. And in a way I could say that I am a master trainer. At least you treat me as a master trainer, and I have my associates. Even if a capable surgeon comes and does some things, there should be the junior doctors and nurses and nurse's aides. So we have many aides to do the operation. But once in the hands of the surgeon, if you are going to take it half way, it won't be a nice thing. Wait patiently until the whole operation is well done.

So be patient. You will have well trained minds. But cooperation is necessary. It all depends upon how much cooperation you give for this operation, isn't it? Cooperation is necessary for operation.

One more thing about the Karma Yoga. When you get a project, the tools and materials must be returned in proper condition at the end of each period. Sometimes we have to say this. You know why? According to yogic teaching every action should be a perfect one. Everything should be treated well, properly, gently, with love. If you are going to dig a hole with a shovel, love the shovel, use it well. Don't hurt it by hitting it over a stone. When you finish the job, clean it. Thank the shovel. "With your help I dug the hole. Thank you."

I have saved myself many times from accidents, from getting stranded on the road, because I thanked my car. Don't think that only animals are pets. You can make your car a pet, shovel a pet, ax a pet. They all have feelings. They all are pets. So that's why when you do something do it perfectly. Bring the tools back. Put them back nicely in their place. That way we learn a little discipline. We learn to love things, at least the things we use. Then gradually we will learn to love other things also. So there is a kind of discipline in everything.

As a whole, we request that you be always indrawn and make your day a continuous meditation. Think that you have renounced. You have renounced the world, or in other words, more drastically, you are dead to the world. Think that there is no Mama, no Papa, brother or sister or family outside. You are dead and you are here in a different world, astral world or whatever world you want to call it. Because only when you learn to die well will you know how to live well. So think that temporarily you are dead to the world. No radios, no newspapers, no telephones. And don't worry about the world. It will carry on. Certainly without you or without us all, the world can still survive, maybe in a better way. So don't worry about it. Have a temporary renunciate life.

Make your day a continuous meditation. This is most important. Think that you are always meditating. Even though on the schedule it says there is a meditation period — that doesn't mean you are not meditating at other times. You are always meditating. When you eat, meditate on your eating, meditate on the food you are eating. Think of it, concentrate on it. Don't think of something else when you are sitting at the table and eating. One thing at a time. That's what is called meditation. And that can be done when you mind is totally in it 100%, and that is what is called togetherness or Yoga. So Yoga is not something that is to be practiced only in the meditation room or only when you do some Hatha Yoga, but all through your life, day and night, morning and evening. Whatever you do, let it be done as a yogic practice or as a meditation. That is the purpose of the retreat in short. And the more you will follow it, the more you will realize the benefit. You will not regret it. I am telling you this today but only after a few days will you know how true it is.

I really want you to enjoy this retreat. I really want every one of you to experience something beautiful, so when you go back to face the world again you will have the proper attitude, with more control, with more balance of mind and body. That is the purpose of the retreat.

It's not that easy. Know that. But all I say is, be patient. Probably within three or four days you will begin to feel, "Ah, that's really good." So be patient and try to cooperate. You will never regret later on.

Again, thank you for your patience and for coming. Thank you so much. I wish you a very, very good night, restful sleep. See you in the morning. Thank you.

Second Day

The Divine Name

Sant Keshavadas

Sant Keshavadas, like Swamiji, is a universal man. He cannot rightly be labeled as belonging to just one particular faith or philosophy; he is not just a Hindu or Buddhist or Christian or even a representative of just the East or the West. He has completely identified with that Cosmic Essence which we call God, which is at the center of every religion. It is with this understanding that he calls his philosophy "Cosmic Religion." But, unlike Swamiji, almost every word he speaks seems to be couched in the terms of the tradition out of which he came, namely Hinduism, and so to understand his message, it is very helpful to have some understanding of the Hindu tradition.

All over the world, Hinduism has the reputation of concerning itself with countless deities, peculiar forms of worship and strange and diverse practices, all so varied and complex as to give the impression of pantheism or paganism. This, however, is not at all the case. The very basis of Hinduism is the concept of the One Ultimate Reality, usually called Brahman, *the unmanifested Oneness or God. Being infinite, omniscient, omnipresent and omnipotent, He (or It) can and does manifest as many forms, in fact, as all the forms which we call the universe or the manifested world. In the aspect of the Creator of the world, the Hindu calls Him* Brahma; *as the sustaining power,* Vishnu *and as the force which is continuously destroying and regenerating, He is* Siva. *As fire He is* Agni, *as wind,* Vayu, *as the Mother Nature He is given feminine names, etc. But however many names and forms you may attribute to Him, He remains as One God. It is this understanding that One Supreme Intelligence is behind all the apparent varieties that gave birth to the science of Yoga. To turn back to that One, to experience and feel one with that Supreme Power, is the aim of Yoga.*

The original scriptures of Hinduism are known as the Vedas. *They are a huge collection of hymns, stories, instructions and philosophy which is thought to have been revealed to the minds of the ancient Yogis during their meditations. In a way, they are supposed to explain God and the creation of the universe, but the Yogis say that actually the vibration of the Vedas themselves created the universe. Just as the Bible says, "In the beginning was the Word and the Word was with God and the Word was God [and] . . . all things were made through It," so also, the Hindu would say that Brahman alone was in the beginning and when He spoke the "Word" (the Vedas), the world was created.*

It is this understanding of the power of the word or sound which is also at the root of the practice of repeating certain mantrams *or sound formulas. The sound vibration is the subtler aspect of any form and gives rise to that form. By repeating the sound, or name, of a*

18

certain aspect or form of God, you awaken the qualities of that aspect in your own system. Eventually your entire mind is tuned to that vibration and you have the union (which is the literal meaning of the word Yoga) or, as is said in the West, "communion" with God. The most basic sound vibration is OM *out of which all the possible sounds come, so by repeating* OM *one could go back to the origin, the Creator, to God.*

The last sections of each Veda are known as the Upanishads, *and the philosophy they contain is called* Vedanta *or literally, the culmination of the Veda. This is the philosophy of the One Absolute Brahman and His realization. The path of Jnana Yoga comes directly out of these Upanishads: to realize the Absolute through direct perception of the Truth of It through the pure intellect. Later other scriptures appeared which depicted the Supreme One as having name and form. The Absolute, in His aspect of Vishnu, the preserver, was depicted as* Sri (Lord) Rama, Sri Krishna, Krishna Chaitanya *and many others. The idea behind it was that, as the preserver, the helper of humanity, God should come in a human form that could be spoken of, worshipped, thought about and emulated. One cannot directly imagine the formless Absolute, but when clothed in human form, with name, form and attributes, as Rama, as Krishna, as Buddha, it is possible. The stories told of these Incarnations form the scriptures of Bhakti Yoga, the Yoga of devotion.*

Two of the most important of these scriptures are the Mahabharata *and the* Ramayana. *The Mahabharata (The Great India) tells of India at the time of the incarnation of Sri Krishna. It tells the story of a huge family feud which culminated in a civil war which was finally won by the side whose leaders took refuge in Sri Krishna. The epic is a wonderful allegory of the human condition, of the internal war of every spiritual seeker between the huge force of bad habits and ignorance and the (at first) tiny force of positive aspiration and faith in God, where the positive force ultimately wins out through surrender to the Lord. One famous section of this epic is called the* Bhagavad Gita, *which is often called the "Hindu Bible." It contains Krishna's instructions to Arjuna, the chief warrior of the "good" forces, where Sri Krishna explains why one must fight against the evil and how to do it with the proper understanding to attain the highest good, namely Liberation or God Realization. The Gita is considered to be one of the main texts on Yoga because it is not concerned with any superficial rituals or religious trappings but deals directly with how to perfect and expand the individual so he can achieve God experience.*

The Ramayana tells the story of Vishnu's incarnation as Sri Rama. Rama's story is that of the exemplary life; He is portrayed as the perfect man, both in the worldly and spiritual senses. He is a righteous King, a perfect husband, a skilled warrior and a sage. When righteousness demands, He gives up His kingdom without a murmur to make good His father's word and again, when righteousness demands, He takes it back and rules it perfectly and with the same ease with which He gave it up.

In the traditional Hindu path of Bhakti Yoga, these incarnations are worshipped as the personal God; their stories are studied and emulated and the devotee takes himself to be separate from the Lord. But the final goal is to merge into God Consciousness or Krishna

Consciousness or whatever name is given to it. As Swami Satchidananda's master, Swami Sivananda, said, "Bhakti begins in two and ends in One."

Sant Keshavadas is a Bhakti Yogi, a man of devotion. He doesn't teach standing on the head, meditating in Lotus posture or restraining the breath. His message, in short, is: Chant the name of the Lord, surrender yourself to Him, feel His presence and become one with Him. Santji (as he is called) communicates this teaching through the traditional expressions of Bhakti Yoga: stories, chants and songs. The stories are culled mainly from the ancient stories of the Incarnations and the chants and songs are either those composed by past devotees or of his own composition. As he speaks, Santji often spontaneously bursts into song accompanying himself on the harmonium, a kind of small portable hand organ. He often requests the retreatants to join him in chanting. He doesn't merely lecture, he brings everyone into the experience. He doesn't so much teach as just pour forth his love of God and humanity.

Santji was born in 1935 in a small South Indian village near Bangalore in Mysore State. As a boy, he tended cows, just as Vishnu's incarnation as Sri Krishna is supposed to have done. At the age of eleven, he was caught in a storm and ran for shelter in a temple dedicated to the Lord as Sri Panduranga, *another form of Vishnu. He spent the entire night there and had the vision (or darshan) of Sri Panduranga, in which the boy was told to spend the rest of his life spreading the holy name of God. He has been doing it ever since. (Though along with this, he has also married, raised a family, taken a law degree and written over thirty-five books about spiritual life!)*

His story seems almost unbelievable, like something out of the stories and myths of ancient sages and saints. But being in Santji's presence is also like that; you feel like pinching yourself to see if you're really experiencing in the normal level or not. Santji makes no pretensions of being a modern or sophisticated person. He is just simple and pure like a child; in short, a saint. And he seems to be able to lift others also to that spiritual level, to know that such things are possible; that even in this modern complex world, such simple, pure devotion and grace is not only a possibility but indeed a reality, at least for this man.

It was largely due to Santji's presence and influence that the entire retreat seemed to be taking place in a world apart from the ordinary: in some divine realm. And it was not so much the philosophy in his words that found its place in the hearts and minds of the retreatants, as the vibration of joy and God experience and the sheer inspiration of this holy man on whose lips was always the name of God and in whose heart always shone the Divine Light. Here was a man who is living Yoga: in the world, serving the world, but never tainted by it.

In this first morning talk, Santji introduces everyone to his elevating vision of spiritual life, calling one and all to feel the Lord's presence through repeating His names. He especially brings out the point that what name you call Him is not important, as "Truth is One, many are the names."

Salutations to the Lord! Adorations to the most beautiful nature and day, people and environment, to Swamiji Satchidananda, Nirmalananda and all the beautiful people arriving from all over the country. I feel as if I am on the bank of the Ganges river facing the Himalayas and all around me are the Himalyan Yogis sitting and chanting and meditating on the holy names!

The Upanishads declare the glory of OM, the most holy name. "O fighter after Liberation, O fighter of lust, rage, arrogance, infatuation and attachment: take the help of OM as your bow; your soul is the arrow, and God is the target. Without any wavering, strike at the Lord, the Brahman, and let your soul be totally dissolved in Him, never to return to the round of rebirth."

This is the teaching given in the *Mundaka* Upanishad. In the Vedas it is said that God is the quintessence of all the essences and the essence of the Veda is the name: OM, Ram, Shyam, Christ, Jehovah, Buddha – any name you want to call. That is why the Vedas say: (Santji chants) "Truth is One but many are His names that the sages have found in their meditations." The Vedas, which are the oldest spiritual record of humanity, declare this fundamental truth: Truth is One but many are His names.

God and His names are transcendental. Jesus said, "Hallowed be Thy name." This divine name is the silken thread which will always bind you to God. You will feel Him in your heart, both within you and without. The repetition of His name is very efficacious. Even if you are constantly in the midst of activities, sing the name of the Lord. Swamiji always teaches: "Hari OM, Hari OM." Those who chant Hari OM will be "hurrying home" to God. Realizing this, let us constantly remember God. "Where thy treasure is, there shall thy heart be also." If God is thy treasure, the heart shall be always filled with God.

God is within, God is without, God is above, God is below, God is everywhere. The sun shines with billions of tons of light every day, bringing us the glory of God. We see it every day, but because it is an everyday phenomenon, we think it is, after all, "just nature." If the sun were to come just a little nearer to the earth than 93 million miles, what would happen to you and me is well known to us. So everything is kept perfect in nature, because of God. Man knows that. During times of troubles he seeks shelter in God, in Nature, in saints. And then like the footprints on the sandy shores of the ocean, which are immediately covered by the extra sand and by the billows dashing against the shore, the *Maya*, the veil, comes and he forgets God. Unless we remain in the company of spiritual people we may forget Him for months and years. So you will know that you are loving God, that you have Bhakti, when your heart feels like a fish out of water when you cannot have spiritual company or when you cannot concentrate your mind on God. That is the test of how much you are loving God.

The Hindu scriptures have an aphorism describing this Bhakti which says that when you are pining for the Supreme you are like the fruit of a certain tree found in India. As soon as it falls to the ground it immediately returns to the tree and clings to it. The same way, if in the midst of some activity the mind is severed from God, it would want to go back to God again and cling there. That is Bhakti: to again and again remember our beloved God until, as the Bhagavad Gita describes, we realize everything is in Him and He is in everything. (*He chants*:)

> "Hey, *Arjuna*, one who sees everything in Me and Me
> in everything shall never lose sight of Me, nor I of him."

This is the description of the highest realization, the highest devotion. From birth everyone of us has wanted love and affection; we give affection and we receive it. You can live without food for some time; you can live without many conveniences but nobody can really live happily without affection and love, for love is God. When we love, we really live. When we can't love, when we find difficulty in loving, when we cannot share with anyone, we find that our hearts have become dry and drained; we feel as if we are dying, collapsing. There is no more charm in life. You may not have much knowledge; you may not have much scholarship. But, if you have love, you have everything. Love is the essence of all the scriptures. We will sing now a *kirtan* which was sung by the great Bhakti Yogi, *Tukaram*. When I sing "Panduranga," you answer, "*Hari Jai Jai!*" (which means, Glory to God!)

(*All sing*: "Panduranga"; *retreatants*: 'Hari Jai Jai!'")

As it says in the Psalms, "Make a joyful noise of God"; from head to toe all the seventy-two thousand psychic nerves should respond, "Jai Jai," "Glory to God, Glory to God!" That is joyful noise. In the glorification of God, the psychic centers (*chakras*) open. When the divine name is chanted, every cell of the human body is divinized.

The great mythological devotee of Lord Rama, *Sri Hanuman*, became immortal, the foremost servant of Lord Rama. Why? Because of constant repetition of His name, "Rama Rama Rama Rama." The meaning of the story is this: Hanuman is your life current, the *prana*. We mainly waste the prana in gossip and other useless activities, but Hanuman sanctified every breath by repeating Rama with every one of the 21,600 daily breaths. When the breath is sanctified, the prana reaches every nerve throughout the nervous system, so that every cell of your body becomes charged with "Rama."

People have tensions and difficulties about various things. Their constant worry brings ulcers and difficulties. We see varieties of tension and diseases all over the world. When you worry about so many things, naturally it affects the body. So why not worry about Hari, about Rama, about the Lord? "Rama, how are you? Rama, where are you?" Feel that realizing God is the real purpose of your life. What is the purpose of life after all? To make some money? To build something? To eat something; drink something? To while away our time?

The musician bhakta, *Kabirdas*, sang, "You ate, drank, slept and snored. And one fine evening, death comes and knocks at the door and you say, 'I am not ready.'" You cannot say, "You are dismissed; get out." He is not going to wait there even for five minutes. Then and there he is going to take you.

"Well, I have not seen my son who is away from here. He is expected to arrive this evening. Please wait."

"No."

"My wife is pregnant. I would really like to see whether it is a girl or a boy. Then I will die."

"No."

"Oh, a wonderful lunch is prepared. I would just like to taste a little. Why don't you join me?"

"No."

"Oh, God of Death, please, I am a very important person for the whole world. If I die, everything is going to stop."

"No."

So, in the midst of all activities, death may come to us. Then we will think of the value of the time we have wasted in gossiping and unnecessary things. At the time of death, when the wind, phlegm and bile get stuck in the throat, how can we remember to meditate on God? We are unconscious that death is approaching us, while we have so much karma which is not worked out. If we die in that state we will die with great fear of leaving all that to which we were attached in life. Before death comes we should learn the art of dying. How? By living in God right now and realizing the immortality of our existence. The soul is immortal. It was there before the body was born and will be after it dies.

Right now, just meditate for a minute. Do you require any proof that you exist? Right this moment, here! Feel the presence. We can just experience it. It is light now. Do you need proof for that? No. Same way, it requires no proof to know that you are. Even in a dark room, does anybody need to tell you you are there? No. You *know* that you are there. You cannot see with your eyes but you know through the consciousness that you are. Moses asked God, "God, what is Thy name?" God said, "I Am. I Am that I Am." We can experience this too. That which sees through your eyes, hears through your ears, tastes through your tongue, smells through your nose, is the "I Am." When you dream you see various phenomena, though there is no physical light, no physical sun, no external moon, no fires, no electricity, no candle. So by what light do you experience your dreams? It is by the light of the consciousness, the "I Am." And when you are in dreamless deep sleep you forget your body, your name, everything is forgotten. Engagements are forgotten. The mind is resting; the ego is not present. There is no dream, no waking, just deep sleep state. For seven or eight hours at a stretch you are enjoying it. What is it that witnesses the continuation of the heartbeat? What is the power which digests and assimilates the food which you have partaken? What is the power that keeps the memory of all the engagements for the next day? What causes the continuity of all the bodily functions? When you wake up in the early morning, you remember all the things you have to do. And to the question, "How did you sleep?" "Oh, very fine, wonderful." It is our experience every day, every day. We are not conscious of this great Witness within us. This beautiful friend, guide and philosopher is always walking with us. You are searching for him elsewhere, rather than in your own heart. "The Kingdom of Heaven is within." God is within; His name is "I Am."

You identify the "I" with the ego and then think the ego to be the "I am." That's the problem. Take the ego away and remember the "am". "Am" is always springing from "OM." Feel this OM pervading the whole body and every cell vibrating. Let the upper lip be the Heavenly Father; the lower lip the Holy Spirit. Feel the Father and the Holy Spirit come together when you chant OM. OM OM OM. Just as by rubbing firewood, the fire that is within the wood emerges, so by the coition of the two lips, with meditation on the sound produced, God emerges from the human soul. Let us chant OM.

(All join Santji in OM chanting.)

The divine name: Om, Ram, Shyam, will give us the key to unlock the mystery which is hidden within us, the real "I Am." Let us sing:

(All sing: I Am that I Am, I Am that I Am ...)

The name gives you strength; the name is the treasure. It introduces you to the Supreme, the Immortal. Once a mongoose confronted a huge serpent and began to fight with it. The huge cobra bit him and the poison that was injected into him caused him to reel. Well, there was a medicinal herb growing on a bush nearby. He knew of it and immediately partook of the herb and got back the strength. So he came back and fought with the cobra again. Again the cobra bit him. Again the mongoose runs to the bush and eats the medicinal herb. More strength comes to him and he fights with the cobra again. Every time the cobra bites and injects the poison, the cobra is losing strength, but every time partaking the medicinal herb, the mongoose is gaining strength. Finally the mongoose kills the snake. This is what the divine name does.

Unfortunately we have *six* snakes to fight. Lust is one huge powerful cobra. Anger, the arch enemy of spirituality and meditation, which can destroy a hundred years of penance in a minute of outburst, is another huge cobra. Arrogance is another great enemy, another serpent: "I am beautiful, I have everything." And jealousy, the most poisonous one which is spoiling the whole world and society. And greed is the doorway to hell. And finally attachment, one of the biggest cobras to work out. *Paramahamsa Ramakrishna,* the great Indian saint of the last century said, "If a man knows that a snake is about two miles away from the place where he lives, he will be scared. If he knows that a poisonous snake has entered the door of his bedroom, unless he is a snake charmer he is really afraid. But yet man happily rests in this world not realizing he has six serpents constantly biting his mind-mongoose within him."

As soon as we wake up, one or two cobras simultaneously bite the mind and we are repulsed; we are reeling. We need some pill, some tea or coffee, something to tantalize. We feel really tired though we have slept eight hours. Some news, some talk, makes us tired again. So why not take the medicinal herb? The mongoose knows that as soon as the serpent bites, he must run to the bush and eat the herb. And that medicinal herb is the name of God.

So, this is the essence of my talk today. You have a medicinal herb. You have no cause for sorrow or fear. Take the holy name of God and you will be strong. You can face the battle of life wholly by the power of meditation on the divine name. Sing the glory of God; constantly hum His name. Let us sing a song which means "Go on singing the name of God . . . " (*Santji sings:*)

> "Gatae Chalo Manme Hare Krishna Rama
> Gatae Chalo Manme Hare Krishna Rama . . . "

And now let us conclude with this prayer:

> Lord, Thou art my Father; Thou are my Mother Earth Divine.

Thou are my relatives, my friends Divine.
Thou are the Wisdom, the wealth of all.
Thou art my everything, O my God of Gods.
Let there be Peace above, Peace below, Peace within, Peace without, and Peace everywhere. Thou art the Peace that passeth all understanding. Om shanthi shanthi shanthi.

Stick To One Thing

Swami Satchidananda

Many retreatants find the first day somewhat strenuous with the early rising, the silence and all the unaccustomed restrictions and programs and if it were not for the anticipation of again being in Swamiji's company for the evening satsang many would probably rather go straight to bed than anything else. But somehow, everyone seems to feel that the satsang is the high point of the whole day. Many even come to the hall early to reserve a space as near the stage as possible and some sit in meditation to be more receptive to the talk.

Sant Keshavadas has already set the mood of the retreat: love and joy and singing the praises of God. There has never been a Yoga retreat quite like this one before. Usually they are quiet and the participants indrawn. The individual and group energy builds slowly over the days while each retreatant goes deep within and it is only towards the end that all begin to collectively realize the vibration of love and joy which has been silently building up all along. But at this retreat the Bhakti spirit is well awakened from the very beginning. Even before Swamiji enters the satsang hall, the whole group is chanting loudly and joyously.

Swamiji enters the hall glowing in his beautiful orange robe and followed by a 'retinue' of (also glowing) disciples in their white and yellow pajama-like clothes. Everyone stands up out of a spontaneous feeling of respect and many bow their heads and fold their palms together in the traditional Indian greeting. When everyone is seated Swamiji begins by leading chanting of his universal mantra, "Hari OM, Hari OM, Hari Hari Hari OM" and everyone follows for several minutes. He then begins the program with a few remarks on the great benefit of satsang or company with spiritual people and practices.

Well, first I would like to ask you a question. How do you like it? Are you getting into the retreat? Are you feeling any hardship or resentment about anything? I know it's a little soon to be asking this, but still, if something is really nice it doesn't take long to know it. There's a South Indian proverb which tells of the great benefit of the good company. Even if you have it for only one day, it says, if it is really good company, it will bring tremendous benefit. It will go to the very depth of your personality. Like a seed sown in beautiful, well prepared soil, it will send its roots to the very core of the earth; such is the benefit of satsang or the spiritual company. So you should be already feeling something after even this one day.

27

Of course some of you may be finding it a little difficult also. Sometimes the enjoyment of good company is like eating sugar cane. Have you ever had this experience? I don't mean candy or sugar but eating the long whole cane itself. The sugar cane is delicious and sweet if you know from which end to eat. If you begin from the top end it will be sour; begin from the bottom, it is so sweet — magic! The good company can be like eating sugar cane from the top end downward. The more you go down, down, down, knot by knot it will get sweeter and sweeter. It begins sour but ends with the maximum sweetness. But the bad company is something like eating the sugar cane from the bottom up. In the beginning it is all beautiful, tasty, fantastic. If someone asks you, "Oh, how was the party last night?" "Oh, fantastic!" If you go to another the next day, it's a little less nice, the next day a little less, and it ends up with a sour taste.

So don't think it should feel all beautiful the first day. Good things can be a little difficult to accept. The human tendency is to go into the ordinary shallow things. The very nature functions that way. If you put a stone on the tabletop, just a little push is enough to drop it to the floor. There's no difficulty at all. But to lift it back up to the table needs some effort. Lifting up is always more difficult than pushing down. The nature always pulls everything toward it. That's its gravitational pull. It's a kind of tug-of-war. The nature tries to pull you down to be worldly, to do worldly things and cater to the senses. It is really difficult to resist that and to pull up.

Even in our modern technology you see this. The moon capsule that has to land on the moon is carried by the Saturn rocket. The purpose of the Saturn rocket is to take the module beyond the gravitational force and the maximum fuel is needed for this. So you spend the maximum amount of fuel just to get out of the gravitation. Then things are easy; you can just float. But the astronauts cannot float within the gravitational force. If by any chance, they should get caught before they get out of the gravitational force, they'll be immediately thrown to earth and get powdered!

So, you see, religion or Yoga is nothing different from science. We are all being pulled by the nature's force which is called *maya* according to the Vedantic scriptures — the illusory force. It's easy to succumb to that but to get out of it we need a lot of fuel, a lot of energy. So, save all the energy you can and fire the rocket when the weather is clear. Once you get away from the gravitational force, you don't need any help, you can just float.

At this point, Swamiji enters into a presentation of the universality, the broadmindedness of the yogic approach. While each of the seven participating teachers was characterized by their broad spiritual perspective, it was clearly Swamiji's function to synthesize the entire experience. This universality and ecumenical spirit was the very keynote of the retreat, but within this context most of the other teachers mainly expounded upon some one particular approach. Santiji and Rabbi Shlomo laid out the path of Bhakti or devotion, Nirmalananda, the path of renunciation and inward worship, Rabbi Gelberman stressed a down-to-earth joyful integration with the life around us (seemingly a direct counterpoint to Nirmalananda) and Brother David balanced the scales with his clear logical approach. But it was Swamiji who, again and again, took the various threads of all these approaches and wove them into a tapestry to show that all the designs fit beautifully into the whole, that all have one common goal, that as the Upanishads *say: "Truth is One but the paths to it are many."*

The point which was particularly stressed in this evening's talk was this: though all the ways are fine, though all are beautiful, we must take up some one path or practice and stick to it. It doesn't matter what you choose, but take it and go deeply into it.

Many people ask me, "What is Integral Yoga? What is *your* technique? You call it Integral Yoga. Is there any special technique?" Everything is special as long as it fulfills the purpose. That's all. If it's not going to fulfill the purpose, it's of no use. Do anything, try anything. If you say, "Well, I don't know what to do."

"O.K., try this."

"Well. I don't seem to like it."

"O.K., then try the other one."

That's why we don't stipulate, "This is the only way." No, according to your taste and temperament, do something. If you like playing the drum and going into ecstasy, singing and chanting, go ahead. Probably within a week or two you might be nearing the gates of heaven! If you are attracted that way, if that's your temperament, fine. But you may say, "Oh, what is this, some crazy people jumping and dancing, I don't understand. I'm not interested in that." Then you are not fit for that. But you don't need to get discouraged. That doesn't mean you are not fit for anything. Your taste is different. You can go to another restaurant.

In Bhakti Yoga you have all the worship and chanting. But in *Raja Yoga* you use the will. Probably you have heard people say, "I can do it myself. I don't need anybody's help. All I need is just a hint. Just tell me what to do and I'll do it all." To such people, I say, "Okay, take Raja Yoga, apply your will, control your senses, sit like a diamond, like the

Rock of Gibraltar. Acquire victory over your posture, your *asana*. Sit for three hours, not even winking."

In fact, if you can do that, you don't even need to worry about concentrating the mind. When I was living with a Swami named Sadhu Swamigal at Palani Hill Temple in South India, he used to tell me, "Don't worry even if you can't concentrate that much. It will all come by itself. Just learn to sit quietly. The control of the mind can come later because the mind is a lot subtler than the body."

See, I can easily control my finger. If I want to close the fist I can easily do it and keep it closed as long as I want. It is easily controlled. But we can't control the mind that easily. So apply the will to the physical part first. Sit quietly in any posture you like. But choose one position and see that you don't move any part of your body, not even the eyelids. If you close the eyes, keep them closed; if open, keep them open; if halfway, then halfway. Any way is okay, but be steady. If you could stay in that one position for three hours, you could easily control the mind. Nothing else would be necessary for you.

So you have to begin somewhere. If you can control one thing, you can easily control the other things also, but you have to begin with something. This is shown very well in one Indian school of thought which is mainly presented in a series of sixty-three stories. These stories are translated into English as the *Sixty-three Nayanar Saints* by my master, Swami Sivananda. If you happen to come across the book, you will see it is just some simple stories, sometimes just one page for one story. If you read all the stories, the one running theme is "Stick to one thing. Decide on one thing and stick to it."

Each of the sixty-three *Nayanar* saints did this. They just decided on something and stuck to that — even at the cost of their lives. Remember this because man loves his life more than anything else, is it not? We all say, "Honey, I *love* you" and "Oh, I treasure the necklace, I adore this." Even: "My beautiful body, I adore it; my fingernails, I must take extreme care of them. I should insure them for ten million dollars."

How many people insure their fingernails? It's fine, but if they treat them as the thing which will bring them happiness, and then that falls sick — say there is some kind of septic in the finger and the doctor says, "You won't survive if I don't amputate" — which will you prefer, your life or your ten million dollars worth of fingernails?

"Please cut it away as soon as possible. Save my life."

He cuts that. If another two weeks pass and he says, "It has gone up into the arm."

"Take it away; save my life."

"It has gone into part of the intestine."

"Cut it away."

"Half the lung damaged."

"Cut it away."

"One eye."

"Pull it out."

What is the idea? What is it you want to save even at the cost of your arm, intestine, lung and eye? What are you ready to renounce all these things to save? *Life*. So which is the dearest honey to you? The life is the most dear, the closest thing for anybody.

But, unfortunately, that cute fellow, God, didn't want to spare even that. "The most dear thing to you is your life so I want you to be ready to forego that; then you will get Me." It is easy to offer a banana or a candy or a flower. Some people see a flower on the way to the temple and pick it and offer it to God. How easy. You have money; you buy some fruits, candies or even build a temple and offer it. But are you ready to offer your life? God wants that. Because He gives Himself to you, He wants you to give yourself to Him totally. Fair business. That is what you see in the sixty-three Nayanars.

Just to give you an example: one Nayanar was a total illiterate. He didn't even know A,B,C,D or E. He would never even take shelter in a school area even in the rain. When it rained, he'd say, "No, I don't want to go there," and he'd run somewhere else, he was such an illiterate man. But he is worshipped as a saint in every Siva temple today as one among those sixty-three, just as we worship the illiterate fisherman apostles who followed Lord Jesus. The illiterate follows the saint quietly, but the literates wonder if he could be a real saint. "He doesn't seem to smile at me. Why should he do this? Why should he do that? He's never written any books . . . " They try to analyze the saints. But the illiterates are like children. This Nayanar was one among them, totally illiterate.

So when he saw everyone going and worshipping at the Siva temple with bananas, flowers and coconuts, lights and palm leaves, he had a curious idea. (It sounds funny, but I'm not making it up; you could read about it yourself.) He said to himself, "Why does Lord Siva want all this oil, honey and milk? Does he need all this? He seems to be wanting only those nice things. Suppose I give him something different? Will he accept? God must accept everything. So I'm going to give him a new kind of *puja* (worship). What kind of puja can I do? The easiest will be, every day I'll take a stone and throw it at Him. Instead of throwing a flower, I'll throw a stone at Him. And unless I throw a stone, I won't eat that day. That will be my puja."

It's something like, unless you finish ten *malas* (rosaries) you won't have breakfast. (I don't know how many people do that. If breakfast comes the mala will go. "Mala is always there; I can do it at the office." It can easily be postponed but breakfast cannot be postponed.) So, many great devotees used to take such vows. They will not eat until they do the thing. This man had decided not to eat until he threw a stone at Lord Siva in the temple. This went on for a number of days and he stuck to it every day. It was very easy to pick up a stone and throw it; not very difficult. After a while he started feeling a little proud. He thought, "I must be very clever, even more so than God."

All of a sudden, one day, the test came. Mysteriously, he couldn't find a stone that day; he saw only huge rocks which he couldn't lift or throw. Sometimes you come across situations like that, eh? Just this morning they wanted to put a stone in front of my tire. My secretary had to spend at least fifteen minutes going around looking for one, even in this rocky area; they were all too big. So, he was looking around and around and no luck. Time passed on and on. His stomach was pinching. He said, "No, I can't eat. My vow is to do this before I eat."

The whole day passed. He felt tired, slept, got up in the morning and again searched for a stone. Days went by; he couldn't eat. Then he thought, "Oh my God, are you testing me? What a fool I am, huh?"

Suddenly he thought, "Hey! I have a stone!" and he clutched his own head. He had forgotten all about the head, hm? "Here I am carrying a stone! I can do it now!"

He tried to wrench his head off and he was almost fainting with the pain, but he couldn't wrench it off. He was almost dying. Then a mysterious voice from somewhere came: "Oh My dear son, I am happy with your devotion. Open your eyes and see Me."

So, he opened his eyes and saw the vision of Lord Siva. "I am happy with you. You stuck to your vow, even at the cost of your life. You don't need to do anything else. You have proved that you care more for Me even than for your own life. That's all I wanted."

So, even today, he is worshipped in Siva temples. Almost all of the sixty-three took vows like this. Simple ordinary vows, but they stuck to them.

So, what is their technique? Some mysterious initiation? "Come quietly, I'll give you a mantram." No, if you really want something, you don't need to even hear about all these mantras and *tantras*. Decide on anything you want. Stick to it and you'll reach the goal.

What is it you want? God? You'll get it, no doubt. "But when?"

When you don't want anything else except God. It's easy to say, "Oh, I want God." But are you serious in your wanting? Are you ready to die for it? Or if you don't get it right away, do you look for an easy way, a short cut, something cheap, someone to give it to you easily without your doing anything? You want everything: your life, your body, your wealth, your beloveds ... and you want God also. What a big dedication, hm? Don't deceive yourselves. If you really want spiritual life, be sincere.

A man once came to Sri Ramakrishna. "Sir, how can I get God? I want God."

"Are you sure?"

"Yes, yes."

"You don't want anything else?"

"No."

"Okay, come with me. Before I give you God, you must take a bath."

So, Ramakrishna took him to the lake and asked him to bathe. In India, before you get initiated you take a couple of dips under the water. So when the man just dipped down, Ramakrishna held his head under the water. The man was fighting for his life, but Ramakrishna kept him there. Almost at the verge of his losing everything, Ramakrishna took his hand off.

"Oh, ah, oh ... hey! What happened?"

"Then Ramakrishna asked him, "What was it that you wanted when you were under water?"

"A little air, sir."

"What happened to your God?"

"Who thought about God? I only wanted a little air."

"Did you think about your wife?"

"Swamiji, how did I have time to think about my wife when my breath was not there!?"

"Did you think of your bank balance?"

"Please, don't bring up all these things. Nothing could save me except a little air and that saved me."

"Ah, so you wanted only air. If you had even one tenth of that urge in wanting God, probably you'd get Him very soon."

See? Otherwise, it's just a modern fancy, like a kind of qualification. Everybody says, "Hah, I do Yoga; I go to this institute, that institute. I can chant; I can stand on my head for ten minutes; I do *pranayama*. And do you know? The *Maharishi* was my *guru*; I took initiation from him. I took initiation from Swami Satchidananda ... " They have fifteen gurus in their diary. "I took initiation from them all."

So, I want to stress this here: decide on one thing, stick to it even at the cost of your life. It doesn't matter what you decide. There you have the will; that's Raja Yoga. You *will* to do something and do it. And you *will* do it even at the cost of your life. But if you feel, "Oh, I don't have that much will; I need somebody's help," then ask for help. Then you are a Bhakti Yogi. And if you say, "No, I don't want all this nonsense, going and asking. What is this God? What is it that I want? I really don't know what I want," then sit and wonder what you want. Analyze: "I want this; I want that. Who is that 'I' that wants everything?" Keep an eye on the "I." Find out who am "I" that wants everything. "Am I the body; am I the intelligence?" You don't need anybody then; just sit quietly and analyze, if you are the analytic type, the intellectual type. That's Jnana Yoga. "Who am I?" Ultimately, you end up with the answer, "*Soham, I am He; I am God.*" By self-analysis, find out that Self.

So, according to your temperament, your capacity, your inclination, decide on one thing. Don't keep on changing, digging wells in different places; you'll never get water. Everywhere, wherever you dig, there is water. But you can't get it that easily; you have to dig deep. By the time you dig ten feet, somebody may come and say, "Oh, stop this digging; do it over there instead; you can get water much more quickly." If you go there and start digging, then somebody else will say, "What are you doing? Over there is much better; leave this and go there." A third man will come and say, "Over there is the best place." If you keep on digging shallow wells, you'll never get water anywhere. The little water you do get will be only perspiration! Decide on one place. Dig it! What you are going to decide, I don't know. It's up to you. Wait till you decide, then once you make a decision, keep digging. And that will bring God to you. I'm positive about it.

If you really try that way and if you don't get God, come tell me and I'll tear off this Swami's robe and walk out. I challenge you, if you are serious. Otherwise, it's just a kind of fun. Go around and enjoy. Only to the serious students, I say this. You must have this firm decision, because the aim is something beyond all the petty things. All these things can be obtained easily: money comes and goes; beauty comes and goes. Even the body comes and goes. What is it that is difficult to achieve in this world? People spend fifty cents and all of a sudden they get three million dollars in the lottery. That kind of thing can come even without your effort, but God cannot come that way. He is the rarest commodity.

So, one again, the point is this: One thing at a time. You say, "That's what I do: this morning I did this; this afternoon I do something else, tomorrow, something else . . . " No. At first, take time, see everything until you desire one thing alone. When you desire one thing, stick to it. You'll get God there — because you have controlled the monkey mind, you have won over it. You tie the monkey to one place; you become the master of your mind. When you become the master of your mind, you *are* God. When you are a slave of your mind, you are man. What is the difference between man and God? God who is controlled by the mind is man. But a man who controls the mind is God. Once you control the mind it becomes beautiful. It's pure. In that purity, you will realize the true God in you. "Blessed are the pure; they shall see God." And that purity is in winning over the mind, not winning over the other man's mind. Win the victory over your own mind.

Questions and Answers on Different Spiritual Paths

Swami Satchidananda

At this point, Swamiji takes up a stack of question papers which the retreatants have written out. Since silence is the foremost discipline of the retreat, this is the main way for various puzzling points to be clarified and specific, personal problems solved. Swamiji reads the questions aloud and then replies.

When we have the feeling of great Bhakti, *should we try to develop just that, or should we keep an analytical attitude also?*

Actually, in this age, if you have the Bhakti feeling you should develop that more. Because the heart does not seem to be predominant in this age. So if you are fortunate enough to use the heart, do it. In the heart we can come together more. Never in the head. Have you ever heard any couple call each other "sweethead"? They always seem to address each other as "sweetheart." At the heart we can meet. Two heads coming together make terrible noise. They're hard nuts, no? But the hearts will melt.

So if you have a feeling of devotion, a Bhakti attitude, develop this. It is really something beautiful. And in Bhakti you can do many things. You can do puja (ritual worship). If you're a wonderful cook you can cook beautiful things and offer it to God. And then eat it! With your analytic mind you will just say, "This food has such and such vitamins. The analytic attitude should be combined with bhakti. Jnana should be combined with Bhakti. Then you know the principle – why you are doing, what you want to achieve. With that principle in mind, do something.

So without Jnana, Bhakti is of no use. You won't know what you are doing, or why; you'll be blind. And without Bhakti, Jnana is very dry. So there should be a nice combination.

Is the path to spiritual realization the same for men as for women? Are they equally fit?

Sure. No difference at all. What makes the men and women? Neither

36

their mind nor the spirit. It is only their physical side. The difference between men and women is only physical. For those who want to take the part of the physical, there is a difference. For those who want to take the part of the mental, both are the same. And spirit is primary because that is above "man" and "woman." Spirit has no sex. So both are equally fit for realization.

It all depends on how you feel. If you feel that you are weak, then you are not fit. This you see in men as well as women. Normally, whom do you call as woman? Not even by the sex of the body. If you are soft, if you are weak, you have the quality of the woman. If you feel the other way, if you do not need any support, you are a man. Man is like a tree, independent. Who is a woman? Hm? Wo-man. See, I am not creating anything. When somebody woos the man, she is the woman. Why? Because she does not want to stand all by herself. She has to woo somebody. She is not independent. So who is who now? If one is independent, then he is a man. He or she is a man. Call it any way you like.

There are many, many great women saints and seekers, both in the West and East. Take Mirabai, St. Theresa, St. Clare, so many. So spirit never distinguishes.

What do you think of the I Ching?

Well, I haven't heard of it that much. I'm sorry, but probably just let me talk about what I *do* know. But if you believe in the *I Ching*, I am not here to disturb your faith in any way. In fact, I don't believe in disturbing anybody's faith. If you have belief in that, then go ahead and do it because ultimately it is not the book which will help you but your belief, your faith in it which will help you. Have faith in something. It doesn't matter so much what.

Many people have faith in the Bible. They just open it, read that page and say the Lord is talking to them, telling them what to do. They believe in that. And if you really believe in that, you will get that. You are a hundred times better than a faithless man.

Even in the case of a faithless man, I say it doesn't matter. He says he doesn't believe in anything, but at least he believes in his *not* believing anything! So there is a hope for him that one day he'll believe a little more. Please don't ever think that I am putting anything down or criticizing. Open up to believe more and more. Let it take you to greater heights.

Please explain the significance of the symbols which make up your Integral Yoga symbol.

They are the symbols of the eight major religions. Some of them you already know. The Star of David — Judaism, the star and crescent — Islam, the Cross — Christianity. The wheel is Buddhist, the fire — Zoroastrianism, the Persian religion. The yin-yang, which everybody knows, is for Taoism, and above that is the symbol for Shinto. That's also a major religion in the East, Japanese. And then the other one is OM, representing the Hindu.

Of course, if you go into the OM you will have thousands of different varieties. It's something like the ocean. If you go into the ocean, you will find a little bit of Ganges water, a little bit of Missouri, Mississippi, hm? And a little of your own New York gutter water, isn't it so? It has everything in it. That's why it's called the ocean. It absorbs everything; it doesn't negate anything. So Hinduism doesn't deny anybody. It has room for everything. It has room even for an atheist. That's why Hinduism is Sinduism. *Sindu* means ocean.

Immediately you'll be thinking. "Ah, now that Swami is coming out with his true nature! Slowly trying to convert, huh? That Swami! See? Ultimately people come out with their own egoism. Conversion, huh?" Your mind can say that to you. In fact, Hinduism is not a religion at all. Or you could say, it is the real universal religion. It has room for everybody. And I say, it has room even for the atheist. Why not Catholic? Why not Jewish? Why not Islamic? That means everything is found in that. That's why it's not just a religion but it is a synthesis of all religions.

But unfortunately, it is not presented that way. If you ask a Hindu, "Are you a Catholic?" and he says, "Oh, no, I'm a Hindu," then he's not a Hindu at all. A Hindu can never deny any other and say, "I'm not that." A true Hindu will say, "I am that also." That's the true qualification of a Hindu. He's everything.

Imagine an ocean. Can the ocean say, "I'm not Ganges. I'm not Missouri. I'm not Mississippi?" It's all of them put together. So why should it think of converting anybody? They're already in it. The Catholic is a Hindu. The Buddhist is a Hindu. And that is the reason why when a baby is born, it is born a Hindu. Anywhere in the world, every baby is born as a Hindu. Afterward, they segregate the baby, baptize it as so-and-so. Until you baptize the baby as a Catholic, what religion does it belong to? He's not a Catholic. Well, he must have a religion of his own then. Every religion has a baptism. Hinduism has no baptism. Why?

Because why should we baptize? He's already a Hindu. Should I convert somebody as a Hindu? No. They're all born Hindus; then they get converted to something else for as long as they want. That's it. Every religion has a ceremony to put you into the religion, is it not? So, until then, can you say that you are religionless? Yes, you are religionless. You have no label. So a label-less religion is what you call Hinduism. It's like the sky. It's everybody's.

I have a personal mantra from the International Meditation Society — Maharishi Mahesh Yogi. Is there any use in my seeking another here?

No need. Stick to it. But if you do not have faith in it and if you cannot cultivate the faith, it is better to forget it and take another one. Probably your decision might have been too quick, because a mantram or any practice should be done with full faith. If you say, "I don't know what I am doing. I do not know if it is going to bring me anything or not, whether I got it from the right person or not or in the right way" – if you have a little doubt, get that doubt cleared or forget it. That's why I say, before you decide something, go, look at everything until you decide on one thing.

The main thing is your interest in it. Any practice without that interest, without that zeal, will not bring good results. It will bring results, but not as much as you want. One should practice with a lot of interest, for a long time, without break. These are the three qualities necessary: long practice, without break, with all the zeal. If you have all three in your practice, you will certainly reach the goal.

The teen-age guru, Maharaj-ji, says that he is the avatar for this Aquarian Age. Do you believe he is the sole avatar? And is the knowledge he says he gives the same as Integral Yoga?

I believe that we are all avatars. We are all the incarnations of God. God made man in His own image. If you do not want to accept this, then you accept at least somebody as the avatar. Then you have hope. But ultimately that avatar will tell you that you are also an avatar. This is enlightenment. Hm? You see yourself as an avatar in that mirror. So whoever you treat as an avatar, he is an avatar to you, because he is in reality an avatar.

Some say, "I am the avatar," after realizing; some do not. But even if they say that, if you don't see them as an avatar, they are of no use to you. So that is why some people do not say it. If they are an avatar, if they are realized, they don't even need to say that, because others will recognize it. Should the candle say, "I am lit"? Hm? People will know if it is lit because it gives light. No avatar will ever say, "I am the sole avatar." An avatar will see everybody as an avatar, because he has that beautiful eye. A God-man will see everybody as God. He will never say, "You are sinners." No. He will treat everybody as equal. He will see the same avatar, that Self, in you. He will love you as he loves his own Self. "Love thy neighbor as thine own Self." And if you have forgotten that, he will help you to know that avater in you.

That is what is meant by avatar. That's why, normally, whoever helps you in realizing this truth, is treated as an enlightened person. And that enlightened person is recognized as an avatar because he represents God. You see God in him. But in others we still don't see that, because it is still a little covered. So, normally, it is up to you. If you have that faith, if you see that, you will be benefited. If not, even if God Himself comes and stands in front of you, you will say, "Ah, that's fine, who made this make-up for you, huh?" You see? So he is no use to you. Who knows to see will see. You see?

Please explain why some Christians say that Christ is the only way. They say that only through Christ will you see the Father.

I also say that: only through Christ can you see the Father. But who is that Christ? A man? The body that got crucified? Christ can never be crucified. When you say Christ was crucified, you are talking only about the body of Christ. Christ is not the body, not even His intelligence. Christ is the spirit. That is the same spirit you see everywhere, in every saint. In one part of the world, that spirit was called Christ; in another part, that same spirit was called Buddha; in a third part, in a different age, the same spirit was addressed as Mohammed. They are all different names of the same spirit. Even recently, when people went to see Ramana Maharshi, they would go there, sit and pray, and then say, "I had Ramana Maharshi's *darshan.*" "Oh, what did you experience? What did you see" "So nice, just with a loin cloth, he was sitting with half-closed eyes." They are talking about the body! The body had a loin cloth; the real Ramana didn't use any cloth. What is called Christhood, Buddhahood, is an attainment. It is not different than any other attainment. There is only one spiritual attainment named in different ways.

Truth is one. People that experienced it, expressed it in different ways. So it does not matter what name you give to the nameless spirit. The only way is to experience that spirit. Because the Christians called the spirit as

Christ, they say Christ is the only way. Because Buddhists called that spirit Buddha, they say the only way is through Buddha. But there is no difference between Buddha and Christ. That is why I say Christ is the only way. If you know the true Christ. So the only way to eternal peace and joy is to realize that Christhood or Buddhahood or Krishnahood. But when we miss that point, we are — in a way — under a hood. Our ego tricks us.

So it is in that sense that the scriptures say, "I am the only Way." Krishna said that, Christ said that, Allah said that. Everybody said that. They all mean that One. So it is a misunderstanding. When you do not understand what Christ is, then you say, "Oh, Buddha is not the way, Mohammed is not the way, Christ is the only way." A real Christian who has realized the Christhood will never argue this way. If ever you hear a Christian saying, "Christ is the only way, all other ways are demonic," know for certain he has not realized Christhood, he is just talking about something which he calls Christ. I feel sorry for such a Christian. They call themselves Christians. They are not really Christians. Probably they are just Churchians.

Are the Yogic systems the only way to reach the God within us? And if not, what determines what system should be used?

We have said enough about the "only way." The only way is to get out of this ego. And that is what is taught by every method — every religion. So Yoga is not something different from other ways. If you think Yoga is different from a particular religion or a particular method, then you lose the meaning of Yoga. What is Yoga, after all? Yoga is union. Yoga is oneness. So to come together is the only way. Not to divide and dissect. How can we come together? Only when we set aside our egoistic "I," "me," "you," and just say "we." And that is what is meant by Yoga.

So it's not a different way than any religion. Every religion tells about Yoga. Yoga is universal. Is there anything beyond universal? No. So the foundation stone of any religion is Yoga. If you dig a little deep into your own religion or whatever faith you follow, you will see the same stone as the foundation. You may have a different name for it, that is all. So in a way we can say, coming together is the only way. And that's Yoga.

The evening program closes with soft "Om Shanthi" chanting lead by Swamiji. The chanting becomes quieter and quieter until the entire hall is completely still, wrapt in silent meditation. This is the culmination of a full day of discipline, study, work and silence, brought to its peak by the intense concentration on the words of the spiritual teacher. The vibration is one of fullness, of oneness, of silence — the human silence within the vaster pervasive silence of the huge black night surrounding the satsang hall.

Third Day

The Three Mirrors

Sant Keshavadas

This second of Sant Keshavadas's talks gives his version of an introduction to Integral Yoga. He gives the classical breakdown of the main branches of the science of Yoga: Jnana Yoga, Karma Yoga and Bhakti Yoga (the path of the intellect, action and emotion or devotion, respectively) leaving out a fourth, Raja Yoga, which along with the other three usually forms the traditional divisions of the Yogic science.

In speaking of these paths, Santji tells of three "mirrors" which can be used to help us experience God realization: the entire Cosmos as the first mirror, the saints and sages as the second, and the various images or symbols of the Supreme (such as the Cross, pictures, statues, etc.) as the third.

But being, as he is, pre-eminently an exponent of Bhakti Yoga, he deals most thoroughly with that aspect in this talk. He goes into quite a lot of detail about the traditional science of Bhakti, speaking of the various attitudes or relationships one can cultivate toward God, and speaks more about the efficacy and glory of the name of God (mantrams and kirtan). As always, this is done through many wonderful stories and songs, mainly from Indian bhaktas of the past.

We hear from the great scriptures, the glory of Jnana, Karma and Bhakti, the three main Yogas. Man is a complex mixture of intellect, will and emotion. For the intuitional light which brings instantaneous illumination he takes to Jnana Yoga. For the culture of will, offering his mind, body, intellect, his everything, he does selfless service and surrenders his will to the Cosmic Will and knows and realizes Karma Yoga. If he deifies the emotion by praying, singing, dancing, chanting, worshiping, obeying, loving, prostrating, hearing, meditating and waiting upon, seeing the Lord of the Universe in everyone, that is Bhakti Yoga. Integral Yoga consists of integrating the intellect, will and emotions. According to what we hear from the Vedas, God is *Parabrahman,* the Transcendental Reality; He is *Paramatma,* permanent, all-pervading Truth; and He is *Bhagavan,* the Personal God when He takes incarnation. These are the three different manifestations of the Lord (though His manifestations are endless).

So through the intellect, saying *"Neti, Neti,"* neither this, nor that, you will reach the Truth which is Self-apparent, known as the Parabrahman. It is always full. This Parabrahman is experienced through the annihilation of the intellect.

The second aspect of God is the Immanent Reality or the Holy Spirit. This is Paramatma, the Cosmic Soul, the Soul of all the souls. The power to experience this will come by seeing this Paramatma without, the whole Cosmos, by developing our will and through gradual surrendering. If a man is married, then he should adjust his ego to his wife. When children are born, both of them should adjust their egos to the children, then to the neighbor, the county, afterwards to the whole country, to the whole world, the whole universe. This will expand the will. "Nevertheless, not my will but Thine be done." This was the key to the teaching of Jesus the Christ. Everything is the Will of God. To reach that understanding, the will must be totally surrendered and our body, mind and intellect must become channels. We become the chosen instruments for an appointed work in this mighty evolution, according to the Will of God. We should purify ourselves so that God may use us as instruments, and we become sweet fruit for Him to eat. Thus we become Karma Yogis. That is why I sing:

> For peace there is a way,
> For joy there is a way
> For all the success and the bliss
> Self-surrender is the way.

> To unlock all mystery,
> Surrender to God is the key.
> For all the bliss and happiness,
> Self-surrender is the way.

> Offer all unto God.
> Make thy heart peaceable.
> For all the happiness and bliss
> Self-surrender is the way.

> The essence of all scriptures
> Is the attainment of Self.
> For the attainment of Self,
> Self-surrender is the way.

This is the offering: day by day, moment by moment, we tame the ego by offering it in selfless service. Through this we really become His chosen instruments.

To develop this selflessness, to attain the Supreme wisdom, the most compassionate Lord God gave us Sri Rama, Sri Krishna, Sankaracharya and all the deities and teachers, the many, many glorious manifestations of God. These incarnations make us realize, as the most blessed Swamiji told us yesterday, that everyone is an incarnation of this Parabrahman. This realization comes to us through various mirrors — the whole Cosmos is one mirror through which God or the Self reflects. And the gurus, the saintly people, the great souls are also wonderful clear mirrors.

If we stand in front of mirrors that are concave, convex, or crooked, we look completely different than we are. The nose will be something like Chinese or the figure will be very tall even though we are short and fat. So this is what happens when we meet with egoistic, egocentric, selfish people who are wallowing only in the physical level; we see, not the real Self, but a distorted vision. It is like when you throw a stone into the lake when the mud is coming up, and you try to look for your reflection, you will have a distorted vision. But when you see clearly, when you reach the highest, you see everywhere the same Parabrahman.

So in the beginning stages, as you are evolving, when you hear the stories and glories of the great saintly people such as St. Theresa, St. Cecilia, St. Paul, James, Peter, when you hear of their great devotion to God, you get strength and the impediments and veils are disentangled and you can clearly see the Way, the Truth and the Life. Through His own example, His self-sacrifice, Lord Jesus showed the Way. So that is why gurus or saintly people are considered as the second kind of mirror to reflect God within us.

Before knowing the third kind of mirror, you should know the third Yoga — Bhakti. Dependence upon the supreme reality in whatever form is called Bhakti. God knows everything when we surrender to Him. He does everything for us. A child need not jump or walk or cook or do anything; a child should just be a child. With simplicity. It knows only one mantram: "Mommy, Mommy, Mommy." Whenever it is in difficulty, only this one mantram. The mother leaves all her work and comes to see if she is really needed. If he is just calling playfully she would just throw a candy, because if she fondles him all the time he'll be always calling. If he is happy with that, she works in the kitchen. Again, "Mommy, Mommy," immediately she gives some toys. If he plays for a little while, wonderful; but the time comes when the child could never be happy with candies or toys. When it cries more loudly she might send some neighbors, friends or relatives or the eldest son. When he is not pacified by that but needs Mommy and Mommy alone and kicks everybody and cries his utmost, it is at that time the mother rushes to the baby, picks him up immediately, holds him, kisses him, embraces him and says, "Oh, oh, oh, you should not cry any more; I am sorry I've come so late. I should have come long ago."

The great saint, Sri Shankaracharya, tells that even an earthly mother would rush toward a crying baby. So could there be any doubt that the all-compassionate Mother or Father would be making us pant and pine and cry if we sincerely wanted Him? No. He tries throwing a candy: the sense pleasures. If we remain for some years like that, He doesn't come to us. Then when we cry out again, he gives us a toy: some jumbo jets. These things are all the toys for the grown-up ones. We play with that and when we are fed up with all those things and pant and pine as all the saints did, as all the great Nayanars did, as Swamiji was telling last night, that indeed brings us God Realization. As Christ said, give all you have and you will have Him. Only then can we actually learn to appreciate the Jnana (wisdom).

So the first two mirrors are: the Cosmos, and the gurus and saints. And now the third one is the Image (*moorthi*). You keep an image in front of you and lavish all your love. This is why in Hinduism it is husband for wife and wife for husband, because in that love the wife should see God in the husband and the husband should see Goddess in the wife. This is a beautiful form of Bhakti known as *Madhurya Bhava*. When we raise ourselves from the physical level to the higher level as St. Bernard or St. John of the Cross who sang of Christ as the bridegroom, we have the bride and bridegroom relationship with God Himself. One of the greatest *Bhaktas, Narada,* wrote in his *Bhakti Sutras (Aphorisms on Bhakti)* that if you want to cultivate this kind of love for the realization of God, follow in the footsteps of the *gopis* (pronounced "go-pees"). The Gopis were the milkmaid devotees of Sri Krishna. They had this Madhurya Bhava. It was by chanting the names of the Lord that the gopis developed their love for Lord Krishna.

Then there is the *Vatsalya Bhava*, worshiping God as a child. Some of the gopis worshiped the *Gopala* Kirshna, the Child-Krishna. Moses was worshiped as a child, Nirmalanandaji was telling me. Madonna and Jesus as a child is very well known in the Christian mysticism. That parental love, motherly love, is the Vatsalya Bhava. You can have a small symbol of Christ, of Moses, Buddha or Krishna and treat it as if God is manifesting in that every day and you will find Him, feel Him as the Transcendental Person. You try to see Him there in your image, just as you offer breakfast for your child, you have to bring breakfast for God, treating him as your child. Suppose there is a child in the chair, you should cover him; same way with God.

Thus, in the great temples of India, they have a feeling that through the mantrams they are repeating, the Transcendental Person is absolutely manifesting *there*. God is everywhere but unless you realize him *somewhere* you can't see Him anywhere. The ocean is all water. Are you expected to bathe in the whole ocean? No, if you bathe just in one corner, it is equivalent to the whole ocean.

The saint, Paramahamsa Ramakrishna, gives a simile. Milk is all-pervasive in the body of the cow. But if you squeeze the ear you will not get milk. Only when you squeeze the dripping udders of the cow can you have milk. So God is everywhere, but first we should realize him somewhere, according to our capacity. That is the greatness of symbols or moorthis; you will see the Self mirrored inside the image. When he was a priest in the *Kali* temple (Kali is God manifesting as the Divine Mother), Ramakrishna would call out, "Ma, Ma, Ma, Kali, Kali," praying to Her image, and the Divine Mother, the Cosmic Mother emerged.

And another immortal south Indian saint, *Nandanar*; was an untouchable. He was not allowed by the priest to enter into the Siva Temple. He had to stand at the gate where his view of the inner sanctum was blocked by the image of the bull *Nandi*, the vehicle of Lord Siva. So he stood at the gate and cried, "Siva, Siva!" becoming completely intoxicated and mad, chanting, "Om Namah Sivaya, Om Namah Sivaya." When you are alone — it may not be here — but when you are alone in your room and you want to realize Siva, slowly begin to chant, "OM Namah Sivaya, Sivaya Namah Om" with all love. As St. Paul observed, when God comes to you He first manifests in the soul as love. As you chant the divine name, His love may come with horripilation, hair standing on end, tears coming from the outer corners of your eyes, clapping, dancing, and sometimes rolling and writhing with the pangs of separation. These are the various signs of His love. So if you want to practice it at home, better tell your parents and other people so that they need not be scared when you do all those things! But when you are in a lonely place, just practice in this way. It is very great. You should feel His presence without and within and every way by the power of the mantram. Let us all chant "OM Namah Sivaya."

(*Chanting*).

So, day and night, Nandanar chanted to Siva and seeing his devotion, the image of the bull *Nandi* was moved aside by the vibration of Nandanar's mantra chanting and Nandanar had divine darshan (vision) of Siva. Such vibration, such feeling. The whole universe is filled with the vibration coming from the sound that is OM, the Word that is God. In Bhakti you are vibrating the divine vibrations of the holy name of God which is transcendental.

There is no difference at all between the name of God and God. The name of God is even *greater* than God. *Tulsidas* says, "Rama, you transformed only one rock into a beautiful lady called *Ahalya* but whosoever chants your name, all their rocky hearts are melted into Ahalyas." Tulsidas further says, "Rama, when you wanted to go across the ocean, you had to employ seven hundred million monkeys to build a bridge, but millions of people need not build any bridge at all to go across this ocean of *samsara* (births and deaths) if they just take your holy name; automatically the bridge is built and you take them across. Such is the power of your name. So Rama, please tell me whether You or Your name is greater?"

Thus Tulsidas questions the great Sri Rama. Such is the right you get in Bhakti. In Jnana you cannot quarrel with God; in Bhakti you can: "Why have you not appeared before me? Why don't you come? How is it that you appear only before St. Paul and Sri Ramakrishna? Are they your close relatives?" Like this the great masters discussed with God. It's really a great fight. Tulsidas was full of tears of joy and at the same time he says, "Hey Rama, I hear from the *Bhagavatam* that when a mere beast, an elephant, was caught by the crocodile and cried, "Ra", before it could chant the second letter, "Ma," between the "Ra" and the "Ma" you appeared and protected that beast. Well, I am singing much more than that, for forty years now, clapping and playing the tambura and crying at the top of my voice with all the melodies possible and you never respond. What is happening? What is wrong with me or with You? What Veda or Upanishad did that elephant know? And I cry at the top of my voice. How is it that you can't hear my prayer? And you are supposed to be the Friend of the Afflicted, Friend of the Lowly, so many epithets you have, so many mantrams and names. We call you the Most Compassionate One who immediately rushes to the devotees. You'd better protect your honor; you don't know — your devotees may glorify you but if you are not coming to protect them and don't give your darshan, they are the ones who are going to beat the drum and tell the whole world with the same tongue. "Don't believe in that God!" We can make and unmake you, my Maker. Be careful!"

So the saints present these feelings. In Bhakti all feelings are sublimated, nothing is spared. As the great exponent of Yoga, Swami Vivekananda says, "You begin in love, continue in love and you also end in love." There is nothing more to be asked except love of God. One saint said, "I have not asked for wealth, nor for property, nor for health, nor for progeny, nor for liberty, nor even for the highest *mukti* (liberation) which you can give. I only want to be at your feet, that's all." What more do you need? That is the cleverness of these *dasas* (servants of God), the saints.

Swami Chidananda was once inaugurating our lecture in Delhi and he said, "Anybody who has the name 'dasa', don't believe him." All the people were looking because I am named Keshava*dasa*. "Do you know why these people call themselves that way? It means, the lowest of the lowly. But when you are totally offering yourself as dasa, God says 'I am *your* dasa.' When you say, 'I am the least of all the servants,' then God says, 'Then I am your servant.' So to have God always near them they call themselves dasas. Don't believe them."

The meaning is the same as when Jesus Christ washed the feet of Peter. Peter said, "Master, what are you doing?" The Master said, "Who is the least among you shall be the first, the one highest among you shall be the servant." This servitude is known as Dasa Bhava.

After the purification, the elimination of the intellect and the surrendering of the will, the sages and masters reach that highest state where the mind is like an unperturbed ocean. So, let us meditate a while and then close.

As the mark of total surrender, please place both of your palms at the crown of your head and chant *"Govinda"*. Now bring both palms to the eyebrow center and salute God, chanting the name Govinda. Bring both the palms to the bosom, feeling the Lord within and without and everywhere.

> Thou art my Mother and my Father.
> Thou art my relative and my Friend.
> Though art my everything, Oh God of Gods!
>
> Lead us from the unreal toward the Reality,
> From darkness of ignorance toward the Light,
> From death and decay toward Thy Immortal Kingdom of Heaven.
>
> They will be done, Thy Kingdom come.
>
> OM Shanthi Shanthi Shanthi

Now seeing the same God within and without, in everybody, kindly open your eyes and salute everyone. I am very beholden to Sri Swami Satchidanandaji and I want to sing the glories of all the IYI people from the different centers where I have been visiting from coast to coast. Again I salute Swamiji and thank you all very much.

The Secret Behind All Religions

Swami Satchidananda

The day of Swamiji's third lecture happens to be Father's Day. Many of Swamiji's disciples think of him as their father since, as the physical father guides you in learning to live in the world, the guru guides you in living in the Spirit. He is the spiritual father. So this evening, besides the usual stack of question papers, Swamiji finds a number of Father's Day cards and presents on his seat when he arrives for the evening program. After looking at them, Swamiji brings out a small cassette recorder which was hidden beneath his robe and plays some songs which a devotee had recorded and sent as a Father's Day gift.

In expressing his appreciation of the spiritual content of the songs, he leads into his theme for the evening's talk which is also the running theme of his entire teachings and his entire life; in a word: selflessness or dedication. Many different practices can be done in the name of Yoga or spiritual life, but the one common principle and most needed thing is the dedication, the complete surrender of the small individual self into the greater Self. This can only happen through the constant practice of serving others, of contentment and loving and giving constantly. In illustrating this theme, Swamiji uses many stories, parables and examples, many of them from everyday life.

In doing this, he foreshadows yet another of the major themes to be explored during this retreat: the two basic Yogic lifestyles of the family life and the life of a single devotee (or monk). Throughout his talks he stresses that the complete dedication must be there to achieve the goal, but he makes it clear that both married and single people can equally be seekers and achieve the goal of Yoga.

Before we begin the evening satsang, I would like to wish you all, from the very bottom of my heart, a very happy, happy Children's Day! God bless you. Because if the children are happy, the father is happy. What could make a father happy? Beautiful children. So I'd like to give you a small surprise for Children's Day and play this tape for you. It was sent to me by one of your brothers on the West Coast, Ramesh.

> From the bed where I lay, I see a clear blue day and a pearly white cross on a steeple,
> Not a cloud in the sky, and I turn my head and sigh as I think of all the lost and lonely people,

51

Who live only for themselves in their tiny little shells, and
who never ever think about their brother.
When we all know the time has come for each and
everyone, to live not for ourselves but for each other.

(*Refrain*)
So let my candle burn, asking nothing in return,
let me live my life for you and not for me.
All the holy Masters say, if we live our lives this way,
A heaven on this earth we will see,
A heaven on this earth we will see.

I see so many beautiful souls like this presenting great thoughts which
can elevate the minds of the seekers. Another example is Carole King.
She sent me her latest album a couple of days back. The words are just
beautiful, saintly words; so deep. That shows the world is changing.
Through proper music we can find peace, joy, God, happiness, harmony,
everything. This is what people who are in the limelight should do.
There is a Sanskrit proverb: "As the king, so the citizens." If the king
follows a certain path, he need not even make it a law, but the people
will automatically follow it. So the music field is something like that.
The yogic boom is so tremendous mainly due to the Beatles; am I right in
saying that? Many of the youngsters did not even know what Yoga is but
when they heard the Beatles are doing it, they all followed it. That's why
I say, if those who have some kind of leadership take to these things, the
world will soon pick it up. And it's happening now. So let us have that
hope and do our parts towards that hope.

Let us make a decision today to make the Absolute One, the Father in
heaven, happy by becoming divine children and proving that we are not
different from Him. We are His descendents. Let us express that divinity.
That should be the aim of our lives. All the rest can be temporarily postponed or brushed aside. Why? Because you don't need to worry about
any other things. Once you get that which is the first and foremost thing,
then everything else will automatically be added. "Seek ye the kingdom
of heaven; everything else will be added unto." The Vedas also say the
same thing. "Know that by knowing which you know everything."
That is the basic knowledge. If that master key comes to our hands there
is not even a single lock that cannot be opened. It can open all the locks,
solve all the problems; it can get us everything. Whether you want things
or not, they will be at your feet. You don't even need to run after
anything; instead they will run after you.

It's like the ocean. Sri Krishna gives this example in the *Gita*. All the rivers are running to the sea. Why should they run? Have you ever seen the sea sending nice golden-lettered invitations to all the rivers? "Hey, come on, come to me. Be happy. Come Ganga; Missouri come, Mississippi come." No. He never sends any invitation to anyone. He is happy and contented. And that is why all the waters yell, "There is a contented man. If we go and join him we will also have that joy. Let's all go and run to him." So, even without an invitation all the waters run towards the sea. Just imagine if ever the sea thinks, "Oh, why not send invitations to these rivers?" If he does it, that will be the end! No river will fall into the sea. Why? Because they'll have a suspicion. "Why does he want us all of a sudden? Hey, there must be something fishy. We better wait and find out what it is." They begin to suspect the motivation. But instead he just expresses that contentment. "I am happy within myself. I'm contented. I am happiness personified. I don't need anything to make me happy." That is the message the ocean gives. And that is the reason why all the waters go to fall into that ocean — to become that.

And another point is that even with all these waters constantly falling into the ocean the ocean still remains the same. It doesn't get excited. "Ha, look at this. How many waves are coming and falling into me. I am really a great man now. How big I am; see everybody wants me; everybody runs behind me." No. He doesn't get swelled up. Even after all the wants want him and come to him, he is still contented; he is not excited over it. That is the state of a contented man, a true saint, a true Yogi, a man of steady wisdom. He is contented; he is just happy. He doesn't depend upon anything.

There is a simple proverb which we hear very often: "Contentment is golden." So where is the gold mine? Not in Nevada, not in Colorado. We don't need to rush there now. The gold mine is within you in the form of contentment. Once that comes in, everything comes. As I said, if you don't want anything, then all the wants say, "Ah, here is a contented man. Let us go to him." Why do they come? Why can't they go to somebody else, to the average greedy man? Because even the wants have intelligence. Everything has intelligence, even your dollar bills. If a dollar bill goes to a greedy man, the very next thing the man does is bundle it up, put in the safe, put on ten locks and hide the key. He wants to keep it for himself. The dollar bill knows that. If by mistake it goes to a greedy man and gets caught, then it is there sitting in the safe: "I made a mistake in coming to this dirty fellow. He has imprisoned me. I don't know, God can't you help me? Can't you send somebody to release me?"

So that somebody comes at midnight and slowly opens the safe. "God sent you, come, take me quickly before that greedy fellow sees you. If he sees you we are both in trouble. I will be back in the safe and you will be in a 'safe' too. So please take me quickly."

So the man who wants to possess everything directly or indirectly imprisons everything. Is that not so? Nothing wants to be in prison, neither your dollars nor your jewels. Not anything. And that is the reason that the more you want to possess things, the more they will run away from you. They do not want to be caught. Even a child: if you want to play with a baby, just sit there, put some toys there, let the baby play by itself and enjoy, but the minute you try to catch the baby it will run away. It won't even come near you again if it knows you are going to hold on to it.

The same intelligence is seen everywhere. That is the reason why a greedy man never can keep things without anxiety and worry. They don't want him. But when they see a contented man, "Oh, there he is. If I go to him, he won't lock me up. I will have my freedom with him but not with that other dirty fellow." That is the reason why all the wealth comes to him. The scriptures say, "In the presence of a true *Sannyasi*, a true renunciate, you will see the Goddess of Wealth on one side and the Goddess of Learning on the other side sitting and waiting on him." Yes, even the ideas; you don't need to read books. The Goddess of Learning, *Saraswati*, will be sitting there, "You want some ideas? I'm ready to give them to you, come on, make use of me." They are ready to serve him. Why? Because he is not after them.

There is a saying: "Even with God, do not be avaricious." You can love God but don't be passionate. What is love here, and what is passion? Passion means for your sake. When you love something for your sake, it is not really love, it is passion. If you love for the joy of loving, it's love. Then it is pure and divine. It is that love which is called God. God loves everybody without expecting anything. He doesn't stop loving. That is Divine Love. Everything else is a kind of passion: "I give to you; you give back to me."

So we should have that contentment, that tranquility or steady-mindedness. We should have a mind free of all kinds of disturbances, anxieties and greed, totally free from everything. That is what is meant by *Nirvana*. When we talk about Nirvana we mean nakedness; there is nothing to color or cover the mind. It is just plain and pure, crystal-like. In that mind you get the true reflection of God. That is the mirror. Whosoever will go before that mirror will see themselves beautifully. So, the essential purpose of all these practices is that you should become more and more contented, more and more settled. You should reduce your wants.

I often give a device by which you can know how close or far away you are from God. We search for God: "Where is He? How am I to catch Him? How much more time have I to wait? How much more ground do I have to cover?" If you want to measure the distance between you and God, the simplest way is to get some paper and a pencil, sharpen it well, and start writing a list of all you call "mine." Everything from the very beginning: "my ego, my intelligence, my emotions, my beauty, my joy, my pride, my education, my degrees ... " Make a full list; search deeply. If your list grows longer and longer, you are farther and farther away from God. If you have a small list you are that much closer. If you have only a couple of words you are close but not there. But when you see that there is nothing which you call yours, then you need not search for God, He is there clear enough. Immediately you can see Him. In other words, a "mine-less" mind, a mind free of what you can call "mine," will know that it serves God.

That is the reason why you can read any scripture, follow any religion. The secret behind them all is: renounce. Detach yourself from "mine," free yourself from those possessions. If you give them in the name of God and say, "It is all Thine; there is nothing more of mine," then you use God to give everything away so that you can be free. If you do not believe in God, it doesn't matter; give them to others. If you do not feel like giving to others, just drop it all. Otherwise they will be bothering you, they will bind you. So by self-analysis you can reject them. But you do not need to push them away or destroy them. The minute you know they are not yours, you have no business even to destroy them. It is not your business. When they are not yours, why should you worry about it? If it is there, let it be. As long as it is not yours, it is not going to trouble you. What bothers you is the feeling that it is yours.

Imagine that you are traveling in a train. You have a small, restless child, who goes and pokes into everybody's suitcases, pulls out everything and makes mischief everywhere. You constantly say, "Please stop it. Come and sit here." Every time he disobeys you punish him. Your co-traveler is not worried about this child; he is just watching the fun. Everybody else watches the fun; only you are disturbed. Why? Because it is *your* child; he should behave the way you want.

Now suppose the scene changes. The child is no longer yours, the child is another man's. Do you think he will sit and watch? He will take up your burden and you will be just sitting and watching. So what is it that bothers you? The feeling of ownership. The minute you think something is yours, you are the owner and you seem to feel the responsibility. You are either excited or depressed. So what is it that needs to be renounced? You should be liberated from the feeling of ownership, not from the things. Let them be around: if you see a plant, give it water if it needs it. If you can't, it doesn't matter.

So then you have that kind of detached attitude with things and people but you do your duty. Detachment does not mean negligence of your duty. If you have a responsibility, if you feel the responsibility, do it. Your own conscience will tell you. If it is in your hands, you must take care of it. So we have a duty to perform, but no right to own anything. Knowing that, our minds will always be free.

That is why we surrender to God and give everything to Him, saying, "It is all Yours." It is all for Jesus. It is all for Moses. It is all for Siva, all for Krishna. I dedicate everything to Allah. He is the Supreme, He is the owner of all. All the religions teach this. Liberate yourself from this ownership. It is the feeling of ownership which binds you; nobody else binds you. You are not bound by anything in this world. God didn't create you as a sinner, as a slave, as a man bound by things. No. It is your own egoism, your own feeling of possession that binds you. If you are liberated from that you are the master. You are totally free. No other freedom will really free you. We are in a "free" country; are we really free? Are you a free individual? Who is really a free man, then? One who is freed from this self-made bondage. That is the purpose of religion. That's the reason why, in the Bhakti approach, the devotional approach, they say, "Give everything to God. Treat everything as God's, not yours, not yours." Even if you do some duties and get some results, offer them to God.

That's the idea of offering fruit to God. The fruit of your life is to be offered, not a couple of bananas or a few oranges or apples. God doesn't expect you to bring Him bananas. If He wants, He has plenty. He gives them to you; you never created a banana. He created it; you go and pick it and say, "Ah, my banana, I offer it to you." He appreciates that also: He says, "You brought me a treat? It's very good, very good, take it." He doesn't eat anything. If our God starts eating all the offerings, nobody will bring anything to Him. We are sure that if we put it there for Him, we can take it back later on.

It's something like with our human papa. Imagine after a couple of days away a papa comes back home with a nice big box of chocolate candies. And his child says "Papa, what have you brought?" "Candy." So the child opens it. In some cases the child says, "Papa, you take one; it's nice candy, Papa." The child takes it and gives it to the papa. There are some children like that. But if he gives more than one, the papa will say, "No, no, that's enough, you eat." Others will open the box and take one. If the papa asks how it is, "Very good, Papa." "Don't you want to give one to me and one to Mama?" "Okay, here Papa." After being asked, he gives one to the papa and one to the mama, or probably he'd take one, bite it into two pieces and give half to each and keep the rest for himself. And then there is a third type of child. He takes the box and runs into his room. He won't even show it to anybody.

Aren't we like that? Papa has given boxes and boxes of candies. As Santji said this morning, jumbo jet candies, television candies, position candies, beauty candies, car candies, so many things. A good child will always take them and offer the box: "You take it." And a real good papa will not even eat. He'll say, "Oh, nice, very sweet, you take it." He'll just imitate as if he's eating some. Don't we see that? It's the same with that Papa in heaven. When you go and offer something, "Oh, that's good. You brought all of this to me? Oh, very good, come on, you take it and eat." He gives it back to us. He only wants to know whether you knew that it belongs to Him and He brought if for you, or whether you want it for yourself.

So, as I said, to renounce does not mean that we should not use anything. Use it, but use it as Papa's. "How great, my Papa brought all this. Papa, only you could give this beautiful rose. Before I smell it, did you smell it Papa? Come on." And then you smell it, and Papa will be happy and give more and more candies. Share them with all the children in the house. That's what we're expected to do. Just know that it all belongs to Him. We are presented with all of these things; we use them; we share them. And when the time comes, we leave them and go. We don't carry anything with us because we never brought anything with us when we came. If we think in these terms and live like this, there is no room for robberies, wars, hatred. But we take the position, "This is mine. This is my area, don't come in." Since man started doing that, he gained room for all his troubles. So in the name of religion or spiritual practice we should open up. Let us perform our duties; let us take care of everything well. And let us enjoy things.

You might ask me another question here. "Okay, then. If it is not mine; if it belongs to Father, should I do anything with that or not? Should I take care of it or not? How am I to use it?" Here, we can take another example, the example of a bank teller. When you produce a check, he gives you the money. He seems to have a lot of money there near him. If you produce a $10 check, he will give you $10. If you produce a $100 check, he will give you $100. He won't even bother about whether you are his enemy or friend. If an enemy comes and produces a $10 check, will the teller give him $8 because he is an enemy? And if a friend produces a $100 check, will he give him $150? No.

Now suppose all of a sudden his old bosom friend comes and says, "Hi, John, I'm terribly sorry but on my way I just lost all my money; somebody robbed me. I'm penniless. Could you just give me $10?"

"Oh, Jack, I'm sorry, I don't have any money in my pocket."

"What? I see so much money lying around and you say you don't have any money?"

What would the teller say? "Oh, you know that's not my money. That belongs to the bank. How can I give it to you?"

"But I saw you giving $100 to the other man."

"But he produced a check."

"But am I not your friend?"

"Yes."

There you get the clue. You are a custodian. You can't just give it away anywhere you want. You give it according to the need, to the deserving people. You don't need to throw it away. At the same time you can't use it for yourself. Even though you have millions of dollars around, you know that not even a cent belongs to you. And that is how we have to transact in the world. When the evening comes, you just close the bank, leave the key there and go empty-handed. That's all. And after you go home, if somebody comes and robs the bank, you don't lose anything. If there is a lot of profit for the bank, you don't gain anything; you only get your salary. So neither the profit of the bank nor its loss affects you. You are doing your duty; you are the custodian of a certain area.

According to your station in life, you are given certain responsibilities. If you are a family man, you are the custodian of your wife, children, parents or whoever is there in the family. If you can have this attitude, then you can easily become a renunciate. But if your interest is in serving others more, then you renounce a small family group. That means, not that you reject them, you just add more to that. You open up your fence and they also become part of the humanity whom you'll be serving.

I know this might create a little doubt in the minds of those who want to renounce and come to the ashram. Take, for example, here is Swami Nirmalananda. If you want to go and stay in his ashram as a would-be monk, immediately he would say, "Cut off all the old associations and family ties. You should not even write to your parents or go there for twelve years." That is the Hindu way of thinking. Why? Not that you hate them or reject them. No. But you still have the old associations. Until you forget that and they forget that, you are asked to be away from them. Once they understand you and you understand them and there are no former ties or relationship and you could take them as one among the many whom you will be serving, and if they could treat you as any other Swami and not as their son, then you can go there or they can come. Until the past *samskaras* (impressions) are erased, you have to stay away. It's not out of any hatred. So all we do is just break that small fence open. But even if you are serving just one small family, you are serving the whole world. As you are loving your small family, you are loving the entire world. It is also included in that. That is the idea of renunciation.

Questions and Answers on Attachment

Swami Satchidananda

God has blessed me with a wonderful, loving family. My feelings for them are so great that the thought of anything happening to them terrifies me. How can I deal with loving too much?

You say that *God has blessed you* with a wonderful family. If you really understand what you have written and you really mean that, you won't worry about it. *God* blessed you, is it not? It not *your* family, it is God's. You call it "yours." But it is the blessing of God. It's easy to say, "God blessed me with the family . . . but I am still worried a little; I might lose it." He gave you; He will leave it with you as long as He wants. When He thinks you don't need it anymore, He will take it back.

We often contradict ourselves. We say, "God blessed me." We don't even mean what we say then. Are you worrying over the family He gave you? He probably thought you were a capable person to take good care of the family. It is something like, God has employed you as a nanny to take good care of the family. God saw you and said, "You seem to be clever enough to take good care of the child. Okay, you be the nanny for My child." That's it. It is God's family, God's children. You are only appointed to take care. Probably He'll take the family away from you one day or even dismiss *you*! He hires you and He fires you, that's all.

Of course, as long as you are the nanny you say, "my baby." You fondle it, feed it at the proper time, take good care. You treat it as if it is your own, *as if* it is your own, but all the time you know it belongs to God. Just like a nanny, however much she fondles the baby, she knows within her heart that it is not her child. "I am paid for it; I am only a servant. I love the child, fine; but it is not mine." That should be our attitude with the family. Nothing belongs to us; it all belongs to God. We are His custodians, caretakers of the house and the family. When He desires to take them away, He'll just take them. He has His own reasons, it is not to hurt you. He may say, "He was in your house all this while and now he has to be transplanted into a different place."

In a nursery you have a plant. The cultivator comes all of a sudden, plucks it and takes it somewhere and plants it in another garden. Should

60

the nursery feel bad about that? No. The gardener knows, "It won't grow here anymore, it should grow there." The same way with children also. The babies are "planted" in the mama's womb. It's not the mama who creates the baby. The Cosmic Consciousness which we call God knows everything. "Oh, you are a soul. You're ready, hm? You need a field in which to grow, hm? Where can I plant you? What are your *karmas*? I see; you must have a silver spoon in your mouth as you are born, hm? Okay, which soil is ready? I see; she is waiting for it and he is also working for it. Fine." He just computerizes it. "Go there; that's your place." And then immediately, "Ah, *I* conceived a baby." It was given to you to take care of. You take care of it within for about nine months and then without for a few years until the child grows up.

One day it says, "Mama I don't need you anymore; I'm grown up. I don't need your advice anymore. Let me learn all by myself even though I'll make mistakes." "Oh, no child, no, no. How can you? You are *my* child". Then trouble comes. The minute the child says, "Mama, Papa, I know what I am doing. Leave me alone, I want to learn by myself," the attitude should be, "Okay, you've grown your wings, go ahead and fly. Anytime you want to come back, come. The nest is open." That should be the attitude of papas and mamas towards their children. If you try to lock them in, they will revolt. You have done your duty. As long as they wanted and needed you, you gave them protection. Now they don't need you any more. Fine. Renounce. You have many more things to do. That should be the attitude. Nothing will happen to them without His Will. Know that. Whatever happens to your family members, happens because God wants it that way for their benefit. It's all for good ultimately.

If we are one another's brothers, shouldn't we try to absorb each other's pain and suffering so that the burdens are easier to bear?

Sure, if you can. If your brother is suffering from a headache, take half of the headache if you can. If you can't, at least give him the strength to bear it. That is another way of reducing his pain. Make him understand the cause for the pain, help him accept it; then you are reducing his pain. Either way you are helping your brother. If the first way is possible for you, do it, take half the headache. But that's not possible. So do what you can. Or find a doctor. If he doesn't have money, spend a little money, get him some medicine . . . there are so many ways you can help.

Please clarify attachment to one's work. I make sculpture and I'm attached to it. I love it. I don't want to give it up.

Well, you don't need to give it up. Do it. You can even be attached to that. But what kind of attachment? Is there any selfishness behind? Or are you doing it for the benefit of the humanity? That's why, again and again, we stress that renunciation or detachment is not from the things. You don't need to run away from things, people, from the world, from your home, from what you're doing. Do anything you want. A porter can be a porter, a barber can be a barber, a doctor can be a doctor, a teacher can be a teacher. You don't need to change your occupation. But the main point is to renounce the selfish approach. If you are a family man and I say renounce everything, does it mean you have to leave your wife, your children and run away somewhere? No. If you leave this and run away, you'll get attached to the new people also, wherever you go. The idea is, think of your motivation. Why are you connected with something or somebody? Why are you interested in something? Why do you want to do something? Why do you want to follow something? Why do you want to learn? If the answer is: "Not for my sake, but to serve the people, to serve the Nature, to serve God," then you need everything. To serve, you need instruments, money, objects, vehicles, you need everything; you need the whole world. So the point is, detach from your personal interest and selfishness.

Even with God some people are selfish. You can build an ashram for your sake, so that you can have a number of disciples around you and you can just sit back and be a big Swami attended on by everybody. Then it's not renunciation, it's not a detached act. But if you are interested in their welfare, and if you do it to help them, to serve them, to accommodate them and to teach them, it's always for them, for them, not for me, not for me. So it is the motive that is to be taken care of. Building a church can be the most selfish act. Everyone will look and say, "Oh look, he is building a church for God." But in the back of his mind, he is saying, "Well, if I build a church, so many people will come and there will be a lot of money coming in and I can enjoy it. Or at least I can get a name for myself: 'So-and-so built a church.' I can put a big label there." If it's for your name or fame or for comforts, then you are not building anything for God or humanity but ultimately for you.

Even then, you may say, "Well, it doesn't matter. I am doing it. Why shouldn't I enjoy the benefit? It's I who did that. Am I not entitled? I'm not exploiting anybody. With my own hands I did this, I earned this, I produced this, why should I not enjoy it?" There you should know that you are not really enjoying it and you will never enjoy it. What is enjoyment? When there is no anxiety, no fear, no worry, no concern behind it. Real enjoyment is not mixed with anything else, it's just pure joy.

In that light, let us look at how you are going to do some business. Maybe you are going to plant an apple tree. You put in the seed. Then you'll be really anxious, "Is it coming up? Oh, the other man's was planted the same day, I see two leaves on his tree. Oh, probably it hasn't started sending the root yet." You may even pluck it out to see. "Oh, no root, better put it back. Hurry." You'll be anxious to see that it is rooted, huh? You're in a hurry to see the result. "When am I to get the fruit?" You're not really enjoying. And if by any chance it gets bitten by some cow or something that comes around, you lose everything. You sit around and moan for a number of days. So, the fear of losing it. And then, the pain of having lost it.

Take any act. When you are doing it for yourself, you will have this anxiety. "Will I get it or not?" Even if somebody comes and says, "Hey, that seems to be nice," you say, "Don't touch it; take care not to break the branches." You're worried. You can take good care of it. But the anxiety is there behind it. You can't escape from that. And when you get it, "Ah, I got it; I got it; I got it." Probably for a little while. Soon after that, "Oh, now I have to protect it. I should not lose it. Where can I keep it?" Or the fear of competition. A man works for months and months to run half an inch more than the other man and get a cup to be the champion for the year. But if he hears somebody is really working hard for the same cup, he may even pray, "God, can't you break his knee? Let me keep the cup for myself." He may even go to extent of praying for the other man's fall. Why? Because he doesn't want to lose what he's gained.

So let there be no personal attachment. I can give a lot of examples. I always give the example of the doctor. Imagine a very capable surgeon. He can perform any kind of operation easily. He can transplant your heart or remove your brain, clean it, tighten all the screws, and put it back very easily. He's a very clever man. Everyone knows, "Oh, he performs operations very well, very easily." Imagine, all of a sudden one day when he comes home, his own beloved honey says, "Honey, since this morning my hand has been terribly painful. I don't know what to do." "Oh, honey, it needs an operation." "Then, please do it." You know what he will do? He will immediately call for his friend, another doctor. "John, please come, she seems to have an abcess. Why don't you come and just cut it out."

Why can't he perform that operation? Because normally doctors do not operate on their own wives and children. It's a known fact, is it not? Why? In other cases he does everything easily, like drinking water. So what is the reason? "*My* wife. I don't want to hurt my honey." There in the operation theater or in the clinic it is just somebody's wife, just my patient. But here it is "my wife." That is the trouble. It is the attachment that makes him almost unfit for that operation. He has to call for somebody else. See, all your skill fails when you have the attachment.

It is the same way with a boy who is just learning to deliver lectures. He will have gotten the entire lecture written out and learned by heart all by himself. In his room, in front of a mirror, he will have repeated the whole speech so impressively: "Beloved friends . . . ." But when he comes onto the platform, "Be, uh, loved, uh, friends . . . ." Everything goes. Why? What happened? Stage fright. Why? He wanted the audience to applaud. He didn't want to lose that. So the fear of losing that applause made him lose everything he had. The same with examination fright also. You know everything by heart. Then you come and sit in the examination hall and get the question paper. All gone. Because of the anxiety.

That's why I say, if you are freed from the personal attachment, you are free from the anxiety, worry, concern. You just do it freely. "Well, this is all I know. I'm just doing it. I don't worry about the result. Whatever comes, let it come. I have done my job." Your duty is to perform the action. Leave the rest to God. And that is why we say that even though you are the person putting all the effort into performing it, please don't expect the result, because the minute you expect the result, even your performance will be failing. You will lose the capacity to do it well, so the result will be endangered.

That is why only a detached man can perform a perfect act. Only a Yogi can do a perfect act. He doesn't worry about the result. He doesn't worry about what others say. He just does what he knows. I don't need to prepare my lectures. I don't even know what I'm going to say before hand. I just go there. If I say something useful, fine. "That is all I have. I gave it to you. If you like, take it or throw it in a ditch and go. If you take it, you gain, if you throw it, it's your loss. All I can say is this is all I have. If it is worthwhile to you, accept it. I don't want your applause. And I'm not frightened of your curse. What do I care, whether you appreciate it or not?"

That's what. Don't wait for the praise or the censure. You know what you are doing. You should appreciate what you are doing. Why do you wait for the other man to appreciate? So this is the fruit of being detached: you can perform any work beautifully. You can be a good wife, good husband, good father, good mother, good student, good teacher, good businessman, yes even a good businessman. You can be a fair businessman. You can plainly say, "Well this is how much it costs me and these are my establishment costs, so altogether it comes to this much. And I need 10% profit so this is the price. If you like, take it, otherwise go." No need to worry about that. You don't need to compete with other people.

It is this competition which is bringing all the troubles now. Even between the countries. Why all these anxieties? Everywhere missiles. ABM, ICBM, anti-missiles. Why? With all this wealth and strength, are we at ease? No. Constantly, we are mortally afraid of the enemies' missiles. We employ a man day and night to sit under the ground and put his finger on the button. You call him the "minute man." What does it mean? Any minute anything might happen to you. Every minute you are in trouble. Your life is hanging on this button. You may think it is the other men's lives which are hanging on this button, the Russians, or whoever it be. But how do you know that there is no "minute man" there? So *our* lives are hanging on *his* button. Even a false signal would make him press the button. Missions fail. Electricity fails. Didn't you all hear the "crick, crick, crick?" [*There was trouble with the speaker system during Swamiji's talk.*] We never expected that. It can happen. However clever you are, there can be some short circuit. So, if he gets a false signal and presses the button, what will happen? And why? "My country must be the super power." Instead we should say, "Come on, this is all we have, let us share. Let's be friends."

So all these calamities, troubles and turmoils are based on selfishness, either personal or communal or national. "My country must survive. Therefore I won't hesitate to throw a bomb on the other country." Do you remember the Japanese suicide squadrons? They used to come in tens of thousands to join the suicide squads. They had to get into a bomb and then the bomb was fired with the man inside. He will direct the bomb, hit the target and get himself killed along with his enemies. "It doesn't matter, even if I get killed; I will be killing a thousand people at least." For that, there were thousands coming forward in Japan. Why? The "national spirit." "I'm dying for my country." They were proud. So it means that his love was limited only to his country. He loves only his country and not the other country. He should know the other man will love his country the same way. He should think, "Just as I love my mother, he also loves his mother. How can I kill his mother?" So the reason for all these troubles is attachment — "Mine, mine, mine! Mine must be the topmost!"

That's why renunciation of this attachment is the basic rule for all the spiritual or religious practices. Without this renunciation, there is no peace at all. Let us not forget that. We can just talk about peace. There can be thousands of peace talks but they will just be "piece" talks. There won't be any "whole" talks. Each one wants to grab something for himself, even at the peace table. How can there be peace then? That is the reason we insist on this renunciation.

Does this mean we are expecting you all to become Swamis? Please don't think that. You needn't become a Swami. But be a Swami for yourself. Swami means the master. Be the master of your own mind. Don't be a slave and get into this attachment. Wherever you are, you should be free from this attachment. Perform your daily duties, free from this attachment. That is all we say. Otherwise, you will always see troubles wherever you are. Even in the family life you cannot be happy without this renunciation.

So the question was from a sculptor. Why should he produce a sculpture? If his interest is to make everybody admire it, then the anxiety will be there. If people don't appreciate it, he may say, "Oh, I worked for six months. These fellows don't seem to have any artistic sense or anything. They don't even know how to appreciate art." He will make them to be fools.

In the same way, if I want you all to appreciate my talk, I'll keep on giving quotations from scriptures and this and that and if I don't even see a smile on your faces or some applause, I will think that you are all fools. "They don't seem to know anything about these things, that's why they're just sitting." See? Because I didn't get what I wanted from you, I make you all to be illiterates.

Fine art is an expression of your joy. A baby smiles; what more beautiful sculpture do you need? And the baby doesn't even expect anybody to look and appreciate. He just smiles. You just sing a song because you feel like singing. It's just coming out. Like a scent coming out of the flower. The flower doesn't worry whether you smell it or not. That is fine art.

So don't do it for the sake of others. Just do it as the expression of your own joy and leave it there. If people want to appreciate, let them appreciate; otherwise, let them close their eyes and go away. You don't need to worry about it. But if you do it for the other man's sake and he doesn't enjoy it, you also lose your joy of having done it. You are unhappy. But if you don't expect that, then you can appreciate what you did, "Ah, what a beautiful thing I made, wonderful."

Why do you worry about the other man? Fine art, living art, means it does not come from the ego, it comes from the soul. All the poetry that lives even to this day, since ages, is the outcome of the spirit, the soul, and not the ego. We've seen and heard many egoistic paintings, sculptures, poems. Where are they now? Gone with the wind. The living books are the outcome of the spirit. That's why man should not write books, man should not compose songs, but the spirit behind should do it. God in man should compose these things and they will live long. They will be appreciated by the souls of the other men. So, if you love it, do it. But not for the sake of the other man's appreciation. Let there be no personal motive behind it. It is very difficult to really live like that. But let us try it.

Phew! I spoke about this for half an hour. This also seems to be an attachment. I want to drive home the idea, hm? Maybe that's why I want to talk too much. I want you to just catch it and go.

Fourth Day

Let Go of the Cat's Tail

Swami Nirmalananda

Swami Nirmalananda is the founder and director of the Shri Ma Anandamayi Monastery near Oklahoma City. One of the few Americans to be initiated as a Swami (monk), went to India in 1962, where he practiced spiritual disciplines under the guidance of his guru, Shri Ma Anandamayi (also called the Mother) — one of the great spiritual figures of our time.

Still young himself, Nirmalananda is appreciated in America not only because he is that rare thing — an American Swami — but because American spiritual aspirants can identify with his background and his American humor. He comes from Oklahoma, from farming country; heavily built and with a very expressive face, he speaks very forcefully and dramatically, with large doses of humor, much of it sarcastic and much of it deriving from a very earthy background. At times his way of making a point strikes home in a heavy way. His famous pig story will be remembered by all those who attended the retreat. And in spite of his sometimes heavy approach, Swami Nirmalananda also has a remarkable quality of sweetness. He is very bright, unpretentious, and his heart is very soft.

As both an American and a Swami, as a person who was raised in the Christian tradition (Oklahoma is part of the American Bible belt) and is now a Hindu, Nirmalananda is a kind of one-man synthesis of East and West. This enables him to bring the Hindu tradition and mythology — which otherwise might be vague and confusing — right down to the everyday level of American living.

Once he is seated on the stage, Swami Nirmalananda sings along with a harmonium which he plays, and he invites retreatants to join in with him. Most of his songs are in English. They are about the Hindu mythology and the devatas (gods). As he introduces a song, he takes the opportunity to explain the meaning of it. Often this gives rise to a lecture. This is the case in his lecture today, which focuses on the Lord Siva.

The theme of this talk is that Yoga is based on what you are, that Lord Siva is not an image of some external god but is a mirror of your own inner being. (This is what would be called a Jnana approach, as distinct from the Bhakti attitude of worship.) And because Yoga is based on what you are, you need not get anything, but only let go: let go of the cat's tail.

There was a young Indian man who was educated exclusively in England, where he went to Oxford, and learned how to theorize. When he went back to live in India, the whole set-up in India was quite a shock to him. Having been raised in a very sophisticated, Western atmosphere he didn't like the idea that these people were going around involved with this god, that god, this goddess, and so on. But for some reason he decided to take up a little bit of Yoga. He thought, "These poor people are superstitious. It's really too bad. But I don't have to go for that stuff. I'll just go for Yoga. After all, with Yoga, you don't have to be involved with all that. Yoga is the *essence* and that's the real inner thing. That will circumvent all this god and goddess business." But, to his utter shock, as he advanced in his Yoga, he started seeing the gods and goddesses!

Once a year in India the feast of Saraswati is celebrated. Saraswati is the goddess of knowledge. She wears white, plays a stringed instrument and holds a book. All the school children worship her, hoping she'll help them pass their exams. The young Indian man thought, "That's silly. Why don't they use their brains? Why depend on some person who's playing a stringed instrument? How will it do them any good?" But one day while in meditation, who did he see? Saraswati appeared before him! There she sat, waiting for him. And that was a shock! Then after a few days he saw another form of God, and another and another. Then he came to realize that all of these forms are really existing in a person's consciousness, and are arising as the individual's awareness moves up to different levels. This is the old principle we have in the West, in Hermetic philosophy: What is above is below. What is within is without. And so he realized, "Yes, the sages saw that in the cosmic mind there are these states, which correspond to what is in the individual mind."

So if a person really looks into it, he finds that every form of God is of course a form of his own self, because that's who God is. And just as the cosmic mind is going through processes whereby these things are arising, so in our own inner being these will also arise. And so we're going to speak on a very, very good subject today. We're going to talk about the supreme Absolute, who is God Siva.

Siva is the one worshipped by all the Yogis; he is liked by all the Yogis. Why? Because he is the utmost embodiment of the real state of our soul. He is our true self. Siva is the depiction of our real nature. When we look at His picture we should realize that we are looking at the picture of some external personality; we are looking at a symbolic form which is saying: "This is you." And it can also be a test. You can take that picture, put it on the wall, and every so often look at it and inquire, "Have I come to that yet?" Because that is your true face.

Let us consider Lord Siva's qualities and how we are a reflection of those qualities. To do this we must guard against the typical pitfall of saying, "Oh, Glory to Him! Isn't He wonderful? Let's just think how grand He is." Where will that get you? The tendency is to say that God is all-pervading, He is imperishable, and so forth. We go on with "He, He, He," and that's grand. But when we are finished we go home empty. We forget that we are made in the image of God.

At this point Swami Nirmalananda begins to play the harmonium, and to sing the song, "There Siva Dances." It is a rhythmic and melodious song, describing the attributes of Siva. Nirmalananda says:

This song was written by Swami Vivekananda. Vivekananda is looked upon as the very embodiment of Siva. So he is the man who should know Siva's attributes.

As Swami Nirmalananda sings, the retreatants join him by looking at the song sheets that each one has. The words are a little strange at first, but soon everyone gets used to them.

> There Siva dances, striking his cheeks
> Ba-ba boom they resound
> Di-mi Di-mi Di-mi sounds his drum
> A garland of skulls from his neck is hanging
> In his matted locks the Ganges hisses
> Fire shoots from his mighty trident
> Round his waist a serpent glitters
> And on his brow the moon is shining
> And on his brow the moon is shining.

Ah, nice isn't it? "There Siva dances." The dance, of course, is the expression of joy. And in dancing, in playing his drum, he is making all the cosmic rhythms come out; all the rhythms are making this whole universe come forth. How does this relate to you? Know that your *jiva*, your individual consciousness, is Siva. Your soul is going through this dance also, and it's the rhythms of your soul that are producing every level of your being: your will power, your intelligence, your capacity to perceive, the sensory mind, your feelings, your physical body. Everything is being projected by you. You're the master. Sometimes we refer to Yogis as masters. But your own soul is the master, the real master. And the nature of that soul, like Siva, is absolute bliss, absolute joy.

The catch is: *There* he dances and we're out *here*. There, in the depths of our being, we aren't sinners who need to be saved. We are ever-joyful beings. But the problem is that we're out here and that is in there. You know, some people do not understand Yogis. They think Yogis are kind of crawling off into a corner, all self-involved, and they couldn't care less about anybody. But the truth is that the Yogi who taps that inner source of bliss, that inner source of joy, feels far more strongly for other people, because he finds that although his external environment goes through many changes, he always has joy. And he is surprised because he remembers one day that he used to be miserable. "That made me sorrowful, that used to depress me, that used to unsettle me." But now things can happen, even more intensely, perhaps worse, and he realizes, "I always have peace inside; I always have joy inside." It's a marvel. So when he goes out on the streets and sees others' sorrow, their suffering, his heart really breaks, because he realizes it's all totally needless. This is what is meant by the ocean of delusion — holding on to the sorrow.

That's the sad thing — all this suffering is totally pointless. There is no need for anybody to suffer. Each person is himself a whole ocean of joy, an ocean of bliss. But the problem is, we are hanging on to our suffering so intently. If you take a cat and you jerk it by the tail and hold it in the air, you know what will happen. You will get scratched; you will get bit. So some people are holding on to the cat's tail and saying, "Oh, why do I suffer? Why am I miserable? Oh, can the church help me? Can Madame Zola the crystal-gazer help me? Can that Swami I read about in the magazines help me?" And all they have to do is let go. All you have to do is let go of the cat's tail. That's all. The cat will stop scratching.

One of the favorite activities in India is to go and visit the local Swami and say, "Swamiji, what can we do for peace of mind?" It's a very interesting phenomenon. And each teacher sort of has his own particular "medicine." If he believes in *Tantra*, he says, "Oh, well, until the *Kundalini* is aroused, nothing will happen." If he believes in kirtan, he says, "Unless you chant every day how will you have peace of mind?" So on it goes. Interestingly enough, nobody ever says, "First, let's look not at what you should *do* for peace of mind, but what you should *stop* doing for peace of mind."

Isn't it true? The secret is letting go. Not grabbing. You see, getting implies losing. This is the whole law. If you get it, you must lose it. So the idea that we need to grab, grab, grab, means only that ultimately, even if we can grab something we're satisfied with, we're going to have to let it go. So why not let go of the cat's tail?

Your nature is bliss, your nature is joy. You're like the most beautiful person in the world, whose got all these masks and all this paint in order to be beautiful. You don't understand that if you throw that junk away then you'll have it. That's inner beauty. Why, then, keep on living here, why not go there, inside? There's no happiness in this world, and there is nothing you can call your own. Everything has to go away and leave you, or you have to go away and leave it. Why then are you hanging on to it? How old are you? Haven't you learned anything in all these years? Haven't you learned that you can't hold even the simplest thing? Your shoes wear out. Your clothes wear out. Your friends wear out. Your parents wear out. Everything in this world wears out.

When I was little, I used to dream that I was in a five-and-ten-cent store. Children think that F. W. Woolworth is paradise. When they grow up, they say, "Oh, that junk store!" Unfortunately, we don't grow up in our souls and we keep clutching for such cheap things. In fact, the things actually get cheaper as we get older. Well, I used to dream I was in Woolworth's. And there were all those things on the counter and so I used to go and grab an armful of everything I wanted. And for some peculiar reason, since birth, I have always known when I'm only dreaming. So I would hold that armful of things, thinking, "I can still have it when I wake up." Imagine! Oh! I would wake up and my hands would be empty.

So don't you see, we are all holding on to these things. "They are mine, they are mine." And they are only dream shadows. Our problem is that we base our lives on the idea that we need something external. And sad to say, we have the feeling that we need someone extra. But the real you is seated deep within; the real you cannot even eat an apple. The teeth chew, glands work, it goes into the stomach, and the digestive tract digests — the real you does not get a dot of that apple. It is blissful because it stands alone. But it is wrapped in layers and layers of these subtle and gross energies.

Swami Nirmalananda is now about to begin his famous pig story.

The parable of the Prodigal Son means this. The Prodigal Son left home and went to a faraway country. And everything he had was expended. So he took care of pigs, and we are told that he wanted to eat the food of the pigs. But he could not. We too are keeping pigs.

Listeners begin to get restless as the Midwestern Swami raises his eyebrows high and imitates supping on something exquisite, saying:

We say, "Ah, how grand!" But it is just pig food. I don't care if

Michaelangelo made all those statues that everyone says are beautiful. I don't care that people are so involved in drawing Venuses on couches and what not, it is just pig food. And these are the pigs.

He points to the eyes, ears, mouth, nose, to all the sense organs.

Of course, there are high-class pigs and low-class pigs, you understand. The low-class pigs know they just like to see a little splash of color and so on. While the high-class pigs say, "Oh, Picasso . . ." Yah, that is high-class piggery. Have you been to the art galleries? Oh, they spend hours looking at all the sculptures, "Oh, look at the colors, oh, oh." They are just pig runs. Yah, don't be deceived. They are the kind of people who say, "Oh, have you listened to the string quartet, you know, by Brahms . . . Stravinsky?" "Have you heard this one's experimental music, have you heard it all?" They listen and they say, "Ah, ah," but it is just slurping at the trough.

Sure, don't be deceived. This is just pig food. You say, "Oh, if only I could just have that nice feeling again, that sensation. Oh, that was so nice; I swam, I played tennis, I did this and that." Just a pigsty refrain, that's all.

People don't like sex – did you know that? That's why they make such a big to-do about it. Books and books on how to get more out of it. How to do the real things to get more out of it. How to do weird things, right? But if the orange was full of juice, you wouldn't have to read a book to know how to get the juice out of it. It is like eating meat. They take steak. Look at all the trash they put on top of it. The steak gets smothered in onions and this and that. The reason is, it is not worth eating by itself. They have to garnish it and garnish it, which shows they really understand the stuff tastes foul. Sure. And that's why people are running after sex – because it cannot satisfy them. If it could satisfy them, they would not run after it. Isn't that right? Think about that. Don't be a fool. Don't be deceived. The very things you run after – your attitudes toward them, your reactions to them – proves that they are, as Krishna said, wombs of pain, not of joy. Not of joy at all.

But instead, we hang on. We want to gnaw at the slop. But your soul can't do it. You will never be happy, never at any time. The parable says the Prodigal Son came to himself one day. He woke up and said, "Hey, wait a minute. Who am I? I'm not one of these people that's born down here in the dirt. I don't have to keep these pigs. What am I doing?" So he said, "Look, I am going home. I'm going to go where I belong. What am I doing down here in the pigpen?" That's all you have to do, just decide to go home. It's so simple everybody misses it.

Just let go. Don't even renounce. Somebody will tell you about renouncing. No, just let it go, that junk will slink away. In one way, a real Sannyasi, a real Swami, a real monk, is not a person who said, "No!" He is a person who simply opened his hands and it all fell away. Easy. You don't know how easy it is.

People don't know how to live life to enjoy it because they are so involved. They worry all the time. Before discovering Eastern philosophy, they used to think, "Oh, the devil will get me. Mama said that if I do that the devil will get me, and when I die, I'll go down there." So then they think they've broken out of that, and they come to Eastern philosophy and they start to think, "Oh, my karma! Oh, God, my karma will get me for sure for what I've done." Isn't it the same thing?

Here, Swami Nirmalananda is talking about the Law of Karma: for every action there is a natural reaction, or as you sow, so shall you reap. So here the word karma refers to the consequences of one's actions, good and bad.

Don't worry about your karma. You don't have any karma. You've been writing rubber checks all your life. Don't think you have to cash them. You don't. Say, "No, that's it." That's all it takes. Just say, "I quit." Think of a situation right now: "Oh, what will I do?" No! Say, "I quit." That doesn't mean that you should head off for Montana. Just say to the worries, "I quit." See what happens.

You don't understand that you can think, "Wow, what will happen next?" And the answer will be real. Instead of asking, "Oh, why did God make the world?" know that He made it for fun. You may ask, "You mean to tell me that all this stuff is for fun?" Yes, if you just know how to look at it. Sometimes I get caught in a tight spot, so I think, "Well, let's see what will happen now." You're the star of your own production. So why not enjoy it? I'm really serious.

Scriptures say, "Be detached, don't want the fruits of your actions." Why? First of all, because that's realistic. You better be detached because there is nothing you can have. And you better renounce the fruits of your actions because there is nothing you can produce. Some people think, "Oh, this Bhagavad Gita stuff, it's such a high ideal." No, it isn't. It's just being realistic. We think, "Oh, I've done bad, and this suffering will come back to me." And we think, "Oh, I'll do that and happiness will come about." But it isn't so. Just move where the stream takes you. Do you follow me? Just live. See what's around the corner. It's nothing you ever thought up. It's far, far more interesting.

There have been times when I thought, "Oh, God, what next?" And then I think, "No, let's see what comes next. It'll be fun; it'll be interesting." Now, I know! I once broke both legs, one in five places, the other in two, but I still sang on my way to the hospital. So I know what I'm talking about. By the grace of medical science, I was given an anaesthetic to which I was allergic, when I was twelve years old, and used to go through unbearable agonies afterward, in damp weather, and when I got a cold and when I got tired – both of which qualities I have at the moment. I had all kinds of internal difficulties too long to tell about, and unbearable pains. At the first sign, I would have "blacks." If any of you have migraine headaches, you will sympathize. It is similar, though it is not the same. I would first go blind partially, and then it began. I used to go home and lie down, and see flashing lights, and feel dizzy, and it was great since I didn't have to go to school. So I just lay there and sang hymns and prayed and I enjoyed it all.

Do you follow? In the midst of so-called suffering, what suffers? The nervous system wavers, the mind receives it, the intellect says, "Oh, I am suffering, I am suffering," but you are not. There's just a picture there. You may say, "How did the martyrs do it?" They had *ananda,* they had joy. They were no longer here. Instead, they were there, inside. This joy comes from within.

That's what Yoga is. Some people have the weirdest ideas about Yoga. They try to make it very mysterious. They talk about the Secret of the Ages, which they say has never been revealed before, but now in our modern times, it is going to be brought out, and we're going to tell you this secret stuff. They like to do that, you know. They say, "Two hundred dollars for the course." So then they think up a whole lot of gimmicks to teach you, to fog up the fact that they could have taught you in about two minutes. Isn't that so?

The truth is that the process is so easy, so simple, people miss the whole thing. Because we're complex, we try to make something out of nothing all the time. It's the easiest thing in the world, but the ego says, "Wait a minute. What am *I* going to do in all of this?" It's like the man or the wife who comes home and says, "What do you think? I heard a lecture today on Yoga, and I'm going to practice Yoga." Maybe some of you have had this personal experience. And the dear wife or the dear husband never says anything, but they think, "What about *me?*" Right? "What about me?"

So the ego says, "What about me? What is going to happen to my personality? And what about our children, all these desires and all these egotistical little ideas? What about our little baby likes and our little innocent dislikes? And what about the patter of little opinions that are running around the house? Are you turning away from all this?"

So the ego says, "What about me?" The good ol' sweet ego, that's what we are wedded to, you see. We are all man and wife. And it's that ego, ego, ego that we are married up to.

What we do is we say, "I remember, I read in that book about that superhard, complex, advanced *sadhana* (practice)." Once, I met this lady who said, "Well, what kind of Yoga do you believe in?" And I said such and such. She said, "We do Kundalini! You must understand, that's really tough stuff. That is for *advanced* people."

People love thinking they are on top of the pyramid; just a little group, you know. "Hah, if they all knew we were up here at the top. If they just knew." And then they have this meditation class. First do this, do that, do that. It becomes more and more complex. "We've got five more things beyond that." That's the gimmick. They love the gimmick. What's the higher technique? "Now, don't let anybody know you do this and don't do it publicly, after all this is a secret." So now the ego is pleased to think, "Ha, I'm doing something not many people can do."

But you see, it won't be Yoga if it isn't something that everybody can do. Yoga is based upon just what you are. Yoga is not trying to make you anything. Yoga is the way to start being what you are. The simplicity of it is the effectiveness of it. The more complex a thing is, the more the energies are split up, the more they are divided. Some people lay on a bed of nails; you know, that's what some people think a Yogi is. You have many nails evenly distributed. You lie there. Nothing pierces, because it's all evenly distributed. But take one nail and that will . . . ouch! So the way to pierce the shell of our delusion is to be one-pointed. That's why we make the mind one-pointed. That's why in meditation we do only one thing.

They say, "How did the Buddha get enlightenment?" Because he knew how to sit. His mind sat, his inner body sat, he sat and merged. It's simple, it's the simplest thing in the world.

What does this have to do with Siva? Siva, who is the real father, the real originator of this universe, is our own soul, our own being. He is the inmost being, the consciousness part of us, who is taking us and putting us in different situations. The ego, the mind, the will — or what we call the will — the senses, the emotions, and so on: these are only instruments. They have no consciousness in themselves. The ego, the mind, the body, are just being put here, there, do this, do that.

So Siva is making his music that way. "There Siva dances, striking his cheeks." That means, out of himself he's creating all these rhythms; out of himself he is making this cosmic manifestation, this universe. That's you. You're doing it all. You've made this body grow; no need to complain, no need to say, "Well, my grandfather had a funny nose, so I've got a funny nose." Your grandfather's fault? No. You decided to have that kind of nose; that expresses something. So all this is under your control. But we like to be cowardly and say, "Well, at the moment, I can't." That's a complete fantasy of the mind. You can, and you will have to one day. Do you understand? You like to say. "I am a victim." He is And He is enjoying his own Self – the thing He is projecting. This is the idea of *leela:* that the universe is for joy.

It's all for joy. The soul is sitting there in the middle and projecting a stream of creative vibration. "Ba-ba boom they resound." And that's what a mantram really is. A mantram is not a magic trick which is given by the guru. The truth is, the guru looks at you, and sees the creative pattern, the creative *shabda* (sound). And then he he tells you. There's a little more to it than that, but basically that's it. In other words, the mantram has been going on inside you forever. But it was unconscious. The guru enables you to make it conscious, and to follow that spiraling power back to the depths of your own being. That's what Mantra Yoga is.

So the mantram is inside you. It isn't that through sound power something is coming to you externally; it is moving within like the yeast in the dough, expanding, expressing, wanting to get out, wanting to bring you to that highest development. The guru comes along, he sees you, what's inside; and he says: "That's it." He imparts a power, he clears out some of those clogged-up channels – which is essential – and then he tells you, "All right, this is your light, this is your song, take it and consciously go on." That's the whole idea.

So Siva is dancing through this mantram and this mantram is the way to enter back into that real state. And this mantra power is coming out from within. That's the real you. It's consciousness. Now the way you're saying the mantram, mentally, it's a kind of sound. But basically, it's consciousness, it's a whole state of being, and as you do your sadhana more and more (but it has to be more and more) the more that calms, the more that moves. Then you will see that that mantram is consciousness itself. It isn't just a sound, something that will soothe your mind, something to just help you calm down, something that will merely aid in concentration. It is itself your inmost being, translated in sound terms for you to take hold of and trace back. Like the form of Krishna, Rama, this God who comes down assumes a form. It is really a revelation of God. He is your own Self. Krishna, Rama, Siva, Durga; they are all your own Self. So the mantram is your own Self; it's your own face. The Guru is just handing you a mirror. And the more you look in the mirror, the more you'll see of your Self. Self-realization. It's like adjusting the eyes to dark or light. The objects are already there; you just suddenly become the perceiver. You don't have to *get* it. So the mantram is to open up that inner eye, so that you'll see your Self. That's the whole idea of it. That's why it's so simple.

Meditation is the easiest thing in the world. You sit and you repeat the mantram. See what I mean? How could I charge you seventy-five dollars to tell you that? That's why, as I said this morning, these Yogis fog everything up: "Oh, if you sit this way, imagine this is happening, the current's doing this in the spine, put your fingers this way, plug your ears this way . . . ." And on and on and on. This method, that method. I remember hearing a lecture one time; I couldn't believe it. It went on for nearly forty-five minutes with one gimmick after another. Why, nobody in their right mind could even hold all those instructions and remember them, much less do them all. So if someone says, "Oh, teach me," then say, "Oh, it's easy. Just sit up straight. Now, just close your eyes, let them be natural, and now mentally repeat a mantram." (*Here, Swami Nirmalananda makes a disapproving face.*) Will that be the reaction? Sure.

Breathing is simple; nobody objects to it. Isn't that right? Nobody objects to it, saying: "Well, I ought to do something more than that." No, people are perfectly contented to just breathe easily and naturally. Sight is easy and natural. Who objects to that? So it ought to be obvious that this sadhana is also just as simple. That's it, that's all you need to know. How long does it take to tell a person? (*He looks at his watch.*) "You sit up, in a straight position, you relax, put your attention at the point between your eyebrows, and repeat the mantram." I said it in nine seconds. How could I charge you seventy-five dollars for nine seconds? That's why they make a big to-do about it. And also, we're rational — but *not* intelligent — so we think, "Well, look it just couldn't be that easy." But why not try?

So that's what we do. We sit in meditation, and we repeat that mantram mentally and we let our mind get soaked and absorbed in that sound. No, you don't fight thoughts, you don't fight memories. You don't bother with those things; that's not your business. Your business is that sound. If you've been initiated in a mantram, you use it. If you haven't been, you use Om, Om Tat Sat, Hari Om, any of these mantrams. You just sit there, you relax, and you just let your mind merge and melt in that sound, and your awareness will start to go where it belongs. And when distractions come up, when distracting thoughts come up, don't push them away and don't try to be more intense. That's exactly the wrong thing.

If you've got a sponge full of water, the tighter you squeeze it, the more water will squirt out. The mind is like that. So hold it in complete relaxation and balance. If distracting thoughts come, it's because you're not relaxed enough. It's just the opposite of what people usually think: "I must control the mind!" Not at all. You will find, when you start remembering something that happened yesterday, that what has happened is that a little tension has come into your mind. You've sort of "pinched" your mind a little to think of that thing. What you need to do is just relax, consciously just breathe out. And the more you relax, especially in the inner attitude, the less the thoughts will come. That's the real path, that's the real way.

The key is TOTAL relaxation. That's why we have *asanas*. Why do you learn to sit correctly? So you can relax 100 percent and not fall over. That's the whole idea of the real asana. That's why *padmasana,* the lotus pose, is considered the best. You will sit, and you won't have a muscle tensed in your body. That's why we say posture is important. It's true, if you're slumped, you tend to go to sleep; it's good to have the spine erect so that currents can flow up and down. But the major idea is to be totally relaxed and not moving. That's the real secret, relaxation, and no worry, no anxiety, no interest to go anywhere because you don't have to go anywhere; no interest to obtain anything because you've got it all, and all you're doing is just becoming aware of it. Then the mantram will take effect. Otherwise, it's like tightening up a muscle. People get muscles all tight and tense; after they come out of meditation, they're all stiff and sore.

You can see this. You can see this in people when they're not meditating right; they're tensed inside all the time. It's as though all the time they're kind of knotted and shifty-eyed. Because they have not relaxed in meditation. *Sahaja* – this is the thing – sahaja *japa,* natural meditation.

You've got lots of distractions in your mind? All right. That must be natural for your mind at that moment. Why bother? Why worry? You follow me? That's where you are right now. So that's natural. Your back aches? That must be natural at the moment. You understand what I'm talking about? Rather than, "Oh, no, I've got to change it," it's better to say, "All right." As soon as you think that, it goes away. It's just like in the water – you reach for something and it moves away from you. When you're no longer interested in it, it floats to you.

Listen, this power of maya is something that we never stop to think about. But we are so totally hypnotized, in every little detail, that it's almost terrifying. We see virtually nothing in the correct way. Nearly every thought in our head is wrong. It's remarkable. I mean, there's such a percentage it's astounding. That's why we just forget that mind — because it isn't us. We don't have to do anything with the mind — don't straighten it up, don't control it, don't do anything with it. You understand? Somebody just handed you this bag of fighting cats. Just drop it. Don't try to make peace. Some people struggle and struggle for twenty years to control their mind. But the problem has not been that their mind was either restless or calm. Neither one amounts to anything. It is that their consciousness wasn't in the right place. In fact, to try and control the mind you have to merge your whole identity in the mind and forget about your real nature. Does it make sense, what I'm saying?

All right. Let's get back to the song. "A garland of skulls from his neck is hanging." The skulls represent all the *samskaras,* all the impressions. Let me explain samskaras. It's just like you go to the store and buy something; you eat it, you don't like it, and you say "nevermore" every time you think of it. Ugh! That's a samskara. It's a habit pattern. It's a thought, an attitude, a conceptual pattern. It all stores up in the unconscious mind. We carry with us every single thought we've ever felt. Isn't that horrible? What a load. Inwardly, subtly, you still have every form you've ever had. Believe me, you're a whole crowd, you're never alone. When you're in a room, and there seems to be nobody with you, let me tell you, there are a couple of thousand people in that room. And when you go inside, you'll be amazed. And that by the way is why we have the *yama* and the *niyama,* the very strict Do's and Don'ts: to make right conduct a habit. Because you are going in and bringing out those old samskaras, and if you don't have a safeguard, where right conduct is almost automatic, you'll be gone; they'll sweep you away. Do you follow me? You can be a person who's never thought of being dishonest and taking anything that wasn't yours. But believe me, you can meditate and meditate and meditate, and you may walk into a store and suddenly think of stealing something. Really. And you'll be shocked. "Hey. What is this? I wasn't that way before." We have good samskaras, but we also have very bad samskaras.

Spiritual practice is called tapasya. It means, "that which generates heat." So we start heating things up in there, and the first thing you know, all these things come streaming out. That is why you find that "religious" people are not so good in Yoga. You know why? Because all their life they've said, "I am faithful. I am following God. I am doing His work." Do you follow me? They are hypnotizing themselves into how well off they are spiritually. Then they take up Yoga and they find out that they're a mess. They've been hiding it. They've been *doing* good, not *being* good. The doing was a substitute When they felt hatred or when they were selfish, they rationalized it or they turned it off from their mind, because it wouldn't be the right thing to feel. So they made it even worse by keeping it bottled up. It has really aged down in there and really gained power. Then they turn the mind within. They find they're filled with hatred, filled with greed, they're filled with selfishness. Nothing but resentments. They are really a horrible picture. "Yoga is of the devil. Yoga is making me evil. It's making me degenerate. I'm falling apart. I quit."

Usually, you have to take people who have hardly any religious training and hardly any religious identification. They don't have any illusions about themselves. They meditate and say, "That's right, I am really number one on the bad list. Yep, that's me, I recognize it." And they improve. Do you realize that in our whole ashram, in our whole monastery, I am the only one that was religious? In fact, sometimes I think, how did I make it? Because when you come across the religious ones — "Ohh, I've been seeking for truth all my life" — well, you'd better watch out, because if they're been searching all their life and haven't found it, there's some kind of subconscious reservation around someplace. So Yoga is not for people who have a grand opinion of themselves.

So all those skulls are hanging around the neck of Siva. That means, there are samskaras there, hanging around your soul, and it's your job to cut the thread of identification and ego. Then they will all fall off. Just because you don't do anything on a conscious level doesn't mean you don't do anything on a subconscious level. Who do you think is making your heart beat right now? You're not sitting here, thinking, "Open, close, open, close," are you? So think of the level of your mind that is controlling every single cell of your body. If you don't think that that doesn't have a lot of samskaras in it to be wiped out . . . . So all of that is lying in there, to be swept away. This is what Siva is saying. That is why we look at his garland of skulls, to remember all that.

All right. "In his matted locks the Ganges hisses." I'll have to go into that story. I'll say this very briefly. The Ganges river needed to come to earth, but the force of the Ganges would destroy the earth. So Siva said, "I will receive this on my head." So the Ganges fell on Siva's head, and he had very long hair, very matted. It's said that the Ganges was absorbed or held in the hair of his head and unable to get out. Now I'll explain that. In the matted locks means in the subtle *nadis,* the subtle channels of energy in our bodies. That very Ganges power, which can wash away all samskaras, which can wash away all negative impressions — and has to wash away all good ones also — which can completely sweep away all delusion and duality in a mighty flood, is locked in there, in those nadis. "The Ganges hisses." That is, it is trying to get out. It's caught there. The idea is, all power is in you. Everything you need is in you. All you need to do is know how to release it, how to release it properly. Some people do the wrong thing and they release just a little atom of it too soon and they just fry up, I think you are all familiar with this, about kundalini rising too soon and so on. So in you is all that power to be unlocked. No external force whatsoever is really needed. You are the source. Understand? This is why Siva is so well liked by the Yogis — because he is reminding them constantly of their inner state. That is all inside, inside, nothing outside. All inside.

"Fire shoots from his mighty trident." There are three gunas: tamas, rajas and sattva. Tamas: the force that brings inertia, heaviness and ignorance. Rajas: the force that causes all kinds of activity and restlessness. And sattva: that which brings harmony and balance. But still a balance which causes us to see duality, though in a much more detached way. All of them must go. *All* of them must go.

Then, of course, in the spine we have three major channels: *ida, pingala,* and *sushumna.* This is also the three-pronged trident of Lord Siva — in which the fires, the pranas, the subtle forces are moving. When these are brought into balance, they sweep away all these samskaras, all these negative things, and give the vision of what is true.

"Around his waist a serpent glitters." Serpent! This is the symbol of the primal *shakti,* the primal power, which is under his control. Not only has it risen but he has tied a knot around it, and he has it around his waist. He uses it for a belt. That which has everyone else under its sway, he is wearing. And just as he wears an ornament too. You could have that mastery.

"And on his brow the moon is shining." The moon is representative of the individual soul. The sun is the supreme soul. The earth's shadow — maya, materiality, gross consciousness — gets in the way and sometimes we see only the tiniest sliver of the moon. That's why we worship the guru on *Guru Poornima Day.* The Poornima Day means the day when the Self is fully revealed, and since it's the Guru who brings about this revelation, we worship him, we honor him, on a full moon day. So the Self is fully revealed here. All the identification with the lower things is finished, and here all is light. That moon, that reflection of the Divine, has even come onto the physical level now. Jesus said, "If you have seen me, you have seen the Father." That seems odd. You mean, if they looked at his body they could see God? Yes. Physically, what is this body? It's just frozen energy, and what is energy? It's consciousness. The body becomes divine. That's why some saints, when they die, never decay. When they took Saint Theresa out of the coffin, they washed her face off, they combed her hair. She'd been dead for nearly a hundred years. You understand? No changing. This is true of many saints. It isn't because God decided to wow the crowd and astound people. "Wow, would you look at that! They didn't rot, isn't that amazing?" No, that's not the idea. The idea is that their body has become imperishable because it has become pervaded by divine consciousness.

There have been cases where, when they opened the tomb, there wasn't any body. Those of you who are familiar with the Catholic religion know this happened to the Virgin Mary. Coming closer to our own time, around the 800's, St. Andrew of Constantinople. When he died, one moment his body was there – and a moment later it just dispersed. When the great Indian saint, Mirabai – she lived about the 16th or 17th century – left this world, she was sitting in a temple singing to Lord Krishna, and before her was an image of Lord Krishna. Everybody there saw her body literally just lose its general form and turn into light that streamed into the image – and that was that. This was witnessed by hundreds of people. It's not like a few people that wanted to start a personality cult. Sri Krishna Chaitanya, also living at that time, went to the temple, walked up to the image of *Jaganath Puri,* and was *gone.* Because that was his control.

We hear of saints that were in two places at once. They were sitting in such and such a place and three thousand miles away somebody saw them. Why? Because they are all-pervasive consciousness throughout this universe. And that's all the body is: it is just consciousness. They could just move it like that – no trouble. It was nothing for them, because they had become everything. And that's who you really are. Aren't you a remarkable person? Then why are you messing around – playing such a puny little role? You are the master director. Why are you just playing a little walk-on, walk-off part, and nobody understanding who you are or where you come from or where you are going? So bring that even onto this physical level.

We hear of saints – somebody who is sick touches them, and they're well. Why? Because their bodies have become that perfect thing which has such a powerful magnetism that any imperfection coming near them must disappear. You see? That's what disease is – it's an imbalance. And that's your state. And that's what wrong with people when they start making a hero worship on any level – because then they start thinking, "Oh, the Great One, and me the little one." And then they stay in that "little me" consciousness for lives and lives. That's what Krishna says,

"He who understands My birth and My task in this life is liberated."
Now, how many people worship Lord Krishna and still come back many
times? There are people who built temples to Lord Krishna, and you
know they died, and they come back; they had a "return ticket." You
see, people want to go on. "Oh, Krishna, Krishna, Krishna, Hey Krishna,
Oh His leelas," and they weep and so on. Not that I've got anything
against Bhakti. Bhakti is essential, but it must be understood that Krishna
was the Self revealed. He showed the nature of the Self. So if you understand the mystery of his birth, that is the mystery of your own birth. We
say, when he came into the world he didn't quite have a physical body. It
was just an appearance, it wasn't even a normal birth. That's fine. But it's
the same truth about us and we should say, "Now, wait a minute! What
about my birth? What about my body?" You understand what I'm talking about? We say, it's just leela for him. He's just playing a game. Okay,
grand, but we should realize that we're just playing a game too. Why
crawl around in the mud, saying, "Oh, poor me. Oh, I can't wait until
I'm a butterfly." This is your real nature. You are Siva. *Sivoham, Sivoham*
(I am Siva, I am Siva). We should sing that, shouldn't we? I am no
mother, I am no father, I am no brother. I am formed of blissful consciousness. I am Siva. Incredible thing. I am not this body. I am not this
mind. I am not this seeming will. No. I have no birth. I have no death. I
have no station in life. No caste. Sivoham. Sivoham. That's me.

We have these ideas in religion. People don't understand. They see a
picture of Siva on the wall and they think, "Oh, they want to get me
into some kind of weird stuff about some really exotic, far-out thing in
Hindu religion. They're trying to convert me to that and make me
worship that strange business." No. The pictures on the wall are saying,
"Here's your face. Do you recognize it?" Or, "Here's the chart. Which
of these qualities do you have? Which of these qualities do you recognize
in yourself? Which of these qualities do you manifest?" That's the whole
idea behind these forms.

It's the same way with the guru. We say that the guru gives light. Each
person's soul is *jyothi,* is light, and you have your own light. If I gave you
my light, what would it be? It would be artificial, isn't that so? You don't
need to realize *me,* but you have got to realize *you.* Why are you here?
Because that light is shining out from inside, not because someone has
shined light on you. Some people don't understand this. They say,
"Why, when I meet certain people, I feel very high, I feel very changed,
and when they're gone, I'm back in the old slump." You tried to take
their light as your light, and tried to be satisfied with that external thing
instead of getting down into your own source. In other words, you were

dying of thirst and saying, "Please give me a cup of water out of your well," not knowing you yourself are a never-ending fountain, and that's what counts. That's what the guru does. He helps you to open your own inner well. Jesus said, "If a person comes to Me, out of his inmost being, rivers of water are going to flow." But people like to get into hero worship. "Oh, the guru is so great, the guru is so high, the guru is so fine." And so they want to say, of the few drops that drip off the guru, "That satisfies me." That way they never have to drill inside and get it. That's why the guru does not pamper us. Sometimes he gives us a good whack so that we'll understand. He cuts us off from this hero worship — not to make us mad so that we go away, but so that we quit this sort of little jig around him, thinking that *he* is "it", when *we* are really "it."

So it is you; it is your growing; it is your truth that must come forth. But the ego, knowing that, prefers you to get stuck in some external idea, external concept, and external form. As Krishna says, "He who knows My birth and My task, he never comes back to birth." But people take a statue and they worship and they worship and they worship, and they build temples and they come back to birth because they still think Krishna's outside. They don't know Krishna's inside. They don't understand that. So this is the thing. All we need is that simplicity. All we need is to know what we are.

Undoism

Swami Satchidananda

The satsang given by Swami Nirmalananda earlier in the day laid a strong emphasis on the renunciation of sensual and intellectual pleasures. But for some of the retreatants, many of whom were just beginning their study and practice of Yoga, his teachings seemed a bit harsh and difficult. So, in this, Swamiji's fourth lecture, he clarifies the concept of renunciation, of "letting go," and how it could be practiced by all. He introduces the idea that absolute renunciation is not possible in the beginning, but that many negative things can be replaced by one good thing which in turn could eventually fall away. Swamiji refers to this approach of his as "Undoism," saying that that is his religion.

In the course of these comments Swamiji also clarifies the idea of sense control. Many retreatants carried away from Nirmalanandaji's "pig story" the impression that the senses and sense pleasures and even artistic pleasures are to be considered undesirable for a spiritual aspirant. Swamiji asks how we could have even heard the Swami's lecture without the senses, the ears. So it is not that we should destroy the senses, but master them.

In closing, Swamiji presents one more important point: the importance of understanding the reasons behind what we do in the name of yogic life — we should not just do something, but should know the ultimate aim behind it and eventually be totally free of all the practices, dogmas, labels, and even organizations.

Following the talk, Swamiji answers questions of a practical nature on sense control and also on repetition of mantrams and other aspects of meditation practice which came up in response to Nirmalananda's extremely helpful comments on the subject.

So, the latest formula is "Let it go," hm? So you think it is that easy to let go? Swami Nirmalanandaji said it's easy. Do you think so? There's a story about Christopher Columbus; have you heard it? An Indian asking you people that! I don't know why I'm trying to sell coal in Newcastle, but still, let me say it. You know, when Columbus discovered "India," almost everybody welcomed him home with all joy and nice feelings. But there were a few people who were jealous of his fame. During the reception they said, "What is the greatness? What is the difficulty? You just sailed and landed in India. Anybody could have done that. It's so easy. Why all the pomp and show and great reception for you?"

Columbus quietly stood up from the lunch table and said, "Okay, let's forget all about the discovery of India. Who can make this egg stand on its end? If you could just do it, fine. Who can do it?"

"What, man, are you crazy?" Who can do it? How can an egg stand on its end? See, the minute you put it, it just rolls. Nobody could do it. Why do you even put this challenge?"

"No, certainly somebody could do it. I could do it."

"Hah! Okay, do it."

So Columbus just took the egg. It stood. How? He didn't just put it down slowly. He plumped the egg on the table so that the egg's curved end got squashed.

Then they said, "Oh, this we can do, anybody can do that."

"Then why didn't you do it before? I didn't ask you not to make a dent in it. You could have done that."

So it's easy if a man knows the gimmick. If you don't know, it's impossible for you. That reminds me of Nandanar, the untouchable saint who stood in the entrance of the temple praying to God, "God I'm an untouchable. The priests don't allow me to come in. But still I want to see you. Won't you bless me with your darshan? You know my heart. The priests may not know. They see me as a pariah, a low caste person. But you know me."

The temples in India are built in such a way that when all the doors are open you can see the *sanctum sanctorum* – the very inner shrine where the light is flickering even from the road. The inner shrine is in semi-darkness so you see only the light, you can't see the image there. But sometimes in big temples they have a huge vehicle of the Lord, a bull or a peacock or a tiger, sitting right in front of Him, almost hiding the shrine inside. So, in the case of Nandanar, when he looked in he couldn't see the Lord; he saw the huge bull right in the middle. So he said, "I know You are all-merciful. You want to show Yourself to me. But unfortunately the bull is sitting between You and me. So before I even ask for Your blessing I should request the bull to bless me and move a little so that I can see You."

So he started singing. He prayed and prayed and the Lord ordered the bull, "Okay, child, move a little. Let him see Me." That's the story; I don't know how you're going to take it. But even today in that temple you can see the bull is not in its proper place. It's moved aside so you can see their God from the road itself. All because of Nandanar, such a great saint.

But still, before he had darshan Nandanar used to sing, "Oh, alas, it is difficult. Alas, it is difficult to get the grace of God." That's what he sang. But Ramana Maharshi, who was a great modern Indian master with whom I stayed for some time, used to twist this song to say. "Oh, it's very easy!" The same song, he just made it easy. We asked him, "What do you mean by this? Nandanar, the great devotee, who made the bull move, sang, 'Oh, it's almost impossible, it's so difficult.' But you say, 'Oh, it's very easy.' " Ramana would say, "I don't know, this is what I feel." Why? To hold the cat's tail is difficult. Let go — easy. Renunciation is not difficult. Holding on and clinging to things is difficult. The simplest thing is to just let go. Don't hold on to anything.

But there is one thing which we could hold on to. As one saint says, "Hold the unholdable feet of the Lord." Cling to the feet of the Lord who has no clinging. Take the support of the Lord who doesn't have any support. Why? To get us out of this other clinging. The one who doesn't need any hold at all is the Lord. So the idea is, to let go of all our holds, we stick to one. By holding this, we can let go of everything else.

Have you ever seen a fox? The fox teaches a beautiful lesson. I'll tell you the story. "Once upon a time . . ." there lived a fox in a jungle. Somehow, it so happened that it got into some kind of trouble with lice. You know what lice are? The small, small insects which come even to the head and creep around. The hair is the jungle for them to roam around, hm? So this fox got millions of lice all over the body. It was a terrible thing. The fox rubbed and scrubbed and did everything but he couldn't get rid of them. One day when he went to a pond to drink a little water, he just stepped in because the water was so low. He placed the front paws in and drank, and then he noticed that the paws which were in the water were free from the lice. The lice had moved up because of the water.

You know, the fox is a cunning animal. He thought, "Ah, here is the trick." He came out, took a small stick and held it in his mouth. He put one end in the mouth and then slowly walked into the water, half an inch at a time. Slowly, all the lice started coming up. All the four paws were inside, then up to the abdomen. When the water touched the abdomen, the lice came up the back and then he slowly went further into the water. Little by little, the fox went down still more. Fortunately the nose is the topmost thing. So he just went down, up to the nose opening, till almost all the lice having no more place, were on the stick. Only a few of them were sticking around the nose. Then the fox took a long, deep breath. Pranayama, hm? He took a slow, deep inhalation, held that breath and went into the water. Even the few remaining lice came onto the stick. And then, gently, the fox let that stick go and walked out. Isn't that a cute thing to do?

So what is there in this world? Everything is nothing but lies (lice).

What is true in this world; what is permanent? Nothing. Anything that is impermanent is false, is a lie. So we too have many "Lies" on our body, physical, mental, everywhere. So, we have to see that all these "lies" go onto a stick. That is what you call practice. Any practice: *japa, (repetition of a mantram)*, study, whatever you like; hold on to that one thing. Let all the "lies" go onto that. Give everything to that.

That is what we do in the name of God. One of the things that Swami Nirmalananda said in one of his articles is, "We renunciates lead a simple life but we do a lot of elaborate pujas at the altar. What does that mean? We don't want anything for ourselves, we want everything to go to God." So God is our stick. We allow all the lies to go onto God, and then one day, even that should be dropped, otherwise we're not renunciates, we're still holding on. All these things are excuses, even your mantram, meditation, chanting and everything you do in the name of practice, because the liberation or enlightenment cannot be attained by *doing* something. The more you do, the more you are involved with trouble. You have done enough. So all you are to do now is just to *undo* what you have done. All these practices are for the sake of undoing. (*Swamiji pauses here and smiles.*) That is my religion. Do you know what religion I believe in? (*Again he pauses and smiles.*) Undoism. (*Laughter.*) Yes, if anybody asks you what your religion is, just tell them: Undoism.

The question is, how to undo. As Swami Nirmalanandaji said this morning, "What can I do? A person who believes in constantly doing something, if you tell him that he doesn't need to do anything, he will wonder, 'How can I be without doing anything?' " Doing is very necessary to be able to undo. Only actions will nullify other actions. So this is a kind of catalytic agent.

As I often say, if you want to get rid of the dirt on some clothing you go buy a piece of dirt, which you call soap. What is soap after all? A piece of dirt that was made good looking and good smelling; is it not so? You pay for it and apply that dirt onto the existing dirt with a little moisture. When that new dirt comes in, the old dirt receives it. "Ah, who are you; where did you come from? You seem to be a nice friend." So they start chumming up and the laundryman knows the exact time when the old dirt is coming out of the cloth and receiving the new dirt and celebrating. At that time he just dips the cloth in the water and takes it out. The poor old dirt, forgetting that the cloth has gone out of the water, is still enjoying the reception. That is how the old and the new dirt remain in the water when the cloth comes out clear. Did you ever want the dirt you paid for to remain in the cloth? Do you say, "No, I don't want the old dirt, but *this* dirt I paid for, it must still remain on the cloth"? No. Because your interest is in cleaning the cloth. So the soap acts as a catalytic agent. Only dirt can destroy dirt. Only an ignorant act will destroy our ignorance.

There is no enmity between the light and the darkness. You go tell the sun, "Oh, Sun, you have destroyed the darkness." The Sun will say, "I didn't destroy anything. I don't have any enemies and I don't know anything about darkness. Without even knowing or seeing an enemy how can I destroy him? If you say I destroyed the darkness, then can you take me to see him or bring him to me?" Can you take the sun to show him the darkness? Or can the darkness come in front of the sun? No. There is no enmity. That is why there is no enmity between the Truth and the untruth. They don't even exist together. When one is there, the other is not. The Truth always remains. What you see as darkness is not really darkness, you only see it as darkness. There is only Light. Self exists; God exists, here and everywhere. If He exists, then where can you go to see Him? If He is omnipresent, in everything and all places, then what can hide Him? The hiding screen should also be God then. If you say, "No, God is not that screen," then He is not omnipresent. Just to know the Truth, that's all you have to do, but unfortunately our knowing seems to be in the wrong direction.

Jnana is wisdom and *ajnana* is just illusion and that has to be removed. Jnana will not come to help you remove ajnana. That is why I said, in the story of the Sun, that the Sun has no enmity; he will not even come to see the darkness. To destroy a country, the political trick is the same. You have to make contact with a person in the country itself. Then it is easy. Only the one who is in the country, who knows everything, can help. Even Sri Rama destroyed Ravana with the help of Vibhishana, one of Ravana's own brothers. Vibhishana knew everything. So get help from someone of the enemies' country and destroy it. There's another beautiful example of this: the handle of the ax. Such people who come from a country and who give all the clues about their country to help the other country's men destroy their own country, we call "the handle of the ax." Do you know why? The handle of the ax comes from wood. Without the handle, you can't chop more wood. See, a wooden handle helps to chop the rest of the wood. So we call such people as the wooden handle of the ax. They are the enemies of their own kind.

So, the same trick is used even in the spiritual field. We have been doing many things. And to un-do them we have to do something again as a catalytic agent. That's why the scriptures say, "Not by doing something do you get the Wisdom, not by karma, not by wealth, not by progeny. Only by dedication, only by renouncing, only by letting go, do you realize the Immortal Principle." But in the Gita, Arjuna asked, "Then why do you push me into doing this? You say all this and then you add, 'Therefore go and destroy the people; therefore fight.'" There seems to be a contradiction, hm? Then Sri Krishna said, "Yes, you have been used to doing things. I can't stop you from doing immediately. To destroy a devil you have to get another devil. Therefore I ask you to do something which will go, later on, along with the other, without affecting you, like a catalytic agent." And that is the reason why we have all these different practices, whatever you want to call them. Everything is to be done as a practice. Do something. You may say, "Let it go; we don't even want any puja or any pranayama or any japa, why not just let go?" It's impossible. So from one thing you go to the other.

That's why Shankaracharya, the great seventh-century Indian philosopher, said, your interest is to liberate yourself, to become a *jivan-mukta,* to live as a liberated being. But to have this liberation or to realize this liberated state, you must do something first. So you begin with the good company, satsang, the company of the wise people. The minute you are with them you will be doing something which will not affect you, which will not add more burden to the existing burden. The immediate result of having satsang is that you are no longer in the *nisang,* the bad company. The immediate result of our ten-day retreat is that you are not in a cinema house or in Las Vegas; you cannot be in both places at the same time. Whether you get anything else here or not, it doesn't matter. Just by being here you avoid so many troubles, is it not? How many packages of cigarettes will be thanking you for not having got burned? That is the immediate benefit.

"Satsangatwe, nisangatwam," Shankaracharya says. There is another meaning to that also. It means you are freed, you are detached. Because satsang means detached-minded people, people who do not have selfish attitudes. Sat is the truth. The one who knows the truth will not be clinging on to anything. He or she is not attached to anything. So when you are in their company you also learn to be detached. So that is another meaning of this *sanga* (company).

So what is the benefit of staying away from nisang? The benefit is that you are no longer deluded. You always get a clear vision of things, what is right and what is wrong. Your eye opens. You know what is. You know what you were doing all these days, with what kind of make-up you were doing, what roles you were playing, what delusions you were pampering. To use Swami Nirmalananda's words, you would easily realize that you were tending the pigs. That means, all the senses are our pigs. You were just taking care of them. Whenever they cried you fed them. There is a proverb, "If you want to fatten your pig, feed it whenever it squeals. If you want to spoil your child, give him whatever he wants." It's an Indian proverb. It means you just tend to the senses. When you want to see the cinema, you must buy a ticket. At any cost, borrow or steal, you must go see that movie. Because the mind wants it. In other words, you go crazy. If you want to eat some pizza, the very minute you think of it you must go and get it. Even if it is five, ten, twenty miles away, midnight, away you go, otherwise you won't sleep. We become slaves to the senses.

Say the boss of a huge factory says, "I am the boss here; I am the master here." A small half-burned cigarette in the ashtray laughs at him. "Hey, who is the boss? Can you exist without me?" An ordinary inert thing enslaves him. How many people go really crazy, lose their entire day, if they don't get the cigarette for the day? So if you think in these terms, how many masters we have. Where is the glory? "Oh, I am this or that, I am free." Hah! Everything enslaves you. Your cigarettes enslave you, your hairdo enslaves you, if you don't have the right dress you won't go to an important function. Isn't that so? How many people miss their church because they do not have the proper dress? As if the Lord is look- ing at their dress and not their "address," hm? Superficial, superficial. This is what you call slavery.

According to Patanjali, the exponent of Raja Yoga, when you control the senses, you can control the mind because the mind functions through the senses. If the senses are restricted, the mind is restricted. To control does not mean to stop. You do not need to kill them. Control them and put them in the proper place. Eyes are not bad, ears are not bad, if you see the right thing, if you hear the right thing. So we should understand also what Nirmalanandaji was saying this morning about pigs. They are not really pigs. If you allow them to be pigs, they are. But if not, they are fine. Because, when he said that the ears are pigs, we heard the same words with the ears, is it not? How could they be pigs then? A pig could not even hear that! So that is not the meaning. Do not allow them *to become* pigs. It is your mind. Train it.

So the entire retreat is for this mind control and sense control. That's why on the very first night I said, you control your tongue, your sense of feeling, sense of touch. It is not just a kind of holiday gathering or festival. Just imagine nice beautiful young couples lying around under the trees, kissing and hugging each other, oh, a beautiful scene will be there! But here we do not even touch each other. Is all that bad? I did not say so. Do it, but with limitations. Everything has its limitations. That's why you are learning to control your senses here. On a retreat, your tongue is controlled, your eyes, even your ears are controlled. However much you want to listen to your rocking and rolling music, you can't hear it here. All the music here makes you sit and meditate! Indirectly you are training or helping to train your senses and the mind. Once that happens the soul is free, because it's the mind that binds. It is the mind that brings in all kinds of feelings: "I want this, I want that." It is constantly getting disturbed. So because of the disturbed mind, you see a wrong picture. If the mind is clean and soft and tranquil, you see the right picture.

It is something like if you see yourself in a clear mirror, you see the right image. If you see yourself in a distorted mirror, you seem horrible. You are not really horrible, you are beautiful, you are the divine Self, the image of God. But unfortunately it is being seen through your distorted mirror. Neither you see yourself as clear nor can others see you clearly because of the distortion of the mirror. Even a small fingerprint on the lens of a camera makes the picture bad, is it not? You shouldn't even touch it. But here, how many prints we have, how many impressions. That is the main purpose of all these practices. So take up something. The fox didn't take a huge log, eh? Within its capacity it picked up a small stick which it could easily carry to the water. Pick up some stick. Temporarily hold it, until all these things go onto that.

That's why even the teachers, or gurus, if you want to call it that way, demand some kind of surrendering or giving up everything, renouncing everything. Don't think that the gurus are getting anything or benefiting or keeping anything. They may even be harmed, if they're not careful. It happens. There's a priest class in the Hindu system which performs the rituals and last rites. The people who go to Benares want to get rid of their sins. So the priests perform certain rituals. And during the ceremony the priest accepts offerings from these sinful people. And the mantram said during the offering means that along with what you give the priest, you give your sins also. So, he not only gets your offering, he will be accumulating the sins too unless he practices well. If you have any doubt, you should actually go and see some priests in Benares. You will see the devil's face in them. If you see their faces you will see they are coming from a black, devilish land. They don't even realise they're being affected. And the person who comes to the rites does it with all sincerity so he is free from all the sins. The priest has taken them and he will have to wash them away.

It is something like a doctor operating on a septic wound. It is a contagious thing, so every time he performs the operation he should sterilize himself, is it not? If he treats a leper, he should not become afflicted. He should take all precautions. Soon after the treatment he should go and cleanse himself. If not, he will get that leprosy. The same things happen in the mental field, the astral field. So don't think it is a joke to receive all these things that the students give to the priests and Swamis. If they don't do the proper things to wash it from their shoulders, they will be ahead of you as a sinner. If you still go to hell as a sinner, they will be waiting there to receive you!

This reminds me of a funny story. There was a man who was constantly called a sinner, sinner, sinner by his priest. When he died, still as a sinner, he was taken to hell. He was put in a room and as he walked in he saw his priest sitting there. "Priest, what are *you* doing here?" And in a whisper the priest said, "Don't shout my name, please. The High Priest is next door!" So that is why it is not so easy to perform these duties. The teachers may tell you to do this, wash this, give everything, surrender everything. But at the same time, they should know what they have to do with that. If I am careless you will be going to heaven and I will be going to the other place.

That is the reason why I say spiritual practice is to be done with the proper understanding. You should know why you are doing certain things. What is the goal? What is the thing you want to achieve? Not that you blindly do it because you were asked. If you just do it, it is better than doing many other things, no doubt. But it is best if you know what you are doing. Then you will know if you are getting closer and closer. "How am I now? How was I yesterday? Am I at least slightly better today?" Then you know you are progressing. That is why Master Sivananda, my guru, used to ask the seekers to keep a spiritual diary. "How much time do I spend in meditation? How much time on my mantram, asanas, pranayama? How much selfless service do I do?" And on the other side: "how many lies I told; how many times I got into fits of anger" — all the things that should not be done. Make a list of those also. So you compare with the past week. First week, ten lies. This week, eight. You are growing. So you should check up on your growth. Slowly clean the dirt by using the soap. One day when everything is over you won't need these at all. You are totally free. You are not bound by anything. Neither by an organization, nor a religion. Nor by certain practices, nor by a label. No. You need not call yourself a Raja Yogi, Bhakti Yogi, this yogi, that yogi, or belong to that institution or country. You are free from everything.

It is sad to see that sometimes even the Sannyasis consciously or unconsciously get into organizations. "So you are not part of the Yoga society in Pennsylvania?" "Oh no, mine is the Integral Yoga Institute in New York." "Oh, you don't go to the Lutheran Church?" "No, I go to the Universalist Church." That is a kind of binding. But, begin with something and then open up more and more and more. Then one day you will see that there is nothing more to open. You are fully opened. You are everywhere; you belong to everybody and everybody belongs to you.

Questions and Answers on Self-discipline and Meditation

Swami Satchidananda

As I was walking today I passed two people sneaking a cigarette. They looked so childish, like a couple of kids being caught in the cookie jar. Please say a word for them and all of us about the importance of gaining control of the senses.

Oh, my sweet children, I am sorry for that. That is what, they are still not strong. They want to control but the "flesh is weak." What can we do? You can't gain the control overnight. So some succumb to that. So we'll even pity them. They are still weaklings. It's not a big mistake but they are not strong. They are convinced that it is not the right thing to do. In fact, everyone knows, including the Surgeon General, hm? And the makers of the cigarettes also know and the man who paints, "naturally refreshes, coooool," he also knows. The unfortunate thing is, the producers want the money. They are slaves of money. You are a slave of your habit. That is the trouble.

So we have to grow out of that weakness. It doesn't matter even if you make a mistake. Afterwards look at it and say, "What did I do? Why should I behave that way? What caused this weakness? Oh, see? I should not have brought the package here." Immediately take it out and burn the whole thing. In front of everybody, even. Then, even though you make a mistake, you are courageous. But pride might stop you from doing it. Who has the packets here? Is there anybody who has cigarette packets here or in their rooms? Hm? Yes? In your rooms? Okay, be true to yourselves, you two. As soon as you go back, take them out and set fire to the whole thing. See, when you want to control something, you can't keep it there in front of you and control it. If you had never brought it here, you would have controlled it. You would have stayed out of it. The unavailability itself helps you in a way. If you are that strong, you can even live around cigarettes and not smoke. But until you gain the strength, stay away from it. Would you mind doing that? No? Good. Go on, do it. Show that you have the strength. Are we slaves? No, we are all heroes. Let us express that. Who are the ones who put the hands in the cookie jar then? (*When no one raises a hand someone in the audience calls out,*

"Probably they're out for a smoke!" Swamiji laughs.) Oh, what do you do with these kids? Oh, God bless you, God bless you.

So that's what. Why do we seek the good company? Because we are weak. If you are strong you don't worry about the company. Wherever you are, you are strong. But as long as you are a young plant, you should have a fence. When you become a tree, throw the fence away, you don't need it. That's why, as long as you feel that you have a weakness, stay away from the thing. And you should even stay away from the people who will induce you or tempt you. Of course, this is all just if you want to. Otherwise, there's no use telling you this.

How often should a beginner meditate?

As often as possible. And do everything as a meditation also. Meditation is a continuous process. Everything should be done with a meditative attitude. Whatever you do, meditate on it. And as a specific practice, you should do it at least twice a day, if not more. The more the better. Morning and evening. You can even make a habit: every time you want to eat something, have a little meditation before you eat. So you'll at least meditate before breakfast, before lunch and before dinner – three times a day. And at least for ten or fifteen minutes, anyway. You can increase up to one or two hours.

At the same time, don't make it a burden or an ordeal or it will frighten your mind. If the mind gets frightened, whenever you think of meditation you'll feel a headache coming on and your mind won't want to do anything. There'll be all kinds of symptoms. The body might get cramps. You'll get all kinds of funny feelings. The brain has the capacity to produce symptoms all over the body. Even hysteria or fainting. So don't force; gently train the mind as you train an animal. You should handle the mind gently and with all affection. Don't be brutal. Something like steel: it bends but it's strong. You should bend to be strong.

I feel guilty when I don't meditate and do asanas regularly. Would you say a few words about guilt?

That kind of guilt is wanted. Otherwise you won't do it! When you do something wrong, you should regret it. But don't just feel guilty and sit there and cry, "Oh, I'm doomed." If you fall down, you're not just going to sit there. Get up and walk further. Your success depends on your failures. The failures are the stepping stones. Don't let them discourage you and cause you to stray from the right path.

Why do my eyes flutter when concentrating on the third eye? How can I stop them?

Probably because you are ignoring the outer two eyes and thinking of the one inner eye, they are a bit jealous. It's to distract you. You're trying to focus your mind on one thing and because your eyes are used to seeing outside things, they get a little agitated. But if you continue practicing, it will go away.

At the same time, I'd like to say, do not strain your eyes. You don't need to roll your eyeballs up in order to concentrate on the third eye. You can do it, but you shouldn't have even the slightest strain in doing that. Otherwise you might hurt the optic nerves. Instead, bring your *mind* there. Let the eyes be half-closed. Think of the spot between the eyebrows. The more your awareness goes to that, the more the eyeballs turn by themselves, without your even knowing or consciously doing. Then there won't be any strain. When you physically gaze up like that, it is called *brumadhya drishti*. But it is a strenuous practice and normally I don't recommend it that much. I would say to concentrate mentally on the third eye and let the eyeballs go by themselves. If the mind goes there, the eyes also will go there. That is the safe method. I have seen many people who strained their eyes by forcing to see the third eye. This should never be.

During satsang I feel a pressure and a buzzing sensation in my left ear. Is there a yogic reason for this?

It could be that you are in a meditative mood and your mind is one-pointed. There is actual meditation. If you do that meditation, you have a beautiful vibration that is built in. Also, it is the atmosphere here, as well as your fitness, that makes you feel that vibration. At first, you may not hear this vibration in other places, but if you develop it within yourself more, then you can ultimately hear it anywhere. Right now it is just in this atmosphere. When you "grow up," then you can create your own atmosphere wherever you go.

Why are mantrams kept secret?

Well, it's not that you cannot say it to anyone but normally we don't. Why? It's not because it is a sin or anything like that. In fact, many mantrams are right in the chants we all do together here. So, it's not a big sin to say it. But normally, if we keep on repeating something easily, freely, we seem to lose the respect for it. Anything that is repeated very often, openly, loses it's charm. "Familiarity breeds contempt," we say.

If there is something which you treasure as a gem, you won't just put it out in public. Your imitation diamonds may be scattered all over the table, but your true diamonds go into the safe. You don't even show them to people unless you know the person is very close to you and serious and sincere in knowing what it is. That is why with anything you revere, something you treasure more than your own life, you just don't place it out easily.

So, that is why the mantrams are kept hidden. Because they are sacred, they are secret too. But, if you know a similar seeker, who has the same interest, who will not just laugh at you, there's no harm in telling him. He will encourage you. That is why even certain experiences, like nice spiritual dreams, are not to be told to everybody. Some people will even say, "Oh sure, you saw God." And then the minute they walk away they will say to their friends, "Is he serious?" So don't tell these things to such people, because they will discourage you. They will laugh at you. If there is something sacred, if someone can appreciate it, it is fine. Otherwise, no. Nothing will go wrong if you repeat or chant the mantram but not all the people will know the greatness of it. For that reason, you are asked to keep it sacred.

Please explain the scientific points about Ram and Rama mantram, especially its effects on the body, emotions, etc. Thank you.

Well, I can certainly touch on a few points. Ram and Rama are the combination of two mantrams: the mantram of Narayana and the mantram of Siva. The important letter of the Narayana mantram and the important letter of the Siva mantram are put together to make "Rama." Na-*ra*-yana and OM Na-*mah* Sivaya. So Rama is the Siva and Vishnu mantram. But here, your question is the scientific points — you may say that Narayana and Siva are not scientific. When extended, the "rum" sound becomes "raam". Scientifically you know the effect of rum, hm? Without the rum and the drum there won't be a war, is it not? When you go to the warfield, you smell the rum and hear the drum. The mantram Ram has the same effect also. It burns you. Ram is the presiding deity of fire. Ram, Ram, Ram, Ram . . . . You summon up certain vibrations in the body that bring heat. And you can pass that heat into anything you want. It purifies you.

What is the difference between the bija (seed) mantrams which are given during initiation and the standard mantrams which we all chant? For example, the difference between the bija mantram of Siva and "OM Namah Sivaya," the standard mantram of Siva? I was told that the bija mantram invoked the qualities of the deity, while the standard one culminates in a direct vision of the deity. Also, what are these deities (Ishta Devatas)?

The Ishta Devata is your mantram personified. If you want to worship a personal deity through an image, you can select one according to your mantram. Or if you just keep on repeating the mantram, the *moorthi* (image) will appear because the name is more powerful than the form. But if you're really interested in seeing the form, you can do so even without the mantram. Even if you forget the mantram, it doesn't matter. You can try to visualize the moorthi. First you try to see it in the picture or statue in front of you. You have to imagine it first. Then the more you bring the image of the moorthi to your mind, the mind accepts it and you get the vision of the moorthi. For that, you do puja with all devotion. It's not merely gazing at the picture. The heart must also be there. You love it; you devote your time to it. You worship it. And ultimately the whole personality receives the form. When the moorthi is well received you can see it whenever and wherever you want. You don't need an external moorthi, then. You have taken the moorthi within. Every time you close your eyes, you will see it. And you see it living. If you continue, you will see it even with open eyes. Without any outside picture or anything, you can talk to it. You can get all the answers for your questions from that.

Sri Ramakrishna used to feel the breathing of Mother Kali. There were many saints who talked to the images on the altar. They were not mere images to them. They had life. Science says that everything has life. Why not the moorthi then? But if you don't think that way, you won't see it. So, if you are not interested in moorthis, or if you find it difficult to perceive the moorthi, stick to the mantram and the moorthi will appear to you by itself.

Now, the bija mantrams are common to many deities. It need not be that each deity has its own bija. They are more direct. Even what you were calling the standard mantrams should ultimately have bija mantrams. So the bija is more important than the mantram. You can repeat the mantram along with the bija of just the bija alone. Without the bija, the mantram is not that powerful. That's why even OM Namah Sivaya is good, but it also has it's bija. If repeated with the bija it is more powerful.

Swamiji, do you give mantra initiation?

Well . . . yes. Somehow I hesitate to say this openly because normally I don't give initiations that easily. I'm a stingy man! I don't even advertise it. If you are somehow interested, you would have found out; you'll be wanting it. Not just because there are some people getting initiated, "Why don't I do that, too?" At the spur of the moment without even knowing what it is, you will come for initiation and then on the third day, drop it here and go. So that is the reason why I don't make announcements or put an ad, "Initiations will be given!" At least, you should know a little information and be familiar with what it is, how it is, why it is done. And you should have confidence in the person from whom you will be getting the initiation. Otherwise it is like getting something from a market.

Still, I can't say no to your question, I do give initiation. It all depends on how familiar you are with these things and how eager you are. It's not for curious people. If you are really interested, probably you could find out more details.

I would like to take initiation from you. I am presently receiving weekly lessons from the Self-Realization Fellowship of Paramahansa Yogananda. Would these two things conflict?

You can use this mantram separately for your japa and practice that also. There is no conflict. These mantrams in particular do not conflict with anything. All our mantrams are *nishkamya* mantrams or spiritual mantrams. There are other mantrams which are called *kamya* mantrams which are repeated for certain personal supernatural powers, psychic powers. Those mantrams, if not pronounced properly or not repeated with all the observations which are stipulated, might hinder your progress. Sometimes they might even harm you, because you are doing it for your own personal reasons. By personal, I mean something to satisfy your own senses or your own ego, not for your spiritual welfare. You can say that kamya mantrams are wordly and nishkamya mantrams are spiritual. With nishkamya mantrams there are not that many restrictions. Even if you make a mistake, it's not going to punish you. But with the kamya mantrams, many people have gone mad by making a mistake. They have a lot of restrictions: dietary, a certain place, certain number of times to repeat. Sometimes you might have to go at midnight to the cremation grounds, sit there in a place where a body is buried and then repeat the mantram. So many things. Sometimes you get ferocious visions. You get frightened. But the mantrams we use here are all harmless. That's why sometimes they take a little time to give the benefit. With the kamya mantrams you can even give the time needed for getting the result. "Repeat this many times, on this many days and you will get the rewards." It's pinpointed. But the benefit of nishkamya mantrams is something superior to these things. You get God instead of worldly things, so you have to wait a long time. You can't get that so quickly. You can easily earn a little money; within a couple of weeks you can accumulate a couple thousand dollars. But with God you can't do that; it takes time. However, the result is much greater.

Can you please comment on the chants? Are they purposeful in terms of sounds and vibrations, or in terms of meaning? Are people conscious of the meaning while they chant? If so, are the words learned as a new language? I am unfamiliar with this aspect of Yoga and feel very uncomfortable with chanting, as the words seem empty. I've practiced the chanting of meaningful prayers and know their powerful effect. What suggestions would you have, please?

Here, I would really like to say something. Basically, there are two types of chants. One type is mainly repeated for their vibrations. Whether you know the meaning or not, they should bring the vibration. Just use certain names, say, "Ram Ram Ram Ram Ram Ram"; you don't even have to know the meaning. In fact, there is no meaning for Ram. There is only the vibration. It was there even before the God Rama, who got the name. Ram is a mantram. Whether you know the meaning of fire, put your finger in and it will burn. It has a purpose. If you honk a horn, the man in front of your car will not ask, "What is the meaning of it?" It has a purpose. So the purpose of these chants is just to build up that vibration more and more.

But, there are certain other chants repeated as prayers. There are even some which tell of God's life, of what He did for others, how He helped His devotees. So you praise the Lord, or you appeal to the Lord as a prayer. With these chants which have the stories and tales and prayer, it is better to know the meaning. If you don't know the meaning, you will never get either the vibration or the meaning; you will just be repeating. And that is the reason why in the Integral Yoga Institutes we don't have too many chants with stories. The chants we use are only for the sake of the vibration. Maybe just a little *Paahi Maam, Raksha Maam,* just help me, save me. Otherwise, they are all just vibrations.

But, if you want to learn more chants, to know the meaning, there are many beautiful ones. With these, you need a little emotional feeling also.

If you don't enjoy the stories, you may wonder then, why should I repeat them? So it is up to you.

Since I've been here, I have had many periods when I wanted to leave and return home where it's easy. Could you take a show of hands of people who honestly have had similar feelings so I will not feel that I'm the only coward here?

Please don't think that you are a coward. You don't need to label yourself like that. When you try to cut a new groove, the mind faces this kind of tension and difficulty. You are trying to put in a new road, a new groove. You are a brave soldier, otherwise you would not have come here. How can you say you are a coward? If you are a coward, you won't even write a note like this. No. You are giving a wrong name to yourself. If half the people raise their hands, it won't be a surprise to me. Why? We are trying to build something. We are trying to follow something. We are trying to discipline. It is not an easy thing. You can't just appreciate it immediately, until you learn. How many people would want to break their pianos when they started learning to play? It's not an easy thing. How many times you would have thrown down your bicycle and walked away. Nothing is achieved that easily. And here we are trying to achieve something which is very high. So this kind of despairing feeling might come. It is not a surprise.

But strengthen yourself again and again. Think of the great thing you will achieve ultimately. Think of the mastery you will gain ultimately. If a girl is going to get disturbed by her pain after the seventh or eighth month of pregnancy, should she disturb something and get an abortion? No, she continues. She carries from the very first month. What kinds of troubles they undergo, all kinds of nausea, vomiting, swelling, varicose veins, lots of uneasiness all the nine months. Why should they undergo all these things; What makes them face all this? "Oh, I am going to have a beautiful little one to carry around. I am paying the price for that." She thinks of that beautiful one. A beautiful soul to come through her. That part will keep you alert, make you ready to face anything and everything.

It is like that here. You are going to get a baby of wisdom. So you should be ready to pay any price for that. If only you remember the goal, you will be getting the reward. Now, I'll ask his question. How many of you feel this way? Yes, some of you. Do you really want to go back? No? See. Your feeling is natural. The mind is not always steady. "What am I doing here? Why all this 'God' this and 'God' that? I can just go back and take it easy. What am I going to get in these ten days, anyway? Is the

Swami going to give me a piece of God to put in my pocket and take home? What is all this nonsense?" No. Perseverance. Wait and you will see, on the tenth day you will be happy that you did this. All the people who raised their hands, remember this. If you wait till the tenth day, then you will know that you have changed your attitude and you did something wise. So, please don't despair.

What is ten days? People work for ten *years,* fifteen years. Nothing is achieved in this world that easily. How many lives are lost in your moon landing efforts? How many lives lost in climbing Everest? Name one thing that you achieved without paying any price. What you are climbing here is a million times more than Everest. Because, if you once climb *this* Everest, you will be in "ever-rest"! Yes. However slippery it is, do it. There are a lot of good mountain climbers here. They'll carry your burden along with you. Tie your belt well; stick to the rope. Even if you slip, others will hold you. See that the rope is well fastened and that you are fastened to the rope. That is what you call satsang. Keep the company. Don't try to climb all by yourself. You might slip. It's a very slippery path. It has a ridge on each side. So keep it up. You won't regret it.

Fifth Day

There Is Only One Light

Swami Nirmalananda

In his second talk, Swami Nirmalananda picks up on a subject he dealt with in passing on the previous day: the importance and meaning of the mantram or sound vibration that can be used in meditation. He makes clear that the mantram is an expression of one's inmost being, one's essential nature, and so its repetition in meditation is a path back to that essential nature. He also points out that the tradition of the mantram can be found in all the different religions.

At this point Swami Nirmalananda changes his focus, from the universality of the practice of meditation to the universality of that inner being or consciousness, that inner light. Drawing upon his own background and experiences, he makes a long and impassioned plea for the recognition of that universality and for the tolerance among faiths that would be a natural accompaniment of such a recognition. It is a plea for an ecumenism based not on formal or dogmatic adjustments, but upon actual inner spiritual realization.

Let me explain two things. First, has anyone explained why we sing Sanskrit words and not all English words? (*from audience: No.*) Okay. Sanskrit is not an evolved language as other ones are. Other languages change through the centuries, even through decades. Words drop out, new words come in, and so on. A parent language will suddenly split, the way the English of England is becoming different from the way we speak in America; and Australian – the way they're speaking – is also gradually becoming separated from English. We can say that if things keep up this way for two or three hundred years, the languages won't even understand each other.

Sanskrit isn't this kind of a language. What it is, is a series of sound translations of the subtle energy patterns of objects, states of mind, and such. That is, these *rishis,* the ancient seers, saw that an object had a subtle energy pattern and they translated that in terms of sounds which, when repeated, would actually reproduce that same pattern. It's a kind of creative speech. It's not to be considered normal human-type speech, in which people have agreed that this symbol will mean that object. Therefore, a person can actually – if they have their intuition developed – repeat to themselves a Sanskrit word and understand the meaning from within. This can actually be done. Therefore, when certain things are said or recited in Sanskrit, they produce on a subtle level the very things spoken about. When you say, "Gaja," in Sanskrit, there literally arises the subtle vibration of elephant. A man who was always truthful, absolutely, with no error in his mind, could literally produce an elephant by repetition if he so desired. This is the idea behind mantram. It is creative speech. The Vedas are the mantrams uttered by Brahma to make this universe. The books we have called the Vedas are just the tiniest pinhole view of innumerable sound patterns that make up the structure of all our worlds. That's what the Vedas really are. Therefore, the Vedas are recited in India not for their meaning but for their vibration, for the psychic atmosphere produced. So we sing a song in Sanskrit because those sounds will help to unlock and evoke that inner state we're interested in. Of course, when we're singing devotionally, it's only good sense to sing in a language we understand, because devotional songs are songs of feeling; we're saying a certain thing to God. But these other songs we are using as vocal mantrams – not only to produce a change in us but also to produce a more obvious change in the atmosphere around us. Let me give an example which I witnessed.

About two and a half years ago when I was in India, there was a function where a scripture – the *Shrimad Bhagavatam* – was being discoursed upon for two weeks by a swami who is considered the expert on that scripture in all of Northern India. Now, the function was divided into two parts. In the Ashram, in an inner room, which had no windows – it was actually built in the center of the building; there were no skylights, nothing -- the *Bhagavatam* was going to be recited daily in Sanskrit. And in a huge tent, about a block away, this speech – explaining the Bhagavatam, expounding the symbolisms, and so on – was going to go on in the Hindi language. Now, for decoration, they take young plantain, young banana trees, about five, six feet tall; they cut them off and put them in various places. Where the Bhagavatam was going to be recited in Sanskrit, they built a platform with four posts coming up from each corner and a canopy above. At the four corners they put these plantain trees, which of course are cut off and will ultimately wither up and die. They did this in the room where the Sanskrit Bhagavatam would be recited, and they did it in the other place, in the tent where the talks were going on. By the end of two weeks the plantain trees in the tent were completely dried up, had turned yellow and were really ugly looking. Why they didn't take them away I don't know. And in the room where the Sanskrit was recited, they were still fresh and alive because of the vibration of the Sanskrit recitation.

So Sanskrit should not be looked upon as a foreign language. It should be looked upon as vibrations, keys to subtle inner states. That's the reason we sing in this Sanskrit. That's why we sing to Rama, Krishna, Siva and so on. Why aren't we singing to the one absolute God, who is beyond the forms? This is for two reasons: one is that the Absolute doesn't have any name but OM, so we would be limited to just singing OM; second, being absolute and beyond identity, that Being cannot be addressed. That Being can be entered in silence, but can't be talked to in words. And third, these forms are considered just the same as the Absolute, but in a mode we can relate to. It's like Jesus. He said, "If you've seen me, you've seen the Father," yet by theoretical definition the Father was called the Absolute, no form, no name, beyond all, unseeable, unknowable. And yet Jesus said, "If you've seen me, you've seen Him." So it is considered that there isn't any difference, and so we sing this way. So that's why we sing in the Sanskrit and use these kinds of names.

> *Song:*
> Satyam jnanam anantam Brahman
> Shantam shivam adwaitam Brahman
> Ekam evam adwityam Brahman
> Ananda rupam amritam Brahman
>
> The true, the knower, the unending God
> The peaceful, the auspicious, the non-dual God
> One only, without a second, God
> Whose form is bliss, the immortal God
>
> (*repeated six times*)

That's really good. And the more you sing it, the more you get into the feeling of it. It's good to know the meaning of the words; you'll think of it. But even more than that, let your mind just get into the sound of it, and you'll come to feel that.

I was told that somebody in New York, a psychologist, is taking *yantras* — those are the geometric forms which correspond to the mantrams, to the mantric and also to the visual forms of the deities — and having his patients just stare at them. And their problems are going away. Not only are they going away, but these patients, who know nothing about Hinduism, are seeing the forms of God. And not only are they seeing the forms of the gods, but they're seeing events which are written about the gods in the Hindu scriptures. They are tuning in to that through the power of those yantras. So these things will bring that state about. He who says "Ram" becomes Ram. This is the real idea. There is the stage where the idea is, "Ram, you're the Lord, so I'm praying, I'm saying Ram, Ram, Ram; I'm trying to think of you." But the real, deep idea is that you *are* Ram, and the mantram has the power to evoke your own Rama – the inner Rama. That's the real Rama we're after, not a Rama outside. And so we sing in this language to help us get this feeling, this state of mind. It's not an emotion, it's an actual state of mind. Okay. Why don't we try Rama Rama. I'll get you all mellowed, then I can holler at you some more!

Everyone joins Swami Nirmalananda in chanting a song to Rama, whose refrain is: Sri Rama Rama Ram, Sri Rama Rama Ram. Then Nirmalananda resumes his discourse on the meaning of mantrams.

We're wrapped up in five major covers. Our "onion" has about five major layers. Actually it has more than a thousand. But there are five big divisions, sort of like continents. And then the continents have countries.

How can we go through these five covers? From the most gross to the most subtle? We need something very subtle, to get to the most subtle level. And that is the mental sound. That is the trail through which we can go back to our innermost being. It's the thread. Remember when Theseus was in the labyrinth; he unwound a thread? He went around all those twisting places, dead ends, and what not, but he found his way back by the thread. This sound is a *sutra,* a thread, on which we go back to the source. Taken into meditation, that brings us to that deepest experience.

And as I said before, that's why we miss it. Because it's so easy. It's so easy you don't try at all. You just sit there, and you say it, that's all. And that's your business. Other things can rise in the mind: feelings, thoughts, aches, pains, people hollering outside your window and so on. It doesn't make any difference. The mantram is more powerful, because that is the inmost part of your being. Being the inmost part, there's nothing it can't possibly conquer and nullify. So don't worry. Just go on saying it. Just go on; ultimately everything else vanishes. That is the path of the saints. The path of the masters is through this subtle word, this name. That is its power.

Vibration and consciousness are interrelated. They cannot be split apart. These sounds are a consciousness – as indeed is the very wood from which this platform is made; but that energy is covering energy. It covers the real nature of consciousness. See, there are two kinds of consciousness in the world, sort of like the up and down escalator. There are some objects which cover up reality, so when we get involved with them we become less and less capable of seeing what is real. Then there are other objects; though they are objects, they lead us beyond this objective consciousness into where we are. That is the trick of it. It's like being in a room with millions, billions of panels that all look alike, and we're trapped, but two or three of them are doors. We have to find out which one is a door, which one will open up when we push, and let us through.

It seems so completely contradictory. "We're to have non-dual experience, we're to have non-objective experience, yet you're saying, take a name, take a mantram, and maybe even concentrate, visualize a form. Well, how's that going to produce this other experience you're talking about?" The thing is, that name, that form, merge, dissolve, and give you that experience which is beyond it all. It's a trick, you see. It's a hide-and-seek game. Who will guess the mystery? We're all so clever. God has said, "Let Me give you a few little obstacles to run, let's see how clever you are." So not many people know the inmost secret. Did Santji tell the story about the man who was initiated into the Rama mantram? Oh, that's too good a story to leave untold.

There was a man in India who used to visit a Yogi who lived far out beyond the reaches of the town, and he realized he wanted to be like that Yogi too. He didn't want to just sit around and respect him. Where would that get him? So he said to him, "Look, won't you give me something, some instruction, so I will be in your state?" The Yogi said, okay, and set a day. The man came back, and the Yogi, taking him into his house, said, "Now, I'm going to teach you something very secret. You must keep this a very sacred matter. It is a mantram, virtually unknown in the world. Hardly anybody knows this mantram, so keep it very hushed, and value it well, because this is the inmost secret." And then he simply told him to say the name of Rama. He gave him, you know, the full form: "OM Sri Rama Jaya Rama Jaya Jaya Rama" or perhaps "OM Sri Ramaya Namah."

Well, the man was very pleased. Walking, he came to a place where thousands of people were bathing, and they were all saying, "Om Rama Rama Rama." He thinks, "Ooohhh," and he goes back to the Yogi and says, "You told me you were giving me something secret, something new. I went down to the river, a thousand people are saying this. Why would you say this to me? You think I'm some kind of a fool that I could never catch on? I want an explanation."

"All right," said the Yogi. "But first, there's something you must do for me." The Yogi went into his hut. He had a bag, and out of this bag he pulled a shiny hard object and said, "Take this, offer it to people in the town. Ask them what they'll give you for it, but don't really sell it, no matter what they offer you."

So the man went. First thing you know, he came to a lady who had some eggplants to sell. So he said, "Look at this, what would you give me for this?" She said, "Well, it doesn't amount to anything. But I've got a little baby. Maybe the baby would like to play with it. I'll give you two pounds of eggplants." "Um, no, I'm not really supposed to sell it," he said, and he went on.

He went into the town and he came to a man who had a little store. He showed the object to him and he said, "What, um, what will you give me for it?" The man looked at it and he thought, "Oooo, that's really a fine, fine imitation stone. Why don't I buy it? Most people will think that it's real; they'll think I'm far more successful than I am. They'll think I do better business than others, that's why I'm rich. Then they'll figure I'm selling better things, that's how I've managed to get ahead. So all in all, my wife will be happy and I'll be happy. People will admire me and . . ." So he said, "I'll give you 50 rupees for it." "Um, well, no."

So on he went. He thought, "Fifty rupees. If this piece of stuff can get me that, maybe I can get even a bigger bargain." So he took it to a man who was a banker. And the banker said, "My God, it's a real diamond! I'll give you ten thousand rupees for it." The man nearly fainted off his chair. Then he thought, "The Yogi must have good sense, even if I was offered ten thousand rupees." So he took it then to a jeweler, who recognized its value, and said, "I don't have enough money to buy it from you, nor does anybody. Don't ever sell it. There is no one in India who can pay what that's really worth."

Then the man was terrified to be carrying such a precious thing around. He ran back to the Yogi. "Here, take it." The Yogi took it and put it back. Then the man said, "Okay, now will you explain to me why you said the mantram was a secret when I see everybody knows it?" The Yogi said, "I have already shown you. Won't you agree that that diamond was always the same, but that each person valued it according to where he was, according to his status, from the woman who thought it was worth two pounds of eggplants all the way up to the man who said it couldn't be bought? So according to their knowledge, according to their understanding, that's how they valued it. Yes, that's how. Lots of people like parrots are saying, "Rama, Rama, Rama." They don't know the value of it. They think it's like a little prayer. But those who are wise, those who really know, are incredibly rare people. Very, very few people will know the real value of this Rama. Therefore, even though millions know it, it's a secret. And that is why I told you it is very secret."

So according to our status, we will evaluate. Once a woman was looking at some things that were on display. She said, "Well, they're just worthless." The man who was keeping them said, "Believe me, lady, the value of these things has already been established. What is being evaluated here is the capacity of the people to understand their value." So the real value has been set. But we tend to think we're it, we know everything, we're the center of the whole universe, and so if it appeals, it's good, if it doesn't appeal, it's no good. If it has meaning to us, it's wise; if it has no meaning to us, it's nonsense. And we don't stop to think that maybe we're the ones who are being judged, that maybe when we say it's worthless, we're showing that our understanding is worthless. So the divine mysteries always remain mysteries, and very few people know them.

The same thing goes for the power of mantram. People say, "Oh, you control your mind that way"; "Oh, well, it's a holy thought," and so on, but they don't realize that it is itself a consciousness which will dawn in the individual as he uses it. And this is the basis of all spiritual practices. Because you cannot do asanas all the time. You cannot do breathing practices all the time, nor can you chant all the time. But all the time you can do this repetition of one of these transforming sounds. Whichever one you like. Of course, when you get initiated, the guru tells you the best one for you. But until then, you can take any one you like and make it a constant repetition. You can eat, walk, run, work, drive a car and keep the mantram going, if you want to. If you think you can't, just remember that if somebody promised you that at the end of this day you would get what you have wanted all your life, there wouldn't be a moment in the day that you'd forget that. And you'd be thinking, "I'm going to have, I'm going to have." Now isn't that something? If you've got a toothache, you don't forget it. If you've got a broken toe, you don't forget it. Or if somebody you love dies, no matter how much work you do that day, you still have that inner feeling of loss. You know why? Because those things are important in your evaluation. If you make this important, if you see this as important, you won't have any trouble. You'll be able to do it. Now to be able to do it in sleep, or while you're speaking, that may take some time. But that comes in time by practice, by application, continually in meditation, so that you do it and say it all the time. Right now, as I'm talking to you, I'm doing japa. In fact, I'm paying attention to the japa because that's far more interesting than what I'm saying. Because after a while it goes into a particular level in your subtle bodies where it keeps moving all the time no matter what you're doing, and you're aware of it.

That's the path. It's easy and your consciousness keeps being transformed more and more. Every repetition is just like a step; it brings you closer and closer and closer. Then one day you're there. The thing with us is, the ego comes in. "That means you can teach the village idiot to do it. What? That retarded person and me? I've got a college degree and I'm supposed to do the same thing he's doing? I'm supposed to be doing something super-advanced so it can be seen that I am on the higher level." But a soul is a soul. A mind is a mind. Therefore, that way will suit all. It's really universal and it's in every religion. The Sufis do japa on the name of Allah. Those in the Hassidic tradition say those names of God revealed in the Torah which are just as much revealed and have just as much power as the names revealed in the Hindu tradition. The Eastern Christians do *Hesychia,* constant calling on the name of Jesus. So the truth, the heart, of every mystical tradition is japa of some sort. It doesn't have to be Sanskrit japa. But in every religion it's there. Every one of the saints have seen, this is it. They're unanimous on this. I have in our ashram an incredibly wonderful book on the name Jesus and its power, japa on the name Jesus, which one day I hope we'll reprint, because unfortunately the Christians are forgetting all about it, and it shouldn't be lost.

Having described the power of the mantram, and said how it is to be found in all the religions of the world, Swami Nirmalananda goes on to say how all the religions have a home and are accepted in India. In developing this theme, he will refer to his own background as a Christian to make an impassioned statement on behalf of the essential oneness of all faiths and forms.

India is a preserver and repository of the religions of the world. Did you know that the only community of orthodox Moslems is in India? They've degenerated all over the world. They've gone down so far in Turkey that they can't even find a person to go up in the minaret and make the call to prayer. They record somebody; they have a phonograph record. They put their finest chanters on phonograph records and then they play them from the mosque. That's how much they've lost their tradition. But the very strict orthodox practices are being carried on in India; yes, I mean India, not in Pakistan. In Pakistan, they used religion as a pretense to get a political dominion – they're not orthodox. The genuine Moslems said, "We don't want to leave India, we love it here," and they stayed. And the fanatics went to Pakistan – those who didn't really care for the religion. And the only Zoroastrians in the world are in India. They fled to India during the persecutions from the Moslems. They came from Iran. The only place to find a community of Zoroastrians in the world is in India.

The oldest, undisturbed Jewish community in the world is in South India! When the temple in Jerusalem was destroyed, two or three decades after the time of Jesus, those Jews came to India and found refuge there. Not only were they accepted, but the *rajas* (kings) even built synagogues for them. How do you like that? We think Ecumenism is something new. In 1969 Indira Gandhi went to the anniversary – I don't know how many years that anniversary was – she went to the celebration of the founding of a particular synagogue. I think five or six hundred years, because when the Moslems came into India they started persecuting, and so the Jews had to go even further south, and there the Raja and everyone took them in and provided for them, fed them and everything. Because Hindus like God. And Hindus like people who like God.

The oldest Christian communities in the world are in India. Saint Thomas the Apostle came to India. You know, missionaries got up and cried in front of their audiences here in America and in Europe, "Oh, poor India. Never heard of Jesus. All in the dark. Oh, give us money and send us there." When they got there they found millions of Christians. Yes. When the Portuguese Christians got there they found millions of Indian Christians living in harmony with the Hindus and that wouldn't do. So they slaughtered tens of thousands of Christians – not Hindus. Isn't that grand? When they went to India they left the Hindus alone and killed Christians. Until a major peace treaty was made between the two, the innocent Indian Christians were being murdered. Why? Because they refused to be exclusive. They refused to hate Hinduism. They refused to reject Hindu culture. Therefore, they were obviously heretics. Just imagine. They found one community just within the past ten years in India that thought they were the only Christians left in the world. They were living in such an inaccessible place they had lost all contact with Christianity. It was a whole city just of Christians. And they figured that, well, that was it, there just weren't any other Christians. And they were keeping up the most ancient traditions from the very days of the Apostles.

When the Tibetans were driven out, who gave them a home? Uncle Sam didn't give them a home. In fact, hardly any of them will be let in by the government because the government is afraid that the American people will start feeling favorably toward Tibet as such and then identify with Communism and be friendly. Did you know that? But the Indians took them in. You know, they like to point a finger and gripe about India: "Why are you so poor, why are you so poor?" But this much I'll tell you. Those Indians will share what they have with anybody. I'd rather be that kind of poor than selfish rich. So what did they do for the Buddhists? They gave them homes, they gave them places to live. The Hindus even helped them build temples. You see? Any religion can go there and find refuge. That's the genius.

Some people, I understand, feel somewhat disturbed by the supposed Hindu connotations here at the retreat. Believe me, you'd better be glad, because it's in the Hindu atmosphere that any religion can flourish, and where all religions are loved and respected. It's India that has this feeling. Indians love churches. You can go into temples in India and find pictures of Jesus and Mary there. How many Christians do you know that have a place, a special room, where they have a picture of Jesus which they worship every day? Hm? I know Hindus who do. How many Christians do you know who worship Krishna or Rama? Oh, not on your life. Swami Sivananda wrote the life of Jesus and had it printed and distributed as widely as possible. Every night in the kirtan when he would sing, part of it was, "Oh, my Jesus, Oh my Jesus, Lord Jesus, come to me." But Christians will never say that because they don't want Him to come. They want Him to stay there and receive their prayers and give them what they want. I don't mean this to be nasty. But I happen to know. I mean, that's what I was raised. I don't care about our theological definitions. "Brother, we want Him to leave us alone. Come to me?" What would happen if someone walked up and said, "Well, Jesus came and talked to me today?" We'd say he was crazy. Pius the XII was a Pope, head of the Roman Catholic Church, supposedly the representative of Jesus. And when he had visions of Jesus and Mary they laughed at him and said that he was nuts. How's that for a system? A system that when a man that should be closest to God said, "Well, I've seen Him," then they say, "Agh!" do you think those people really believe in God? No. They believe in hallucinations. They believe in their mind. And if they get a little mystical, they believe in the Devil and they say, "You'd better watch out. The Devil may have appeared." But not God. They have a hard God, a horrible God that never appears, that never talks, that just sits there and couldn't care less. What an awful God. There is no such God. I'm glad to tell you. There is no such God as that. That's only a projection of their own hard-hearted paranoia.

You know what I mean? "Jesus is God. Anyone who worships God must worship Jesus." My own guru said, "He who worships Jesus worships all the Gods." He who worships Jesus worships all the Gods, because Jesus is the embodiment of all the Gods. Everything is in Him because He's God. Hm? God isn't chopped up. A little bit of this and a little bit of that. You worship any one form of God, you've worshiped them all. As my guru said, "There's no difference between Him and our Siva." No, there is no difference.

Why am I telling you all this? Because in one way there is no such thing as a religion called Hinduism. There is *Sanatana Dharma* — the eternal path to God. And every path to God is a part of that. The path that St. Theresa of Avila trod, that's ours too. All these saints are ours. God is ours. If you're for God, you have to be for God and take Him as He is. But, "Oh, no, He's Allah. Don't say He's Elohim." Right? Or, "He's Buddha. Don't say He's Jesus, no." "He's Jesus, but don't you dare say He's Krishna, oh no." Listen, God is one. People say, God is one. Well, if He's one and only one, he's united, and if there's a speck of Him you reject you've rejected the whole thing, haven't you? Somebody once came very proudly to a Swami. He thought he was sophisticated and grown beyond Christianity, you know, and he liked this Vedantic business. So he came to the Swami and — thinking the Swami would congratulate him — announced that he did not believe in the divinity of Jesus. The Swami said, "When you've rejected that which is infinite, what is left for you now to accept?"

You do not worship Jesus and love Jesus and deny Krishna; you do not worship and love Krishna and deny Jesus. You take the whole thing. He's total, and it's all or nothing. So he who will not worship God everywhere and in every form, every name, and will not love and revere all those who are going toward that divine life, has nothing to do with God.

This is not Ecumenism. This is good old hard-line Hinduism. And all religions say the same thing, when you understand them. Just like Jesus, Siva said, "He who believes in me . . ." But here's the catch. In Greek you have two words: one means "in" and one means "into," in the sense of merging, joining. In the Greek it is always the word "into." But they try to make it like, "Well, you believe in Him as an historical person, or you ask for His divine grace." But it says, "He who believes *into* me will not perish." That person will become one with Him, enter into Him, his real source, the God from which he came. That person has enternal life, not people who just believe. After all, the demons believed in Him, didn't they? They said, "Jesus, we know who you are. Go away." According to some, they would be good Christians. They believed — fervently. So you must become one with Him.

I had a very interesting experience. Just before leaving India in 1963, after having having become a Swami, I stayed at the Salvation Army Hotel in Calcutta, where all the missionaries who were coming and going stayed. So I was the Swami amidst all the missionaries — it was an interesting thing. To one lady, I said, "You say you follow Jesus. Let's take the case of that woman they caught in adultery. Now, if they brought her to you, the first thing you would do would be to get out the Bible and read her passages about what a bad thing she had done and convince her that she had sinned. Then you would tell her all about hell and you would urge her to repent and ask God to forgive her sins. And then you would tell her to get baptized, right? Yes. And then you would tell her to join the church. Yes? Yes." I said, "Well, Jesus didn't do any of that. He said, 'I don't condemn you.' He changed her life. You understand? It wasn't that He didn't care. But He changed her life." I said, "All right. Sri Ramakrishna lived right here in Calcutta. People would come to him and say, 'Help me, I am bound by these low desires, I am bound by this habit.' Alcoholics came, people addicted to morphine came. 'Help me.' All right, from then on they were cured. So who," I said, "was the Christian?"

One can find similar instances in the life of my own guru. People who are criminals, I mean real professional criminals, have been made to go to some function where Mother was. They went against their will; they didn't want to go. And when they walked in the door and looked at her, their life changed. Well, how many people here were really living down in the dregs? Then they took just one look at Swami Satchidananda . . . So who are the Christians? Do you understand?

We mistake the shell, the container, for the contents. When God appears on this earth, that's just the container. God's inside! You see? That's what you should be after: crack that shell and find God inside. But people get enamored of the shell: "My shell came two thousand years ago. When did your shell come?" Both of them empty. No experience.

This is what unites us in our Hindu religion. We have a multiplicity of saints, a multiplicity of views, six orthodox systems of philosophy and then elaborations on those — but no wars, no fights, no hatred. Why? Because we know that only one thing matters: where you are at. And that you're going to that absolute status. That's the only thing that matters. Who cares how you describe it, who cares what name you give it, as long as you're going toward it. Isn't that right? Who cares whether you call it water, or call it *aqua,* or call it *pani.* Who cares? As long as you're drinking out of the river. What matters is going toward that goal. And as all the rivers flow toward the sea, so all lives come in the end to God. In Hinduism, they ask, "Are you flowing?" If you are, good. If you're not . . . . It doesn't matter what name you call yourself, as long as you're really flowing. So the test of a man is his state of consciousness, not his dogmatic definitions.

When a man dies they write a book and talk about his life — no need for books while he's there. And everybody adores the books: "Oh, my

God, the Pentateuch, the Torah, the Koran, the Bible." The Hindu religion alone says when you adore God all those books are trash. It's the only religion that tells you to go beyond books. Now the saints in all the religions have told you to do that, but actually every common man in India is told. Every day in the *Gita* he hears, "As a pump is useless when the whole countryside is flooded, so the Vedas, the highest scriptures, don't mean anything when you've got knowledge of God." You see? This is life. That's what real religion should be; it should be life.

There is only one light, and he who is glowing in that light does not deny any place where it shines. Not ever. Now obviously people are going to follow different paths.I can easily see a person saying, "Well, frankly, Hinduism bores me." I mean, I can understand that, because Hinduism doesn't fit them, doesn't suit them. Why should it? There are other approaches. I mean, there are some religions in the world that bore me. From a philosophical standpoint, they bore me. The saints don't bore me at all; their worship, their devotion, don't bore me, but their philosophy bores me. It just doesn't seem to ring a bell, But that's because I just don't have the capacity to see it. It's a blindness on my part, not a fault of the religion. I see that. But for a person to say, "Oh no, I'm devoted to such and such form of God. I'm devoted to such and such form of religion, therefore I can't have anything to do with any other;" that is not so. Because if you're really devoted, and you really have love, you will respond to whoever you like. Isn't that right? A man who's out looking for gold, believe me, he'll take it whether it's in the streams, whether it's in the mountainsides, wherever he has to go to get it, he'll take it. There are not many in this world who are out for God. They're out for ego, they're out for religion; but those who are out for God, they will take any little drop He gives anywhere.

So that's what we should try to be — people who are out for God, people who like God, because God's enjoyable. Believe me, He's the only enjoyable thing. You can't get tired of God. Everything else you can get tired of. It might take you 50 million years, but eventually you will get tired of it. Why not forget everything else, and go for Him? Just say, "Just me for God, God and I." One of the saints in the desert used to say, "Unless you say, just God and me, alone in this world, you will never know God." You don't say, "Okay God, stand in line. First I've got to satisfy this person, I've got to satisfy that person, I've got to fulfill that ambition." You say, "Okay, c'mon, you first, you middle, you last." Don't put anybody on your list, just God, alone; not God first, but God alone. That's what it's all for.

The Tenth Man

Swami Satchidananda

In this fifth satsang, Swamiji speaks about Vedanta — the pinnacle of philosophical thought, the description and explanation of the highest spiritual experience, the direct perception of the Truth or Brahman or God. Couched in simple direct terms and many charming parables, Swamiji places before the retreatants this highest goal, and after four days of inner discipline, they listen with rapt attention. He has sown the seeds the previous evenings with his talks on discipline, sense-control and dedication and now he clearly expounds the goal of all these. And in equally simple words and more delightful stories, he expounds upon the one obstacle which prevents our direct and immediate experience of this Truth: the ego.

Because Swamiji was a little late to satsang this evening, it was preceded by a period of exquisitely beautiful chanting of "Satchidananda" to the tune of "Greensleeves", replete with beautiful and spontaneous harmonies and sung like a round.

So you've been meditating on your "Satchidananda?" Don't think that Satchidananda is just the name of one person. You're all Satchidanandas, not just me. I am called Satchidananda simply because one who saw Satchidananda in everything saw it in me also. In fact, everybody and everything is Satchidananda. You should never miss that. Existence (*Sat*) knowledge (*Chid*), and bliss (*Ananda*) is in everything. Everything exists. This flower exists. And then, it expresses itself. That's the knowledge. Without the expression, you may not know what it is. It just exists. So the Absolute One, which just exists with ease, is the Brahman. Brahman is. But if He is just going to be at ease, He's of no use. So everything should express itself.

The microphone crackles loudly.

Yes sir, yes sir, you are expressing. You learn from these electronic things how to concentrate and meditate so the energy will be well channelized and well insulated. If the concentration is exposed, there are short circuits. Keep it well insulated, well channelized, fixed at the point, then the flow is easy. That is what we do in the name of meditation. Communication is possible only if the meditator and the meditated on are well connected with the electrode of meditation. If the meditation is not

121

fixed well between the meditator and the meditated on, there will be loose connections and you will have disturbance. So the process of meditation should be well insulated from outside influences. Otherwise, if anything comes and touches it, it will be short circuited like an uninsulated wire and heat will be produced. The whole thing will get fused. Or in your case, con-fused. So it's all scientific. It's not just mere theory or hallucination.

Coming back to Satchidananda. We were talking about the flower. It is the absolute Brahman (Sat). But it should express itself. The knowledge of it (Chid) comes only then. And through the proper knowledge comes the joy, the bliss (Ananda). So all these three are permanently established in everything — Satchidananda. Take anything you want — even this material of my upper cloth. The original stuff, the silk, exists. Then it expresses itself as silk thread; it is put together to make some material. And then the wearing of it brings you joy.

Now, over and above these three qualities, there are two more. You call it an upper cloth because it has the form of an upper cloth. If you cut it and make it into a shirt, you call it a shirt. So the name shirt and the form shirt vary from the name upper cloth and form upper cloth but in essence there is Satchidananda in both. So what is the difference between the upper cloth and shirt? Name and form. And what is common? Satchidananda. If you make the silk into a small piece and tie it around, it becomes a scarf. So the name and form vary between the different objects. But the Satchidananda is the common thread.

Krishna says, "In a beautiful necklace of all kinds of gems, I am the running thread. If I am not there, they all get scattered. So I am the thread running through all these names and forms." Without that, all these names and forms will not even exist. The name and form is the superficial part. So what we see in the common world outside, with the common vision, is the name and form. We do not usually go into the Satchidananda part. The minute you say, "Oh, it's a flower, I know. Oh, it's a microphone. It's a piece of paper. Oh, that's so and so," you're talking in terms of name and form. If you could see through the name and form, it's all of the same essence: Satchidananda.

So, in the name of spiritual practice, we are not asking you to forget the names and forms or call everybody Satchidananda. Then there would be chaos. But *see* everybody as Satchidananda. *Know* that everybody is Satchidananda. Only for the sake of convenience you can put different labels on things and call them different names. It's something like a house where several children are born, all into the same family. If the mother and father are going to give the same name to all the children, it will cause a lot of trouble. Whenever the mother calls, "Hey, Jacob, come here," all the boys will run. Even if by chance you do give the same name, you have to have Jacob Senior and Jacob Junior or some kind of difference for convenience sake. If all the houses have the same number, the mailman will wonder where to drop the mail. So just for the sake of receiving our mail properly, just for convenience, we have all these different names.

But behind them the essence is the same. That is why the entire world is called the name-form world, the *nama rupa prapanjam*. It is the names and forms that make the world. Beyond that is Satchidananda. The essence makes sense, hm? So, if you see the essence, you are in sense. But for this nonsensical world we should just show a little nonsense, hm? But do not miss the sense behind it. So, we have to have double vision. In the one vision, all is Satchidananda; all are essentially the same. *Atman,* Self, God, image of God, anything you want to call it. Satchidananda is the Holy Trinity: Father, Son and the Holy Spirit. Father, the existence, is Sat or Truth. The expression of the Father is the Son, or the knowledge, Chid. And the result you get from the two of them is the Spirit which functions everywhere and bring all kinds of joy, Ananda. So the Trinity is Satchidananda.

How can we see this Trinity, this essence, in everything, in everybody? To see everybody as their essence, as God, we must see them as their spirit. It is not possible to go into all the names and forms. For example, if you want to see everybody wearing yellow, you can't force everybody to wear yellow. Everybody may not even like the idea. But whether they wear it or not, if you still want to see them wearing yellow, there is a way to do it — through a gimmick. Do you know the gimmick? Wear yellow glasses. It doesn't matter what I wear, you'll be wearing yellow glasses and everything will be yellow for you. Like jaundice. Change the color of your eyes or the eyeglasses and you'll see everybody and everything the same way. That is the clue. So if you want to see everybody as spirit, you should wear spiritual glasses. Get a pair of spiritual glasses. Where? At the heavenly supermarket. The price? Nothing. It is not that you have to go and buy them. They are already within you. You are already wearing spiritual glasses. But unfortunately they are tainted, discolored and foggy. So when you see through the foggy glasses, you see everything as foggy. All you have to do is just clean the glasses. Just rub them with tissue. Blow a little steam over them. All this rubbing, cleaning is what you are doing in the name of spiritual sadhana. Sadhana means cleaning that cover of the spirit, the veil.

In the *Saiva Siddhanta* school of philosophy there are four great Saivite saints who are known just as The Four. They don't even use their names; simply, The Four. In one of their songs of praise they sing, "Lord, I didn't know the way to Liberation. I was bound and was involving myself in all kinds of undesirable things and people. But all of a sudden one day you took pity on me. You just took me out of it. *You* did it, because I didn't even have the devotion myself. I didn't have Bhakti; I didn't even know any chants. You taught me a little bit of devotion. In that way you helped me in getting rid of the old karmas. And then you just removed the tarnish from this beautiful mirror. And thus you made me Siva, just by cleaning the dirt away. Who can say His greatness? Who is able to say what has been done? It's impossible. I am just saying within my own limited capacity, you see. The blessing He has given me nobody can say."

So all we have to get done is to have the covering taken away. Let it be rubbed off. It all depends upon how deep and thick it is, how old it is. If it is just simple dirt, just a little soap is enough. If not, you may have to add some powerful detergents. You'll have to take it to a clever laundryman. You can't do it yourself. It all depends upon how much you have accumulated all these days. That's why the results of your practices vary. It takes time. But the main thing is that all this tarnish can easily be removed in a second if the base over which the tarnish has accumulated is eliminated. What is that? Ego. All these karmas affect the ego and the ego is right there in front of you. Instead of rubbing out the karmas little by little, little by little, destroy the whole ego. Then the spirit comes out and expresses itself.

In a way it's very simple. Even the words show you this in *Tamil*, my native South Indian language. "Sivan" and "Seevan." Sivan means the individual soul. Seevan means Siva. So the only difference is in the "i" and "ee." In Tamil to make the "i" you have a line and a little horn or loop. For the "ee" you must leave the line straight. So what is the difference between "sivan" and "Seevan"? One is a little crooked. A crooked horn makes you sivan. If you straighten yourself, you are Seevan. All that is necessary is to just get straight. Don't you use that term? "Oh, he's straight." So, he's no longer sivan, he's Seevan.

Of course, all this "sivan, Seevan" language might seem a bit complicated. You have a much simpler thing in English itself. Just one stroke makes you "I," is it not? Just one stroke and you are produced. It doesn't take much of an effort to make you. "I" is the simplest letter in the entire alphabet, is it not? All the other letters need a few other strokes or curves and this and that. But "I" is simply one stroke, see? To make a man is very easy. Make one stroke. Then you stand upright. "I am!" Really you are great, the big "I." Because one stroke means the big "I," the capital "I." But unfortunately you don't stop there; you want to add something. Put a dot over it. The minute you put a dot over it you are no more the capital "I." What happens to you? You become the little "i," is it not? You add something and it becomes smaller. It's a kind of new mathematics.

What is the dot? Some people call it the "beauty spot." It's beautiful for the world but it's the most ugly thing in the spiritual realm. So it is just that dot makes you small. Erase it and you are capital again. Just like the "sivan" and "Seevan." It's that simple. But unfortunately, that dot has accumulated so many things around it that you can't even reach that dot easily. So whoever can erase that dot can instantaneously enjoy and experience that spiritual bliss. Jnanam, liberation, is that quick; simply erase that and you are liberated. You are free. Not that you *become* free. But you feel that you are liberated. With the dot you feel you are bound. So it's all in the feeling.

In the *Ashtavakra Gita,* Janaka the king had many saints and sages around him. One time Janaka wanted a certain point clarified from the scriptures. He said, "The scriptures say that you can give enlightenment within a fraction of a second. The scriptures do not lie, so it must be true." So then he asked, "How is it, even after years and years of practice, people don't get enlightened? Is it because of the students or because of the incapacity of the teachers? Certainly, if a teacher wants to, he can do that. He must be capable of everything." Then Janaka announced, "Whatever master can give me enlightenment within a second, I will really be happy." So he invited all the great sages and saints. Everybody failed and he was still waiting for somebody. Then one day a saint by the name of Ashtavakra came to the country. Ashtavakra had heard of these things and wanted to come to the king's court. The court was filled with many different sages and saints, both men and women. The famous women saints Gargi and Maitreyi were there. (Would you call them saintesses? No. Just saints. There is no feminine or masculine in saintliness; saint is saint.) So they were all sitting there.

When Ashtavakra wanted to come in, the gatekeepers just laughed at him. "What is this? What are *you* going to do in there?" They asked this because Ashtavakra had a peculiar body. He couldn't walk straight. Every time he took a step, his body bent like an eight. Ashtavakra means "eight curves." His body was crooked; and even that had a reason. I'll tell you that also.

When this saint, Ashtavakra was conceived and was still in his mother's womb, he used to listen to his father chanting and worshiping every day.

The father used to recite all the *Puranas,* all the holy verses. The mother used to sit by the father's side whenever he performed all these pujas, so the child in the womb used to listen to all these spiritual things. And one day, all of a sudden the father heard somebody laughing at him.

"Who is laughing at me?" he asked his wife. "There's nobody here but us; is it you?"

"No. I didn't do it. Why should I laugh? It's not a proper time for laughter."

"Then I know who it is! Hah You fellow! You haven't even come out of the womb yet, you are still inside that dark chamber and you are laughing at me. What is the reason you laughed?"

Ashtavakra spoke from the womb, "Papa, you're not reciting properly. You make so many mistakes."

"Dirty little fellow!" cried the angry father. "If you are going to criticize me even while you are in the womb, what will happen when you come out? May the whole world criticize you! I don't want you to be born with a proper body. Let it be as crooked as possible." That was Ashtavakra's curse. That's who he was born as an *ashta vakra* (eight-curved one) and was named that also. Everybody recognized him as that.

Yet, even in a crooked body, saintliness cannot be crooked. Nobody can curse that. Only the body can be cursed. So during his life, Ashtavakra became well known. Unfortunately, those gatekeepers didn't know anything about this. When he said, "I must see the king," they laughed at him. He looked at them with pity. "Well, that's why you are here and not in there. Otherwise you'd be sitting inside. Poor fellows." When Ashtavakra looked at them that way, they got frightened. They just stood there and so he just walked in.

Unfortunately, as he walked crookedly towards the king, everybody there in the court also laughed at him. All those saintly people sitting around laughed at him. "Hm, Okay." He just discarded them as though they were dust and came straight to the point. "King, I heard you had some problem."

Immediately the king recognized his greatness. He got off the throne, received him and made him sit. "Yes, my Lord," he replied. "This is my doubt: the scriptures say one can impart the wisdom within a fraction of a second. I really want the wisdom but nobody seems to be able to do that."

"Aha, you really want to experience that?"

"Yes."

"Okay, certainly I can do it. But it's just between you and me. I don't think these butchers can understand anything. Ask them to clear out of the hall or let's go somewhere to a quiet room."

Oh, you should have seen those people sitting there! How dare he call them butchers! Then Ashtavakra said, "Don't be angry. I'm only telling the truth."

The others demanded, "King, we want an explanation from this man. He is insulting."

The king asked, "Will you please explain what you mean?"

"Sure," said Ashtavakra. "What is the nature of a butcher? You bring him a goat — what will he look for in the goat? The soul? No. His interest is in the physical features and the weight of the goat. The butcher is not interested in the spirit of the goat. What is it that you did just now when I walked in? What is it that you saw to make you laugh?" When he said this, they understood their mistake immediately. "Yes you saw only the body; you didn't see me. The body consists of skin, bones, flesh. So you were interested in only the flesh like the butcher. What is the difference, then, between you and the butcher? You can just go out somewhere; you're not fit for anything." They realized their mistake and felt ashamed.

Then he spoke to Janaka. "Okay. You read that point in the scriptures. But did you read the previous *sloka* (verse)?"

"I did."

"What does it say?"

"It says, 'Sannyasyam sravanam kuryat.' — A seeker becomes ready to hear the truth when he is totally renounced."

See, the wisdom is to be imparted by hearing. You use the *Maha Vakyas*, the great secret mantrams. With just one mantram the wisdom is imparted and the seeker is enlightened. Do you want to know that mantram? Then you will all become enlightened. (We'll have to end the retreat! If you don't ask for a refund, fine!)

In the Hindu Vedas we have four Maha Vakyas. One is "*Tat tvam asi* — Thou art That." All the guru has to say is, "Tat tvam asi," and the seekers are enlightened. I'll give you enlightenment. "Thou art That." Understood? "You are not all this; Thou art That." But then, one must know what That is. That's the trouble. So although we hear this Maha Vakya, most don't get the enlightenment so easily.

So Janaka says, "I know. That's why I'm asking you. There must be a different way to say it."

"No. There's no difference in the saying, but there should be a difference in the hearing. That's why I asked you if you'd read the previous sloka. What does it say?" "A seeker becomes ready to listen when he is totally renounced, when he has dedicated everything, when he is free from ego. Only after total renunciation does one become ready to hear that."

"Have you done that?"

"Not yet."

"Then how can you understand? Renounce everything. You must offer everything, one by one. Then you will hear."

So he did. "This is my kingdom; all that I can say as mine I offer at your feet. And then there is still one more thing, but I can't offer, you have to take it."

"What's that?"

"I have offered everything to you, but *I* still remain."

So the offerer has to be accepted. Then he can be totally free.

At that point, Ashtavakra said to Janaka. "Thou art That," and Janaka understood the truth. It's something like looking into a mirror; you immediately get the reflection. You don't have to wait: "Now I cleaned the mirror — reflection, please come." It's simultaneous. When the light comes, the darkness is out. Not that you bring the light and say, "Darkness, the light is here, are you ready to go?" You don't need to say that. It doesn't even say goodbye to you. This coming and that going is simultaneous. You cannot even separate it as two different acts.

That is what is meant by, "When the disciple is ready, the guru comes." What is discipleship? It is deciphership. As long as you feel you're a hero, become a zero. The truth that is Satchidananda will reveal itself to you. You will know the truth once the dark veil is taken off.

It is like, every temple has a screen in front of the deity. It is not always open. Only at the time of the camphor light offering is it opened. So you should become a piece of camphor. Burn yourself totally. Then the screen will also be opened. All that will remain is the deity. It means that you get absorbed in that. You don't see the difference between you and the Cosmic Consciousness. You become one with it, feel one with it.

This is expressed in many different ways. You might say, "When I renounce everything, why should somebody have to tell me, 'Thou art That?' Can't I understand myself?" Remember, there is still a trace of ignorance there. The pure sattvic ego is still there. And that is what is meant by saying that the renouncer is still there. Though you have renounced everything, the "I" who did the renouncing is still there. The spirit is not the one who renounces. The spirit is never affected. It remains always clean and pure. It is the ego, when it accumulates all kinds of trash, that becomes an impure, unhealthy ego. By renouncing all these things, the ego becomes healthy. And when the ego becomes that pure, it says, "I have renounced everything but I am still here; I am still the same person. Having renounced everything I am pure, I know, but still I have not seen anything behind me. I haven't realized the higher Self."

At that point somebody must tell you, "Look back; turn around and see. There's no difference between you and Him now." When everything is cleaned, you are not different from that higher Self, because you were produced by that higher Self. You have the same purity. In Patanjali's Yoga Sutras, which are the main authority on Raja Yoga, you come across this sloka, "When the Purusha (individual self) attains the purity of the Cosmic Purusha (Cosmic Self) then he attains *kevalya* (liberation)."

This again is explained well through a story — the story of the "tenth man." Once ten friends went for a picnic. It was a rainy day and they had to cross a river which was in flood. So they decided to cross holding each other's arms. You can easily cross a river if you hold one another. So they did that. With great difficulty they crossed over and reached the other shore. Then they wanted to make sure that they were all there, that none had slipped in the river. So one said, "Okay, stand. I'll count whether we are all here now." They all stood there. "One, two, three, four, five, six, seven, eight, nine. Hum, I don't know what happened; the tenth man is not here any more. We are only nine now." And that's all — they all sat there and started to cry. "We lost the tenth man, we lost the tenth man, oh my sweet tenth man!"

While they were crying like this, another man walked by. "What has happened?" he asked. "Oh," they said, "when we started to cross the river, we were ten, but as you can see, now we are only nine. We lost the tenth man."

"Are you sure you lost him?"

"Yes."

"No, you haven't lost him," said the stranger. "The tenth man is there among you."

"What?" they cried. The minute they became curious, they stopped crying. You know what curiosity does. "Who's the tenth man then?" No more crying, the crying completely stopped. There is a time when a man stops crying and becomes curious instead. He wants to know.

So the stranger said, "Okay, stand in a line. You count."

He named one of the men. The man counted, "One, two, three . . . nine. See! Again there are just nine."

"Okay, I'll find the tenth man," said the stranger. He took his horse whip and said, "I'm going to give each one of you a lash but see that nobody gets a second one. You can count the number." He didn't want to give the information so easily. When you get the information easily, it is easily forgotten. So he started hitting. "One, two, three . . . nine . . . now see that none gets a second lash." And then he hit the tenth man who'd been counting the other nine.

"Oh," they cried, "the tenth man, oh thank you, thank you."

They were happy. They went on with their picnic. The tenth man never sat there saying, "I'm the tenth man, I'm the tenth man." He never meditated on it. Just like when you are given the mantram, Soham or "I am He," or Sivoham, "I am Siva," why should you keep repeating it: "I am He, I am He?" It's something like, "I'm the tenth man, I'm the tenth man." He had forgotten himself. He was always looking outside. He forgot to look within. He was always knowing other people. "I know him, and I know him but I don't know me." That is why I tell you, "Know thyself as the tenth man." That is where you need a teacher. And when you're really ready, the teacher's business is really easy. Otherwise he will have to start from the very beginning.

Questions and Answers on the Philosophy of Yoga
Swami Satchidananda

If we are God in reality, how did we come to think we are limited?

How it came about, that is the question now. We are trying to find out the origin. But it can never be answered to your satisfaction intellectually. It can be understood only when you get out of this individual ego. As long as you are still within the shell of that ego, that understanding will not penetrate. It is something like being asleep. You are having a world of your own within that shell and you think that that is everything.

It is like the beautiful example given by the scriptures: the sea frog and the well frog. All of a sudden one day, due to a flood or something, a sea frog fell into a well. There was another frog there already, the well frog. The well frog looked at the sea frog and said, "Hey, a stranger! Where do you come from?"

"From the sea."

"Sea? Is that water?"

"Yes, the sea is water."

"How much water?"

Then the well frog jumped a few feet and said, "Is the sea this big?"

The sea frog just laughed, "You can't measure the sea within this well."

"What? Okay, I'll jump a little longer distance and show you." He jumped a little longer distance. "Is this how big your sea is? Can it be bigger than this?"

The sea frog said, "No, please, don't try to understand the sea within the well; it's impossible."

"Nonsense, you come here and tell me that! Now I am going to show you the longest distance it could be." He swam across the well diagonally. "Certainly you will see it cannot be bigger than this."

The sea frog laughed. "Well, I'm a fool trying to make you understand what the sea is. I shouldn't even attempt it because you have not known anything other than the well you are in. Get out of the well and come with me. Then you will see the sea. As long as you are inside the well, it is not even possible to tell you how big the sea is."

131

Like that, we are in the small shell of ego. Within this we want to see the whole universe. We say, "Is it this big? Can God come into this test tube or this big flask? Is He like H$_2$O?" That is how we try to measure Him.

One day I was walking on the beach and I saw a little doll near the shore. It was a cute little doll. So I said, "Hi, what are you doing here? Who are you?"

"Oh, people call me the salt doll."

"Salt doll? Are you salty?"

"Yes, I'm made all of salt."

"Where do you come from?"

"From the sea."

"Aha, do you know how deep it is?"

"Well, I've never seen the bottom but if you wait, I'll jump in, measure the depth, then come back and tell you."

And the doll jumped into the sea. And I waited and waited and waited. Finally I got disappointed (because I'd made an appointment that the doll would come back and tell me!) Then later on I realized that when the doll jumped into the sea, it got dissolved and became the sea and thus understood the depth but could never come out to tell me.

If you want to understand the sea, become the sea. The rule of understanding is that. The rule of perception is that. If you want to understand a sinner, become a sinner. If you want to understand a dog, become a dog. There is a proverb: "Only a snake will know how another snake crawls." We can assume all the theories about how the snake could crawl but we have not experienced it. It is just theory. To experience how a snake could crawl, you should become a snake. Likewise, to experience a saintly life, you should become a saint. To know God, you should become God.

Until then, you have not known God — you have just imagined in your own way. God made man in His own image and man is making God in *his* own image. There is nothing wrong in it but we should understand that we all make our own images of God. God gives room for all these imaginations and He goes beyond them also. If you understand that, then it's fine. But when will we really know God? Only when we get out of this limited imagination. You can never know the unlimited as a limited person. To know the unlimited is to become unlimited. If you cannot, then limit the unlimited to one thing. And then, expand. The more you expand, the more you will see that it is also expanding.

That is why, still being an individual, you cannot understand how you were before and why you came down like this. But you know that you are like this now. You know you are in a shell. How are you to break it? It's like telling someone who is sleeping and dreaming that he is only dreaming. In his dream he gets frightened, and he kicks his pillow and shouts. You will say, "Hey man! There's no tiger. Why are you kicking the pillow? You are only dreaming." But he's not hearing you; he's still dreaming. The only way to make him understand that he is dreaming is to give him a nice kick. Wake him up. "Arise, awake!"

So give him a nice big kick. Break the nut, the shell of the coconut. Then the true kernel comes out. "Ha, I didn't know I was this pure, white, sweet kernel. I thought I was a hard nut."

So the egoistic nut should be broken to bring the real you out. Until then, this question can never be answered to your own satisfaction. We can only guide you how to break the ego. Whenever you see the ego, try to give a hit. If you can, do it yourself. Or follow somebody. That's all. Something like a laundryman. Let him wash your cloth. He won't just wash it gently. If the dirt is too much, he will apply all kinds of things, squeeze it, rinse it and even then, if there are still wrinkles, he'll iron it. So you should get ironed. If you are interested, put yourself in the hands of a good laundryman. He'll take good care of you. But allow him to do his job. Before he even applies a little soap, if you say, "Ooh, you are smearing all kinds of things on me, I don't want that . . . ," he can't do his job.

If everything is eternal, how does the yogic ideal of Ahimsa, *or trying not to cause death, fit in?*

Hm death, I see. Do you mean that when you pull up a flower, you destroy it? Well, there is no death as such. Nothing dies; everything is eternal. Death is the wrong word. That is why it is very much misunderstood. Nothing is destroyed. You can never destroy anything. And you cannot create anything. What is, is always. What is not, never was and never will be.

So then what is death? Change. Change is what you call death. A piece of log gets changed into some furniture. A lump of clay gets changed into dolls. Gold ore is changed into nice ornaments. Paper pulp gets changed into sheets of paper, sheets into books, books into paper, paper into ash. That's why there is a proverb: "Nothing is lost when a candle burns." So you don't destroy anything; you only change one form into another.

Even your name. You were a "baby"; now you are a "boy". What happened to the baby? Where is the baby now? He is no more. Can you say the baby died? The baby *changed* into the boy, the boy into a man, the man into an old man, the old man into a dead body. So there are all these changes. There is nothing but name and form in this world. The whole world is made up of name and form. If you just ignore the name and form, you will see that the essence behind is the same. That is why you come to the omnipresent One.

Even according to the scientists the whole world is filled with nothing but electrons, protons and neutrons. Everything is made up of that. Even the space between us is filled with that. You are nothing but a bundle of electrons, protons and neutrons. I'm not different from that. Then why do you call me the Swami and yourself as Jacob and the space between as just space? We give things a name. They only appear like that, like the waves appear in the sea. In the sea there is nothing but water: big waves, small waves, bubbles, foam; it is all just water, different forms of the same water. And the water is nothing but the chemical compound, H_2O.

So the entire universe is nothing but one essence. But the One appears to be many, like the many waves of the sea. You give them different names. Even the names vary according to the sea; you don't call things by the same name everywhere. So death is change. How can the body decompose if it is not alive? There must be some energy functioning to decompose. We say, "*He* is dead and gone," but "*that* is lying six feet underground." You don't mean "he" is dead. When he is dead and gone, *he* is gone but *that* is lying six feet under. Actually, nothing is dead. It is a part of the essence. How can that God change?

As such, we expect changes. Where there is life, there is change. We expect it. Seed changes into plant, plant into flower, flower into fruit, fruit into seed again. So what is meant by death? People who can understand death are not afraid of it. We should welcome change. If you are afraid of dying as a baby, you won't grow up as a boy. You are happy growing to be a boy. Death is something welcome.

In trying to be the silent witness, I find that I am judging myself instead of just witnessing. Is judging part of the process? It seems to be getting in the way of purely witnessing the mind. How does one get beyond judgment and how does one get beyond feeling guilty?

If you really tap the witness, you will know that it never judges. A witness will not judge. The judging is done by something else. What is it that judges? Your intelligence, your discriminating faculty. "Is it good, bad, right, wrong?" The analytic mind judges. It analyzes the case, picks the right from the wrong. But even behind the analyzer, there is somebody who knows that something is judging, is it not? And that is what you call the witness, the self-awareness. The witness will never get involved in anything. If the witness gets involved in a case, he is no longer a witness. So he is only an observer. That's why his words are so powerful, hm? Without a witness, the case cannot be made. See?

The Self is that witness. Your Self is constantly witnessing everything. It dosen't say anything. And that is what you call the real conscience-ness. It doesn't tell you what to do or what not to do. It is just there. If you care to look back and say, "What is it, am I right or wrong?" you will see yourself reflected there. It is something like, is my face clean or dirty? Where will you go to see? You will stand in front of a mirror. The mirror will not tell you whether your face is beautiful or ugly. It is just there to show you to yourself, so you know whether it is beautiful or ugly. You don't need to thank the mirror at all, "Thank you for saying I am very beautiful." The mirror is just there to reveal yourself. You use the mirror, but it doesn't even demand that you should do so. That mirror is the Self. It constantly reflects everything. It is just there. That is what you call the antar Atma, the inner Self.

Sixth Day

Wholeness and Holiness

Rabbi Joseph Gelberman

Rabbi Gelberman has spoken at Yoga retreats before – at Annhurst College in 1970 and 1971 – and is an old friend of Swamiji's, going back to the time in the 1960's when Swamiji still had been living in the U.S. a relatively short time. As Rabbi of the Little Synagogue in New York City, he and Swamiji each year have given a joint talk, open to the public, called "The Swami and the Rabbi." This was perhaps the first Ecumenical exchange between these two traditions, and helped to open up new and wider appreciation both of Yoga and of Judaism. Also, as someone who has himself taken an interest in the teachings and practices of Yoga, Rabbi Gilberman has over the years been very helpful in mediating misunderstandings when the families of young Jewish students would become upset at their children's involvement in Yoga.

Up to this point in the retreat, the guest speakers have spoken primarily in the language and symbols of the Hindu tradition, though Swami Nirmalananda's Midwestern Christian upbringing helped tremendously in the translation of these into terms that Americans could readily understand. But with the appearance of Rabbi Gelberman, the retreatants enjoy an approach more immediately familiar. Rabbi Gelberman is, of course, a representative of the Jewish tradition, but more especially of two aspects of that tradition: the Hassidic, which represents the mystical side of Judaism, and the Kabbalistic, its esoteric side. Rabbi Gelberman incorporates both into his approach (he often calls himself a modern Hassid, in the tradition of Martin Buber) and both lend themselves to an appreciation of the universal truths common to all traditions.

In addition, Rabbi Gelberman is also a practicing psychotherapist. This psychological approach to the question of spiritual life is the most prominent feature of his talk this morning. Again, it is an approach to which many of the retreatants can immediately relate, and it gives the talk the down-to-earth quality which is characteristic of Rabbi Gelberman. In this talk, he mainly stresses that one must integrate all aspects of life in the spiritual path, so that one becomes a whole person as well as a holy person. Probably it is this understanding which brought him to appreciate and work with Swamiji, as Integral Yoga (as the name implies) has always emphasized too that all aspects of the individual – physical, mental, emotional and spiritual – must be harmoniously developed.

Shalom. In true Hassidic mystical tradition, I should like to begin my discourse with an affirmation. I remember when I was a very little child, the minute we knew how to put words together, we learned a prayer, a morning prayer or an affirmation for the day. Those of you who come from a Jewish background remember it. "To praise the Lord who in His loving kindness has returned the soul within me." You see, we used to believe that the soul departed during the night to do some bookkeeping in Heaven; to write in the Book what happened the day before. And in the morning, surprise, I'm alive! My soul is still here. My body can move. I'm aware. So we begin the day with this affirmation which sets the mood, the foundation for the whole day: "I'm going to be joyous." So let us begin with the affirmation, expressed perhaps in different words, in the form of a chant.

The chant will say that this is the day that God has created, a day of light and a day of joy, a day of peace and a day of harmony. You know what we are talking about – you have been here six days. So I'll chant a phrase and I'll ask you to repeat the chant after me. It's in the Hebrew but this is the message, that this is *our* day and it's a day of joy and delight.

(*Chanting*)

Believe me when I say that I envy you for being here at this retreat. I'm also glad you chose this place, because evidently it was named after me: my first name is Joseph. And it's a possibility. And interestingly enough, this is the theme of my discourse this morning. That this Joseph may become a saint; in fact any Joe can become a saint.

To begin with, I would like to state, one, that sainthood is not an exclusive club. You can get into it. It's open and free to all. And two, to become a holy man means to be wholly a man. Martin Buber once said, "God does not want you to become an angel. He has enough and He has His troubles with them. But He wants you to be a *Mensch*!" A Mensch, meaning a person. So to be a holy man means to be wholly a man. And three, a simple definition of holiness is readiness.

Those of you who are familiar with the Bible, it says, "Ye shall be holy, for I, the Lord your God, am Holy." And for a long time this passage didn't make sense to me. Because God is holy I shall be holy? For God it's easy, he's God! He has no wife, he has no children, he has no job to worry about. What about me? And then it came to me that to be holy meant to be ready for holiness. The getting ready is the thing. And to be ready means to choose. All of life is actually a choice. A Hassidic master once said that life is like a big department store, say like Macy's, Gimbel's and Korvette's put together and a little bigger. And it has many floors, including a basement. You can get anything you want in this department store and you have to pay for it. To be sure, not with dollars; there they are worth even less than here. No, you have to pay with the self, with discipline, with awareness, with joy and peace. And what a pity, said this master, that most of us spend our time in the basement getting some cheap, second-hand things, when we could climb to the highest floor and get the finest. But life is a choice.

Now, with this simple introduction, I'm going to suggest that to reach this awareness of holiness, or wholeness, we'll have to do it on three levels. On a psychological level, a theological level and finally a metaphysical level. Don't get frightened about the words, I don't know myself exactly what they mean, but we'll struggle through it as we go on together.

It is vitally important that we understand the self, psychologically, before we can express spirituality or oneness with God. I'm going to suggest some psychological musts you need to learn so that you can reach the "I AM." These are the first two words that God uttered in the Ten Commandments: "I am the Lord . . ." And I am a part of that "I AM." But to reach that, I must mature emotionally.

What is the psychological preparation to be a holy man? I am going to suggest several triads. The first is what I would call the three basic needs: food, shelter and love. These are the needs in order to survive. Now, I have a friend who "needs" to eat in the most expensive restaurants, to live in the most expensive Park Avenue home. So we need to distinguish between the needs and the wants. But sometimes we are foolish enough to think we need nothing. We are foolish to renounce too much of the world or to want nothing. We have this notion that we please the Lord when we renounce everything. I know a man who needed a car. Every day he would spend hours in meditation and prayer. "God," he said, "I don't want much, just give me an old car." The day came when he needed the car for his new job. He looked out the window and sure enough there was a car in front of his door, an old car, but he was happy and joyous — a miracle had happened. He gets into the car, turns on the ignition. He rides and he sings — he's happy. All of a sudden he hears a voice, the voice of God, telling him, "To tell the truth, I had in mind giving you a Cadillac, but you insisted on an old, broken-down Ford." The point is, who am I to tell God what he should do for me? By what right? By what arrogance? By what right should I renounce the joys of life? I have to sanctify it. Buber said again, "The difference between the holy and the unholy is that the holy is waiting to be sanctified." Otherwise, there is not, there cannot be ugliness in God's world, by definition. Is this clear? It's clear to me. If God is Love, and God is Joy, and God is Peace, would he take pleasure in my depriving myself of what I really need? For what purpose? For what reason?

So, first, the idea is to understand these three drives, and to distinguish between needs and wants. And there's nothing wrong in wanting as long as I know they are not my needs — and as long as I sanctify them.

A second triad is the three basic concerns of man. They are the fear of death, the fear of loss of self-worth, of being unloved, and the fear of unfulfilled desires. First, the fear of death. We all unconsciously are afraid of dying. Even though I'm certainly not consciously aware of the fear of death, I know every day I'm dying a little bit. That's true. But every day I'm also living a little bit. So we're simultaneously dying a little, living a little. And that's good. And here Yoga or Hassidism or Kabbalism is a tremendous help — because I'm not my body anyway. Let it go (As a matter of fact, maybe I'll get a better one in in my next life. I sure hope so.) So, that which is alive in me — the energy, the soul in me — can never die. It is going to a higher life, a higher form of life, in my next incarnation.

Then there is the dread of loss of self-worth — "I'm a nothing." In the old time religion we said, "I'm a sinner, I'm a worthless nothing." "Nobody loves me." Psychologically we know better. Man cannot be a worthless nothing. David, in one of his Psalms, puts it so beautifully. He said, "Even if my father and mother would leave me" — and this is the highest form of rejection, the very people who are supposed to love me — "but Thou, O Lord, never will." And Kabbalistically this means that there is an unbroken cord, an uncut umbilical cord with which we are all attached to the overall universe.

As far as the unfulfilled desires are concerned, maybe I'm talking to the wrong audience. Perhaps you have no desires any more. Do you? I hope you do. For this reason: all the desires — the good and bad — come from the same root. If you kill the desire for so-called evil, you also kill the desire for good. And then you become a zombie — a holy zombie. So desires are good too. As long as we are not hung up in desires or attachment.

Let me say a word here about attachment. I'm talking about being attached to things. I'm a product of the Western society, and I'm sure it will take many more lives to overcome that. But the idea is to be realistic about it. Let's give a simple example. Have you ever been to Miami? You haven't? Or the Bahamas? (There are ashrams there now, all over the place.) You've seen the beautiful palm tree, have you not? Can you imagine going there and seeing this tree and saying to yourself, "I'll get one and bring it home and plant it near my house and have a palm tree"?

My contention is that for those of us born and bred in this culture — we cannot go along fully and completely with the concept of non-attachment. In our lives we have all kinds of needs and wants: number one, number two, number three. But there is a way. I can say attachment is no longer number one in my life. I can do without my apartment. I can do without my car. I can do without money — and this has been proven. I can do without a job. I can do without anything. But I decided not to. I made a decision and for this reason — because I am called upon to be a partner with God in Creation. Now what kind of a partner am I if I am not involved with life? So, I drive a car like everybody else; but maybe I meditate and the people around me notice it. And when people talk to me, I consider it a blessing, whatever face they give me. You see, I have a little mechanism in my mind called a converter. Whatever they say to me, I convert it into a blessing. I'm grateful for it. The concept is beautiful and it can be done. Each one of us has to work it out in our own way.

So the criteria for emotional maturity, then, is that we deal in reality with the challenges on an earthly level. The great historian, Toynbee, suggests that the reason why some peoples, nations, are wiped from the face of the Earth is that they do not respond to the challenges presented to them during their lives. Another criterion is to have the capacity to change. Doesn't nature change? At least four times a year? So man has to have the capacity to let go, to solve the problems in joy, as an adventure, to learn from everything, to realize that life is a coin which has two sides, and that he can choose.

The next criterion is to free the body from symptoms. And here Yoga is a tremendous help. It hasn't taken on me too much as you can see — but I'm working at it. I'm definitely convinced that you are what you eat. And it is vitally important that you respect the mechanism and not overload it with junk and with unnecessary overeating — with all due respect to our beautiful mothers: "Eat a little more, eat a little more . . . ." And we must free the body from tensions due to unresolved anxiety as well. You can't say, "All right, forget it," as your next door neighbor would say. The tension must be resolved. Otherwise it causes a broken heart, or a heart attack; it blows your mind, to use the language of today. We get strokes and all other sicknesses, including cancer: research has been done that shows that even cancer is created through negative thinking and through unresolved anxieties.

Another criterion for emotional maturity is to find satisfaction in giving. To be a giver and not just a taker; and to love in wisdom is to know when to give and when to take. Another criterion is to direct hostility into creative channels. Suppose I have some hostility and anger in me? Anger wastes psychological, creative and spiritual energies and therefore the result is guilt and separation: "I'm ashamed of myself." But sublimated and transmuted anger has the energy to heal and to create.

The ultimate criterion for emotional maturity is: to love. But to love means to take risks; even though I might be rejected, to go on loving; to yield up some freedom here and there and take my chances; to assume added responsibilities, to be committed; to sacrifice if need be; and to let the other be as he wants to be.

These then are the psychological necessities for wholeness. And we must do these effectively, pleasurably and freely. And, maybe, here is where I may differ in my attitude from all the other teachings. In Hassidism we lay tremendous importance on the concept of joy. I have an idea that God created man in a joyous mood, but something happened to us on the way of being born and spoiled it. We need to become happy, joyous, without tensions, or at least as little tension as possible. This equals mental health. And the ultimate goal is: to have the identity with the I AM. I know who I am because I am part of the overall I AM.

The second level on which we have to achieve wholeness, or holiness, has to do with the way we have interpreted the Bible. I'm going to take three short passages and tell you where we made a mistake. First of all is the Commandment: "Thou shalt not kill." In the Hebrew it's even shorter. It doesn't say, if they happen to be un-American then you can kill them. It doesn't say, if they are of a different race or color or creed then it's all right to kill them. I think we made a tremendous mistake of daring to reinterpret this one Commandment. And it has been sanctified by the churches and the synagogues. We have chaplains in the Army. We even have chaplains in Sing Sing. Taking a man to be killed, there is a chaplain saying prayers. Isn't that unbelievable? How dare they to make God a partner to this ugliness of man? Thou shalt not kill. Period. And it also means, Thou shalt not kill the sensitivity and the need of the other who approaches you with love. That's also killing. If my mother wants to love me her way – her way – and I reject it, I am also killing. The Commandment is very straight and simple and to the point.

The second error is the sentence in the Bible where the Commandment is given, "And thou shalt build me a sanctuary so that I may dwell in it." This has been interpreted through the years, and still is, as meaning to build big buildings. How many of you come from the Island? Long Island? Manhattan Island? You notice they just don't put on symbols of churches and synagogues? Neither a cross nor a Star of David. That's too – what? Too religious. After all, we have to go with the trend. So how do you know when you are passing by a synagogue or a church? Ah, look at the architecture. If it cost over a million dollars, you can be sure it's a synagogue or church. And what do we do? We build these beautiful huge expensive buildings with many locks and we lock God in there. And we say, "Stay there. Leave me alone. You be there and I'll be here. Once a week I may come. Once a week, maybe once a month. You have a nice house, so stay there. That's for you. "While if we understood the text — I wish you could understand Hebrew here — you could appreciate it better. The text says, "Thou shalt make me a sanctuary so that I may dwell among you." Instead, people wanted something they could touch. They wanted a fund-raising committee with a chairman. The sanctuary was for the vanity of the people. But God said, "Build me a sanctuary within your heart and soul, so that I may dwell among you."

The third error is — the Psalm, a part of which we sang earlier as a part of our affirmation, says that this is the day that the Lord has created to be joyous. And we interpret this to mean — on the Sabbath, on church day, on a wedding day, on a *Bar Mitzvah*, on a birthday. And yet the sages who had insight into these things asked a question, "Which day?" And in unison they answered, "We don't know which day — therefore, every day!" We don't need any excuse to bring flowers to the one we love, or to say something beautiful, or to put ourselves into a holiday mood. "This is the day!" I have news for you. We may not have the next day. Therefore, this is the day. Somewhere else the sages said, "Return unto the Lord the day before your death." Again they asked the question, "Which day would that be?" And the answer is, since you don't know which day, every day. It could be today; tomorrow may be too late. So I'm suggesting that to be holy means to sanctify and to affirm every day as the day, the day of the Lord. The day I can express my oneness, my wholeness with God. And create a more joyous, more harmonious world.

And finally, on the third level, the metaphysical understanding of life may give us an inkling how to achieve wholeness and holiness. I'm going to take the very word "life." In Kabbalistic interpretation, not so much the sentence is used, not so much the word even, but each letter of each word carries the true message. So take "life." Some people will say, "Eh, I'm living." Others will say, "I'm alive!" In the very way we say it we give away how we feel about it. Now, the first one, who says, "Eh, life . . ." would spell it with a small "l" — which stands, since he feels that way, for loneliness. He is not very happy with life, because the "I" in his life is tremendous. He's selfish, he doesn't trust anybody, so the "f" stands for fear; he's afraid of his own shadow. The "e" is his diagnosis — emptiness. He's an empty person. He's just existing. It's like Professor Barker of Columbia University used to say, "The epithet of the average American may read: Died at 40, buried at 60." He just *exists*.

On the other hand, take the one who exclaims, "Life!" with a capital "L" — he is ready to embrace the world. Can you see the big "L"? The one who writes "Life" with a capital "L" is ready to embrace everything. There the "L" stands for love. He starts out his life like that, not worried about rejections, about disappointments. So what? That's part of life.

Now the "i" in there is a little "i" — secure, at peace. He doesn't talk about himself; he is included in everybody. Which reminds me of a little story. There was a newspaperman who was constantly talking about himself, and his friends were sick and tired of him already. One of them had the courage and said, "Listen, John, we're all sick and tired. You're constantly talking about yourself." He was a writer and had written books and so on and he said, "Oh, I'm so terribly sorry. This has been going on for years. All right, I'm going to change it right now. Let's talk about you. How did *you* like my latest book?" But in that other kind of life, the "i" is little; there's no need for him to be pompous, to be blown up. He knows who he is. His "I" is a part of the overall "I".

The "f" in that kind of life stands for freedom. He's a free man, he comes and goes. He's the kind that's at home in paradise, and the world for him is paradise. Wherever he goes, he doesn't have the hangups, "Well, I'm Jewish and I'm not Catholic. I'm Catholic and I'm not Jewish. They're different." Different? Who said so? I would like to see the first person who said this. If you study the Book, we are told when Adam, the first man, was created, God went around to take some earth — Adam means earth — from the four corners of the Earth, so that nobody would ever say that my stuff is different from yours. But all of a sudden there is this snobbery that goes on in the world. "I'm this, you're that. I'm white, you're black. I'm Jew, you're gentile." Who put up these man-made barriers that get in the way of our loving each other, embracing each other? Who? And why? There's another Watergate. Maybe this should be discussed. Who is responsible for this cover-up? And finally, in this "Life" with a capital "L" the "e" is also the diagnosis — this man is excited about life. This man is alive, this man is joyous.

To summarize, then, there is a way, I believe, to rededicate our lives, to change our lives, and to experience rebirth. We must find that way. So I rejoice in the fact that there are young people, men and women, who take time out and become researchers of life. You're all scientists, you know. You're just not on anybody's payroll, because the government is still not interested in this kind of thing. But you are scientists, researchers, searching for a better way of life, and I tell you there is a way. But be careful. If to experience spiritually or to cleave unto God can by symbolically described as climbing a spiritual ladder, then I would say that this ladder, like the ladder in Jacob's dream, although it reaches up to the highest heavens, is rooted in the earth. This ladder has many rungs, and you must climb it rung by rung. You can't jump and you can't rush it. And you may get air sickness if you stay too high too long. Friends, do what the angels in Jacob's dream did. Move up and down like an escalator. Up and down. And take somebody with you; never alone. Because ultimately, the object and purpose of man is to be a partner with God, to create a better world, a more peaceful world, and a more joyous world for all men to live in.

You are very kind. I hope I'll have a chance to meet with you personally, to shake a finger . . . and rejoice in your smile. I would like to conclude with a little chant. It's a simple song, a love song. It is a sentence from The Song of Songs, a little book in the Bible. How many of you know this book? Read it, it's a beautiful little song. And the sentence goes, "I belong to my Beloved and my Beloved belongs to me." Belonging meaning not in a property sense, like an attachment, but belonging meaning like my arm belongs to me. We're a part of each other. Of course, this is to be understood on two levels. On a human level, we have a beloved, and on the divine level, God is our Beloved. The Hassidim would read this book every Friday afternoon as a preparation for the Sabbath, because the Sabbath is Love. Sabbath is symbolized as a bride and Israel is the king, the bridegroom. The wedding takes place every Sabbath. So they prepare themselves with the beautiful poetry. Again, I'll sing it in Hebrew, one line, and I'll ask you to repeat after me. This we'll do in the Hebrew and the English.

(The program concludes with the chanting.)

Internal Cleansing

Swami Satchidananda

One of the important aspects of Hatha Yoga are the kriya practices, which the retreatants will be experiencing the following morning, in place of the normal Hatha Yoga class of postures and pranayama. To prepare them for this experience, Swamiji begins this evening's satsang with a short talk about these cleansing techniques – a talk which makes everyone enthusiastic to learn them, whereas normally they might have been a little hesitant.

Afterward, Swamiji answers a wide range of questions having to do with Yoga and health: questions on diet and fasting, postures and pranayama, as well as specific health problems.

I'd like to say a few words about the kriya practice we will be doing tomorrow. As you probably know by now, the entire practice of yoga or what you call spiritual practice is based on cleaning the coverings, the tarnish, from the body, the mind, the society – wherever it is. Because of the undersirable elements that come and accumulate, we seem to have lost our purity – like dusty mirrors. So the entire aim in all these practices is this cleaning. The kriya practices which we'll do are based on cleaning. The literal meaning for kriya is an action, that's all. Any action is called kriya – from "kri," which means "act." But these particular practices are especially called Kriya Yoga because these actions are performed to clean certain impurites from the system.

Six kriyas are given in the Hatha Yoga texts: *dhauti, basti, neti, kapalabhati, nauli* and *thratakam*. Dhauti is to clean the stomach. There are again three types of dhauti: jala dhauti is just using water; that is what you'll be doing tomorrow. It's a very simple practice. This dhauti kriya is done by the doctors also but there they do it in a different way: they insert a long rubber tube through the mouth down to the stomach and then one end is like a funnel. They just pour water into that. The tube will be a forearm's length outside; half the tube will have gone in. So one end will be in the stomach and the other end way up over the head. They lift up the tube and just keep pouring water until the funnel is full and then all they have to do is drop the funnel down; then by the siphon system,

147

the water will come back out. You don't need to do anything. But it's a painful thing to insert the rubber tube down to the stomach.

That is the Western medicine. But in the Eastern, yogic way, you don't need to insert that; you just drink water and throw it out. Drink as much as you can, maybe six, seven or even ten glassfuls — as much as you can up to the throat. The water should also be a little salty; it helps in the cleaning. After you feel that if you drink anymore the whole thing will come out by itself, then the dhauti is made easy. You don't need to do much then. All you have to do is run to a ditch, hm? Then bend down and the whole thing comes out. Sometimes, people try to throw it up after drinking only two or three glasses. That makes it difficult. Drink as much as possible, the more the better. If it still doesn't come up, you can tickle the back of the throat with a little salt and the whole thing will come out easily.

Maybe in the beginning only water will come out. Later on, you'll see thick water, like saliva — the mucus coming out. Maybe later, if there is some bile in your stomach, you will see that the water is yellowish. Occasionally there may be a tinge of blood also — reddish colour. But there is no need to get upset over it. It may be a blood clot or ulceration in the stomach which is getting washed out. And before throwing up, it is better to shake the stomach a little, tapping and rubbing the stomach as much as possible. Shake the whole area so that it will get mixed up well; then you throw out. And if there is a little water left over in the stomach, you don't have to worry about it, because ultimately it will pass through.

This dhauti can also be done with cloth. We don't usually give it at the retreats unless you especially want to go and learn by yourself or by special appointment because it's not really necessary and it's not good for everybody. You take a thin muslin cloth, two or three inches wide and about fifteen feet long. Roll it, soak it in water, then take one end and slowly swallow it. You can sip a little water along with it. The whole thing goes down into the stomach — only keep the last end outside. Then bite down on the last end. You don't even need to hold it in your hand, just keep it bitten. Then shake the stomach well and then pull it out little by little. It's something like the way we clean a bottle, by putting a cloth into it and cleaning it, then pulling it out. It will get wiped out well.

And there is still another way. In India they use the banana leaf, the tender young leaf, rolled like a tube. It is very soft and long, so they cut it and insert it into the mouth down to the stomach. But tomorrow you will be using only water. That is enough. The other two things I don't really advise very much — they are only for demonstration. Just water is enough.

The basti is sucking water through the anus. According to the yogic kriya you don't need an enema bag. You can have control over the anal ring which can contract and expand at your will. So you just sit in a tub of water or in any shallow river, just open the anus ring, create a vacuum in the abdomen with the *uddiyana* (stomach lift) and the water will rush in to fill the vacuum. Those who cannot control the ring are allowed to use a small tube. Insert it, sit in the water and suck it in. But even that could be eliminated and made easy by using an enema bag – because its purpose is the same. So mere enema using water can be considered as basti kriya. We won't do that here, because you all know that and can do it at home. It's good to have the colon cleaned occasionally, at least once a week. You don't need to do it daily and make it into a habit, but once a week will help a lot.

And now the neti, the nasal cleansing. The best and simplest thing, which I do often, is just take a little water in the palm, close one nostril and then sniff a few drops. It will irritate the nose a little and the tears will come and all the mucus will be released and come out. Then do the same for the other nostril. Another way is to fill up a glass with salty warm water up to the brim, then put it to the nose and make a pumping suction; it will come to the mouth and you spit it out. It can be easily done without any danger. And even if it goes down into the stomach instead of through the mouth, it doesn't matter. But still, even if you could do that, I would prefer the sniffing method because the water gets sprayed and goes in more, to give more irritation, and all the mucus comes out very well. Or you can use a pitcher, like a teapot, fill it and then put the nozzle into one nostril, tip the head, pour it, and then slowly it will pass into the other nostril. Open the mouth and breathe through the mouth as you keep on pouring. Then change nostrils. It's good during warm days, if you do this, you will feel the eyes cooled as well as cleaning out the mucus. By neti you can get rid of this sinus trouble; even the hay fever can easily be cured by the neti kriya.

The last three kriyas are done in the Hatha classes in the mornings and afternoons and in the varied sadhana classes so I won't explain them here.

Questions and Answers on Health and Diet

Swami Satchidananda

How often should we do these kriyas?

It all depends on how often you need it. It's not necessary to do it regularly, maybe once a week. If you take care of your diet, you don't even need to wash the stomach. Maybe once a fortnight, when you find the need, you can do it. It need not be a regular part of daily practice.

Are the asanas and regular walking sufficient exercise to help remove the stagnant toxins from the body or is regular rigorous exercise like swimming also necessary?

Asanas and walking are sufficient. Exercises like swimming do help but aren't necessary. They strengthen the muscles. They do help in that respect. If you like to do them there is no harm, but do not over-do them. If you don't have time to do those things, just stick to asanas and walking. Even if you don't have time to do walking, asanas and some Sun Worship — *Soorya Namaskaram* — is enough. If you want to make yourself alert in the morning, do a few rounds of Soorya Namaskarams and then do the asanas. If you still want to combine both exercises and asanas, as I said in the *Integral Yoga Hatha* book, do the exercises first, relax, and then do the asanas afterward. End up with asanas. Instead, if you do the asanas first, and then the exercises, you will disturb what you have built by the asanas.

I like to run at least three miles a day. Will this conflict with my asana practice? Running seems to tighten the muscles, especially in the legs.

In a way it will conflict, because in asanas you are trying to relax the muscles, relax the entire body. A little running is fine, but in running more than you need you will build up the muscles. That means your energy, your vitality, is brought to the muscles. If you pull your energy toward the muscles, you develop the biceps and other muscles at the cost of the inner glands, the inner person. The vital force should be evenly distributed. Man is made with a certain strength of the muscles. That nor-

150

mal, needed strength will be given even by your asanas. But, if you want to be an even stronger man, then you do it at the cost of your inner man. It is difficult to have both. To keep the muscles tense you have to have more vitality coming in, more circulation there, more nourishment there. So it contradicts. But, if you are interested in both, then do it. You won't lose the benefit of asanas, no doubt. Certainly, you should do the asanas, because at least then you'll get some form of relaxation, along with your exercise.

I started my menstruation today. Should I discontinue Hatha practice? What poses could I do?

Well, if you have been doing them for a long time and you are not a beginner, you can do some simple poses. Relax more and do more alternate nostril breathing. There's no need to practice strenuous asanas or violent breathing like bastrika or kapalabhati. But you can always do alternate nostril breathing. And practice more simple postures.

Please explain why women are told not to do asanas during and after menstruation. Personally, I feel better when I exercise during menstruation and don't get all stiff.

So many people have asked this. You see, normally during the menstrual period, the body will be a little weaker than the normal days. There is no doubt about it. There is certain drain from the body. So one feels a little weak, dull.

And not only the body, but even the mind is a little weak during that time. It's a very subtle difference, you may ignore it, you may not know it, but still it is there, mentally and physically. So to give enough rest and not to do strenuous practices, we say take leave for two or three days. That is the Indian custom. During the menstrual period women don't go to work. They don't even come into the house and cook. They just stay in a room and meditate, relax, lie down, read. They take a good rest.

It's a wonderful opportunity. But somehow, the West doesn't seem to be thinking that way. But the fact is — at least all the women folk tell me and this is what I hear from many people with whom I've spoken — during the menstrual period, not only the body is weak, even the mind is weak. Weak means it functions more on a lower level. It's kind of like a cow in heat. Please don't misunderstand me. I'm just giving you an example. Don't imagine that I'm putting you in that category. You should admit we're all like animals. In what way are we different? We also have the hunger, interest in survival, sensuality. But particularly during the period, the lower nature will come up to the surface a little. Mainly for that purpose, in India and other places in the East, the woman is allowed to stay quietly, not even to mingle with men folk during that time. Why? Because even a gentle touch from the other sex will create certain feelings. And if it goes beyond a limit, then it is almost uncontrollable. Then one has to strain oneself to stop it. Otherwise one will get lost in it. And during that time a sexual relationship is very dangerous. It will really drain the person a lot. So to avoid all these things they take rest, not to mingle with the other sex those two, three days. But of course, I'm not asking you to follow this, I'm just giving you the reasons why some follow it. Even in India and Ceylon, not that many people follow it anymore. If you think there is some meaning, some purpose behind it, and some benefit, do it; otherwise, it doesn't matter. Not that you're dirty, or ugly, or unfit. I would never say that. It's a natural phenomenon.

And that is the reason why you can do your normal simple postures, alternate breathing, but not violent kapalabhati or bastrika with them, because even the menstrual flow will get agitated. To be on the safe side, stay away from the postures for a few days. Or if you are confident, practice some mild postures and alternate breathing. Do a lot of meditation, take rest. Don't think, "Oh, they are making us weak." It's a kind of cry, "Oh, why should they think that we are weak?" Whether they think so or not, you should know whether you are weak or not, physically and mentally. It's time to rest. It will be very beneficial.

Most of the psychological problems can easily occur during that period. In fact, in India, during the menstrual period, if a girl rests in a room they will even put a broomstick and one or two old worn-out slippers outside the door, thinking that during that weak moment certain evil spirits can easily affect her. The mind is weak, the body is weak. At that time a spirit can easily possess the body. So they say, you put out these things so that any spirit who comes and sees these things will think, "Ah, I won't walk into that." That spirit has its own pride, no? So to keep the spirit away they do certain things like that. It is a known fact in many cases that those who got possessed by evil spirits got possessed during that time. You're more susceptible at that period. So these are all some of the reasons why there are these customs. At the same time, it's a nice way of getting a little rest!

I used to practice Hatha Yoga and was fairly advanced in the practice but have not done it now for some time. Now I find that even the simple postures are very painful. This is very discouraging.

If meditation and Hatha are not done for a long interval, when you begin again, remember that you are a beginner now. In the case of Hatha, begin as a beginner. You might have been in a very advanced level before. When you stop for a long time, your body falls back, so that you have to begin again slowly. That's why we say never to strain yourself in Yoga practices. If you feel a little strained, don't go further. Do something, keep on doing it and the body will get relaxed again. You will be able to do more and more, better and better. So neither run like a rabbit or be passive like a tortoise. Go in between. Moderation is very necessary. Sometimes even the pain might stop you from progressing. You should know whether it is a real pain or an illusion created by the mind. So watch carefully. Do not stop until the goal is reached.

Two years ago, after forcing a bit in the head-to-knee pose, I developed disc trouble between the last lumbar and the first sacral vertebrae. After that, I didn't practice Yoga asanas but now I am slowly going back to it. What are the poses to avoid and what are the ones which are beneficial?

Well, you learned a lesson. That's why we say never to over-exert, never to strain. Don't go beyond your capacity. Thank God, at least you are back to normal now and doing a few asanas. Don't think that by always performing difficult poses you are going to achieve something. You will break your body. So do it gently. So now, when you begin again, think that you are a beginner and watch carefully. Particularly, watch the spine. Once you have dislocated the disc, there is every possibility of doing it again; because once weakened, it would take a very, very long time to get strong again. So you must be very careful. Even when you are doing it, put your awareness there, and see how you feel. If you feel even the slightest tension, stop. That's enough. Even if you don't touch the toes, it doesn't matter. Touching the toes is not going to help you in touching God.

That is the reason why some people, once and for all, condemned all these Hatha Yoga poses. If you go to the Ramakrishna Mission people, they will even say, "We don't believe in Hatha Yoga. Don't do it." So we should learn to do it in a moderate way. If we don't do it, we'll lose the benefit. But if we do it excessively, we'll get the trouble. We can easily say, "Okay, no Hatha Yoga. Don't do it, it's dangerous." But do we stop walking across the road because it is dangerous? Tell me one thing that is not dangerous.

(*Someone points to Swamiji as being one thing which is not dangerous.*)

No! Even that is dangerous. You probably don't know how dangerous

I am, hm? Come near me, you'll know. If you come too close, you'll get burnt! If you go away, you'll feel chilly. I'm like fire. Did you hear Swami Nirmalanandaji say, "He's a dangerous man. He's here to break all your egos, to give you nice hits and blows."

How many people think, "Oh, I was so pampered, I was always praised when I was away from him. When I visited him just once in a while, he appreciated everything: 'Thank you. You're wonderful. You're great. Nice, honey, dear.' But now I'm coming closer and closer and getting more and more knocks."

That's what they say. The closer, the more knocks. If you don't give the car to the garageman, if he just sees it and you ask, "Oh, how is my car?" he will say, "Oh, beautiful, wonderful." But if you give it in his hands, he will undo every bolt and nut. Is it not so? Then he will say, "That is wrong here; this is wrong there." If you do not desire to put it in his hands, why should he pinpoint its mistakes? He'll say, "Oh. beautiful, nice car, where did you get it? Wonderful, keep it." Once you bring it to him, then he will say hundreds of different things. "This bolt is loose, this screw is loose . . ."

My body is very stiff in the morning. I can barely touch my toes or do the shoulder stand. By afternoon, I can easily take the intermediate class! Why the tightness in the morning? Is it due to unrelaxed sleep or to the body fighting subconscious dreams? Why does one wake up tired?

Generally the body is stiff in the morning, whether you dream or not. But it doesn't matter. Even if you cannot touch the toes as you do in the evening, you can still do the Hatha. It's not how much you bend that's important. Hold the positions for a least a half minute and if you keep on doing that, you will see that after a few weeks you will be more relaxed even in the morning. That's the only way. If you have time, do it in the evening also. But morning is the best time. Though you think that you can do it in the evening, very often you don't get the time to do all these things. In the modern life, evening seems to be constantly occupied. The morning is the best time, before you come out and face the world.

And, of course, if you don't sleep well, you wake up tired. So, you should learn to sleep well. Prepare well for your sleep. Forget all the worries. Don't think of anything. Think that you are dying. If you are alive, you'll wake up tomorrow. Yes! Just say, "I've done my job today. That's all. I don't know whether there will be a tomorrow or not." Going to sleep is like death. Waking up is like birth. It's simple, yes. Because when you are asleep you don't know what's going to happen. In whose care are you? You may have all your doors and windows locked, your watchman sitting there outside, your gun under your pillow. But when you are asleep, the very same man can come and point the very same gun at you! Nobody is going to help you.

So you don't know if you are going to wake up. If God desires to wake you up, you will wake up. Actually, everything comes to a stop when you sleep. A real good sleep is that. So why worry about tomorrow? If there is a tomorrow, wake up and then worry about it! So just lie down like a baby, suck the thumb. Feel that you are a baby. Feel that you are lying in the lap of the mother, Mother Earth. Say to Divine Mother, "Mama, I am just sleeping in your lap. Take care of me. If you want me to do something tomorrow, wake me up. If you think that I am just a burden on this earth, put me to sleep once and for all." Why should you live if you're not going to be useful? Because you are wanted to do something, you are awakened. Otherwise, it is easy for Her to put you into a long "sleep." We all exist here to perform Her duties. We are all Her many instruments. She functions through us. But our egos don't allow us even to think of this.

So, just lie down. Relax. Don't see all these horror movies, or T.V. or read novels. When you do those things, you'll have the same kind of dreams as that. If you don't feel sleepy, lie down, repeat a mantram. Or do some chanting or read some nice spiritual books, lives of the saints. Then you will be well relaxed, getting up refreshed. Another important thing is, don't have late dinner. You should finish your eating at least two hours before sleeping. And it should be a very light meal. Lunch could be a heavier one if you want. You must digest your dinner before sleeping. If you go to bed with food in the stomach, the stomach will be still functioning. This is another cause for all kinds of bad dreams and restless sleep.

I have terrible pain in both hip joints and just under the bottom front of both knee caps as well as the outside of each knee in attempting to sit cross-legged for even a short while. I am unable to come anywhere near a lotus position. I have been taking classes from the Integral Yoga Institute for two months, and progressing greatly in all other postures. What can I do to help my terrible condition?

I would like to tell you that the lotus pose is not that absolutely necessary. Even the people who invented all these asanas had just one thing in mind – to make the body healthy, as supple as possible, so that ultimately they can just sit in *any* posture. "Stheeram sukham asanam" is the definition according to Patanjali. What is a posture? The definition is, anything that is comfortable and steady. Stheeram and sukham. If this posture is comfortable and steady for you, and you can sit for an hour, or two or three in it, this is the posture for you. So you don't need to worry about the lotus pose. But if it is possible, do it.

Of course in the beginning you might have a little pain here and there, but don't hurt yourself too much. It's a good position, no doubt. It has other benefits also. It makes your posture easily and quickly steady. And it does something to control the turbulent vibrations inside, to harmonize the vibrations. And it helps the circulation and the vital energy to flow more along the spine than into the extremities. There's a lot of benefit in the lotus pose, no doubt. But that doesn't mean you should break your knees to do it. No. If it is easily possible, do it. Otherwise, it doesn't matter. Just sit in any pose.

There are many other postures. Sit in the tailor pose, or in *vajrasana* (on the knees). Even if vajrasana is going to hurt your ankles, sit on a cushion, it doesn't matter. Use a small cushion, like the Zen monks. Whatever way you sit, it doesn't matter, but make your seat comfortable and see that your spine is erect, because that helps a lot in your meditation. And even in other postures, if you are going to hurt any part of the body, don't do it. Do the rest. Gradually you will become loosened. Then you will be able to do the other postures also. Rome was not built in a day, hm? We have allowed our bodies to become rigid by not giving proper exercise and by not eating the right food. So we have to undo gradually. We can't loosen the joints in one day. So you don't need to feel bad about not sitting in the lotus posture. Sometimes I say, even if you cannot do Hatha Yoga, does it mean you are unfit for spirituality? It's an aid, not a must.

But it helps you take care of the body. The body will help you to go free in your other practices. Otherwise the body will constantly distract your mind. So to liberate the mind's attention from the body, you make the body healthy. It is something like a healthy child will not distract you much in the house. If the child is sick, you can't attend to any other thing. It will be constantly crying, "Mama, Mama, Mama." Same thing with your body. It becomes a burden then. The minute you sit, "Oh, oh." Where will you be meditating, on your hips or on God? But if you sit comfortably and forget the body, then your mind is entirely on what you are doing. That is the idea.

So don't think that if you don't do Hatha Yoga you are unfit for anything. If by any chance you cannot do it, or if you have certain handicaps, you don't need to feel bad about it. Even if you can't sit, it doesn't matter. Relax and meditate. Spirituality is attained by the mind, through the mind. So don't put the body always as a predominant thing. It's only an aid.

No matter how much I may relax, I still produce a loud sound when I breathe through the nose. I have practiced pranayama for two months with no lessening of the sound. Could this be psychological or just due to bad breathing habits?

There may be some kind of mild curvature in the nose itself, or some gentle growth in the passageways. The passages are thick and if the hole is rather narrow the breath rushes in and you'll get that noise. Probably, if you try some more of kapalabhati, the quick breathing, that might allow the nose to clear. Do a little water neti also. If nothing helps you, it doesn't matter, still you breathe, the air goes in and out. Or maybe you're not doing it slowly enough; do it more gently. If you do it gently, it won't make that noise. If you allow the air to come forced, any nose will make that sound. So instead of controlling the breath at the nose, control it at the throat. Learn to have the control at the throat. In the epiglottis, they call it. When you breathe, making the hissing sound in the throat, then the nose will not be affected that much. This will help you a lot.

I have a visual defect which, with other problems, leads to despair and a feeling of only awaiting death. What do you suggest?

Oh, what a pity. Why should you await death? No, don't think that the vision is so important. If it cannot be corrected, then better forget it. You don't need to see things. You think people are happy with their good eyes? In a way you are fortunate. I tell this even to blind people. They're fortunate in a way. So much trouble is saved. Not that we have to go and pick out our eyes, but if for some reason we have lost our eyes, we have still the inner eye. Physical senses are not that important. If you have them, use them well; if not, forget it. You still have your beautiful mind, beautiful soul. How many people without total vision do many good things? You shouldn't be discouraged. I don't know if there is any cure for this. Is there? (*Someone in the audience replies that there may be an operation.*) There are operations? Well, if there is any possibility, try that. If there is no possibility, it doesn't matter. Accept it as what God wanted you to have. The minute you learn to accept, nothing is that troublesome. You can live with anything and everything. Haven't you seen people in worse conditions living happily? It's all in the mind. If you just accept it, it becomes very easy, very light. If you don't accept it, even a small pimple mark on the back of the neck . . . nobody would even see that but you'll be constantly thinking of it. If you want to feel sorry you have so many hundreds of excuses, but if you want to be happy, you can be happy without any of these things. It's crazy to worry about all these things. After all, it's just a body. And it should not spoil your joy. "I'm not the body. I'm not even the mind. I'm the Spirit." If there is a dent in your car, do you go mad? If you can't repair it, it doesn't matter, leave it. The car still runs. Laugh at it, and be brave.

Swamiji, about ten years ago I had a retinal detachment, requiring surgery. Also, I have had eye surgery three times altogether. Last year after meditating for 3½ months I had another retinal detachment and again more cutting surgery. Are there any asanas which I should not do? Also, will you please share more information with us regarding the eyes, their connection with the soul, and how to make them healthy.

Physically, I would suggest if you feel any strain in doing any of the practices, your eye exercises or something, then you should avoid it. But if it doesn't strain you, you can do it gently without going beyond the limit. Then that will strengthen the eyes. But you should be a doctor for yourself. You should know where to stop. And by way of meditation and even pranayama, when you do pranayama, do alternate pranayama and even when you do a little retention — *kumbaka* — you can imagine that you are sending that prana to the eyes. You can recuperate them. You can rebuild them by your own awareness, by sending the prana there. At the same time do not abuse your eyes. Don't use harsh lights. Don't work too long in very bright lights. Don't keep awake at night too much. Save your eyes. And you can rebuild them.

And, of course, the connection between the eyes and the "I" is understood by the very name itself. The "I" and the eye. The eyes are very powerful senses. If you could train the vision within, to look within — not, as I said the other day, to turn the entire eyeball inward, but to use the mental eye, the awareness, to go within — then you could realize the true Self. Otherwise there is no particular relationship between the Self and the eye. The eye is only part of the body, as any other part. You can use it to develop the Self by seeing the right thing, by seeing within towards the soul.

Since coming here, the gums of my lower jaw have become more and more painful. A nurse was kind enough to check them out and she said I had new wisdom teeth coming in.

Wisdom. What else do you want? You are lucky. So, without pain, you can't have wisdom. Pain is followed by wisdom, hm?

"The nurse advised washing my mouth with warm salt water. Do you agree or would you suggest something else? The pain is disturbing my meditation since my mind is at times more on the pain than on the meditation."

See? You have proved what I said earlier. If you have a pain, you can't meditate well. But you must learn to accept the pain. If you learn to accept it, it won't bother you anymore. There is no shortcut. Some people even do an operation to bring the thing out. It's premature. It's something like, if there is a pain, you just make an operation, bring the child out. There is a delivery here. The child of wisdom. The wisdom tooth is a child, just trying to come out. It's being built within. So this is also a conception. We can't just operate and bring the child out prematurely. Warm salt water would help or maybe if it's too painful take a little Vick's Vaporub or a little Tiger Balm, some kind of balm. Apply it there on either side with a little cotton. Keep it there. Then the saliva will come – spit it out, and that will relieve the pain. You can even have a little warm application.

Are there any methods in Yoga for curing allergies? I've been suffering for years, taking shots and pills and they do not do much good.

I have to tell you a story. I was in Hawaii some years ago and there was a radio announcer, a disc jockey I met there. Probably some of you would have heard of him. He met me and said, "I am allergic to almost everything. The doctor told me to not eat this, not touch that, not to do that, because so many things aggravate the allergy. I really don't know what to do. What can I do?"

I said, "Add one more allergy."

"What is that," he asked.

"Doctor allergy." I said.

"Do you really mean that?" He said that because he came to me as a skeptic. "What will happen if I stop taking all these pills and things?"

"Nothing will happen to you. Just follow a proper yogic diet."

He was a bit on the heavy side, so I didn't even ask him to do any yogic postures, but only asked him to do the breathing and follow the diet. Within ten days, he was seeing a marked difference. He was a thoroughly changed person. He came as a skeptic, but the treatment made a big change in his life. Since then, the entire radio station almost became mine. I could just go there, any time, and he would let me have the microphone when he saw me coming. Every time he knew I was coming to Hawaii, he could start announcing my arrival ten or fifteen days before. And soon after getting his healing, he had an interview with me. I ended the interview with Om Shanthi and he just picked it up. And ever since that time, almost every day before he closed the station at night he would say, "Okay, everybody, let's close the day with Swami's Om Shanthi. Please join me: "Om Shanthi, Om Shanthi, Om Shanthi Om." Every day on Radio K-POI he would do that.

So, you don't need to be allergic. Train the body and mind. Yoga is the answer. Don't just fill your body with all the toxins. Take care of your diet, have a strict yogic diet. Practice Hatha Yoga and pranayama, or just pranayama, and then spend some time in meditation also. In short, if you try to be a good Yogi, all these allergies will disappear. They will become allergic to you.

In Indian medicine there is a system called the Ayurveda. It gives a simple formula for natural health: "Boiled water, melted ghee and diluted buttermilk. If you take them as your diet or with your diet, even if your name is uttered the diseases will run away." See how they put it, hm? If people have a diet like this and somebody says their name they say they will be cured. It is an exaggeration of the benefit; but see how they put it. That's why if you practice Yoga, even if somebody says your name, they will get rid of the allergy. I can guarantee it. Your name itself will have a vibration. You don't need to be afraid of all of these thousands and thousands of diseases. You don't need them!

Yet, people seem to be accepting. Haven't you heard people say, "Oh, this is just a common cold."

"How do you feel this morning?"

"Oh, just the usual morning headache, that's all."

In the same way, "How are you?"

"Oh, the monthly cramps."

Why should you have cramps? There is no need. In fact, until I came to the West, I never even heard women folk complaining of their menstrual cramps. They never had cramps. But now if somebody has the menstrual flow without cramps, it's news to make the headlines. See how we slowly get hypnotized by all of these things? You begin to feel that without all these things, you can't live, you're not normal. Whenever I say: "I don't even get a common cold," people say, "What? You don't? But it's natural for everybody." We can surely just get out of all of these things.

For several years now I have had painful appendix attacks. The attacks are more frequent lately. My only relief from pain is Yoga. Doctors say I need an operation. My question is: Will Yoga heal me?

I know of miracles. Eternal love and joy are the miracles of Yoga. But Yoga need not wait for miracles. You just do what is necessary. Personally, I would say if the appendix is not an acute one, you can be helped by the proper yogic diet and by doing more of *sarvangasana* (shoulder stand) and the fish pose. You should do a lot of deep breathing. That will help you a lot. But if it is really acute, in the state of bursting any moment, don't wait for Yoga. It is better to get it operated upon. I would advise that. It's not a major operation. It's a simple one. If it is not acute, certainly by your pranayama practice you can direct your energy, your flow of prana, to the diseased part and get it healed. It could be helped even by the transfer of prana by someone who is practicing well. Having a lot of prana stored, he can even give you some gentle massages. That can help because, in that way, he'll be rubbing his prana into you, he'll lend a little current to you. It's all scientific. If it's an acute attack, however, don't wait for these things because any time your appendix might burst. That would be a terrible thing.

For the past few days I've been experiencing pain in the lower back of my head, on the top of my head, around my eyes and forehead. Also from time to time, I feel weak. Please explain and what do you recommend?

Well, it's not possible simply to cure it. First, we must find out the cause. Why do you feel that tension? Is it due to your over-eating or over-tiring the body? Or is it because of your practices or pranayama or meditation? You should find out the cause. Is it due to constipation? This too, could cause a pain. Find out the reason and stay away from it. If it is due to meditation, it's even better to stay away from this too, until you again feel at ease. That is the importance of timing. At the same time, take care of your diet. It is best to fast for a couple of days, until you feel light. It's more or less a symptom of congestion. It could be due to many things, however.

I use my voice a lot in my work. I have been afflicted with a constant irritation in my throat for many years, which forces me to clear it constantly. In my profession, it's a great handicap. Is there a yogic way to eradicate it?

If it is due to excessive use of your vocal cords, then you have to reduce the use, because there is probably inflammation. Allow the inflammation to heal. If it is due to some kind of mucus trouble, then you should take care of your diet and have a mucus-free diet as a remedy. I knew a well-known musician and singer and he found this remedy beneficial: I asked him to use some honey and a little black pepper powder mixed up and rubbed in the throat. Then gargle it and spit it out or swallow it. Pepper and honey – it helps a lot in clearing the throat. Very good for your voice. The proportions you can choose any way you want. If it's too hot, add a little more honey, and if it is too sweet, add a little more pepper. Take it, make into a nice paste, put it on your finger, rub it in the throat well and rub it all around. A lot of saliva will be produced. You can swallow it or spit it out and it will help the inflammation and improve your vocal cords.

I tried to become a vegetarian, but feel that I need meat at least once a week or else I end up eating too many sweets. Do you think eating meat occasionally will retard my spiritual development seriously?

People ask, "Oh, how can I get my protein?" It is only a weakness. You say that if you don't eat meat you will end up eating too many sweets. Do sweets give protein? It is just a weakness, a mental weakness. You have to get rid of that weakness. You don't need to eat only vegetables. Even the lentils, seeds, nuts, beans, have a lot of protein. When you still need protein, use dairy products. For the sake of protein, we don't need to eat something that is already dead. What is meat, after all? It is dead matter. It all depends upon whether you have the tongue under control. The rest is only an excuse.

Of what does a fruit diet or fruit "fast" consist? Some people seem to include not only fresh fruit but dried fruit, nuts, milk, yogurt and even bread! Please explain the purpose and benefit of fruit diet.

Well, everything that is said here is good, but not all at the same time. I always like to advocate a monodiet. Eat one thing, just that one thing, at a time. If you eat a fruit, even an apple, eat an apple – that's all. Or two or three. Only apples. Don't even mix it with canteloupe or another fruit. If you eat canteloupe, only canteloupe. Vegetables also like that. If you eat carrots, only eat carrots, at least for that meal. Next meal you can eat something else. Then your stomach will be thankful to you, because it just has to have only one thing to do. And the digestion is easier, quicker. And that is what is prescribed, the monodiet, by most of the nature cure methods. So eat just any one thing, or if you really want, two or three at the most. Not too many things at the same time. All the entire list is good, no doubt, one at a time.

I have been following a mucusless diet: no dairy, eggs, butter, or meat for almost a year and have noted a general cleansing of my system, especially breathing. There have been no ill effects so far. Yet, I know a yogic diet includes dairy products. I have been told that cultured milk products such as yogurt and buttermilk are easier to digest and that goat's milk is better for you than cow's milk. The mucusless diet says that dairy is too rich for human's digestion and tends to block it up. Are there true benefits to eating dairy or is it just a matter of personal taste? Also, how can you tell if a certain diet or fast is good for your body, when you fall back periodically due to toxins dissolving in your system?

Of course, the dairy products can produce mucus if your system is weak. If your system has more heat and good digestive capacity, you can digest milk products as well as fruits and vegetables. If your digestion is bad, then you should stay away from mucus diets. Not only from mucus-forming foods as mentioned but from anything which forms mucus in your system. Even ordinary rice or bread or even an apple can produce mucus. After all, what is mucus? Anything that is not digested well will form bile and produce gas and the gas produces mucus. If the digestive system is good, it can digest anything and everything. So you should select your diet according to your digestion. That's why milk may be good for one person who has a good digestive capacity, who can burn up everything, but another whose system is very weak should not take any dairy products. Each system has to choose its own food. One has to select what one should eat. That is why we say, "One man's nectar is another man's poison."

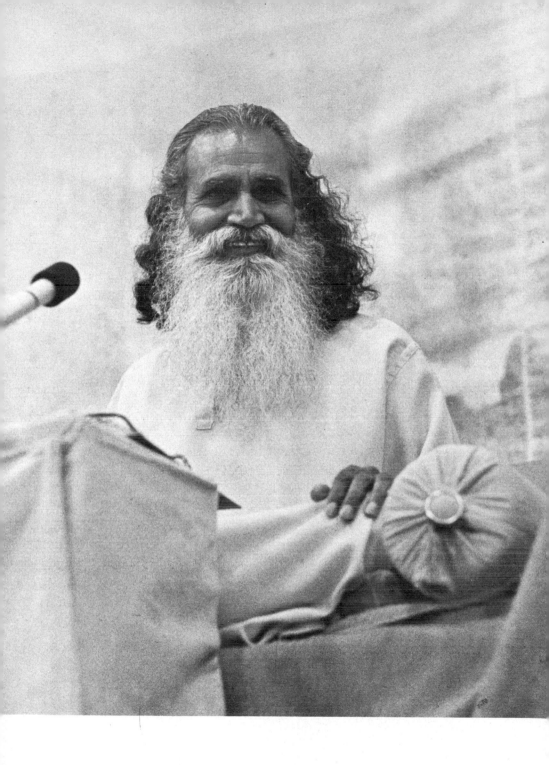

SRI SWAMI SATCHIDANANDA

SWAMI NIRMALANANDA

RABBI SHLOMO CARLEBACH

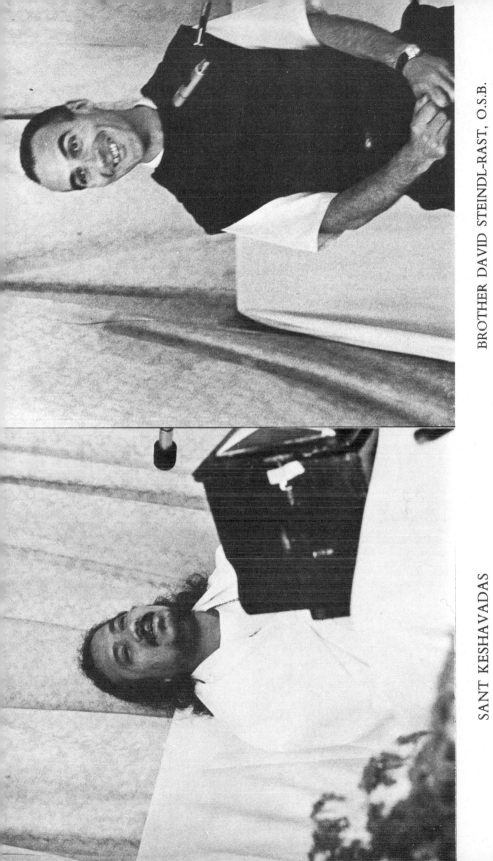

BROTHER DAVID STEINDL-RAST, O.S.B.

SANT KESHAVADAS

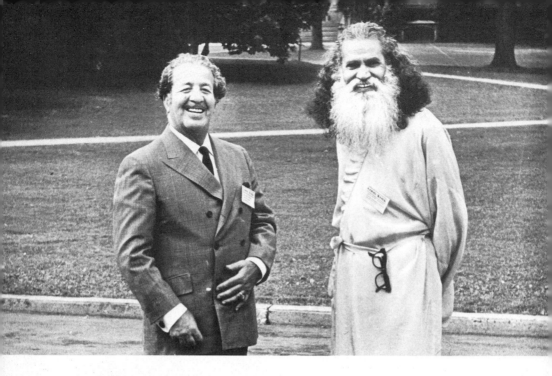

RABBI JOSEPH GELBERMAN AND SWAMI SATCHIDANANDA

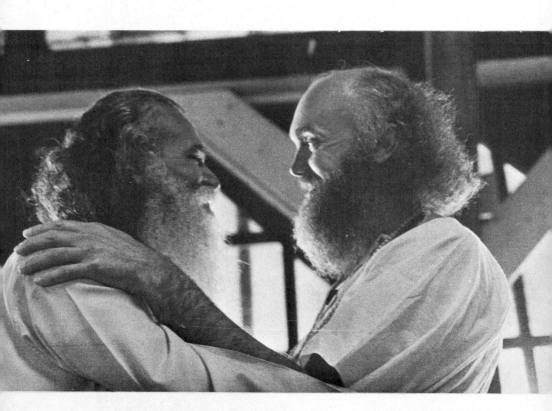

SWAMI SATCHIDANANDA AND RAM DASS

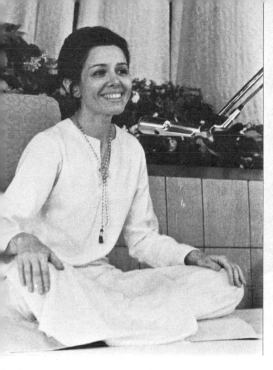
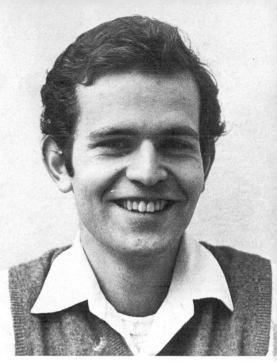

DEVOTEES OF SWAMI SATCHIDANANDA: **Top Left**, AMMA; **Top Right**, MADHAVA; **Bottom Left**, HARI; **Bottom Right**, SISTER HAMSA.

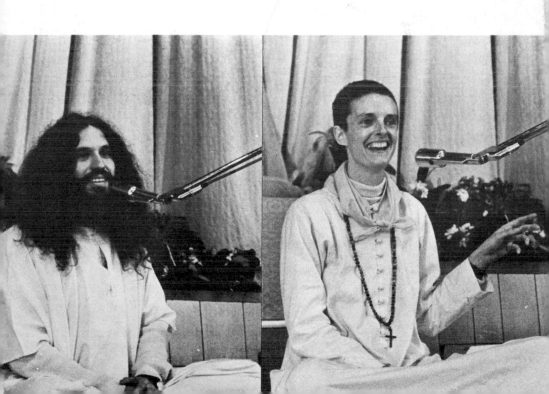

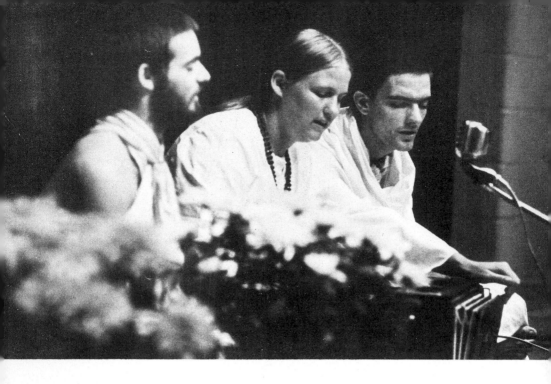

STAFF MEMBERS CONDUCTING KIRTAN (CHANTING)

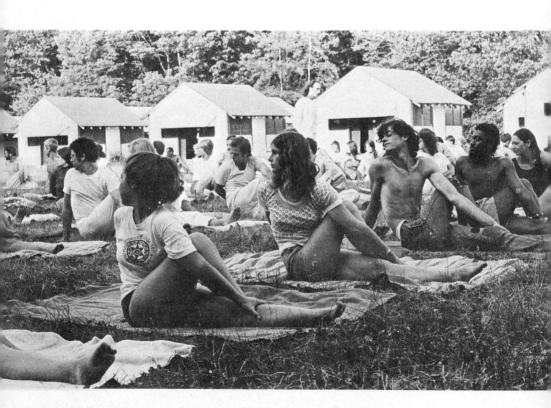

A HATHA YOGA CLASS

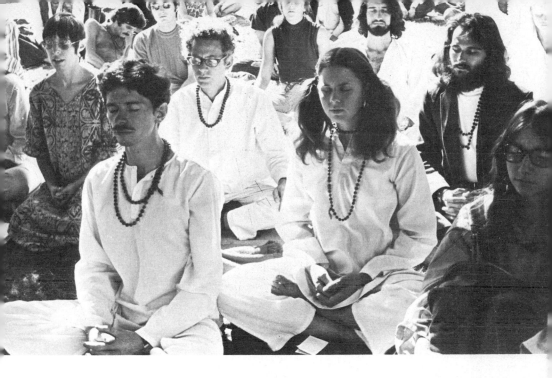

A GROUP MEDITATION

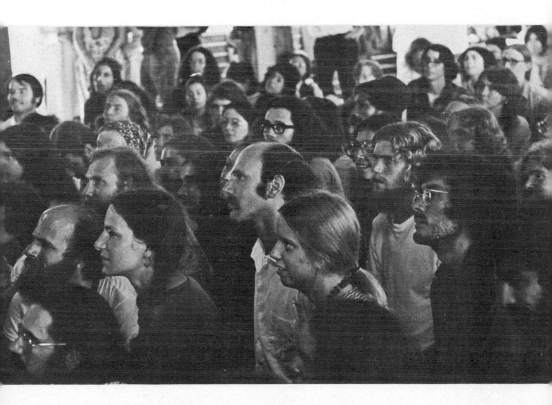

RETREATANTS LISTENING IN SATSANG

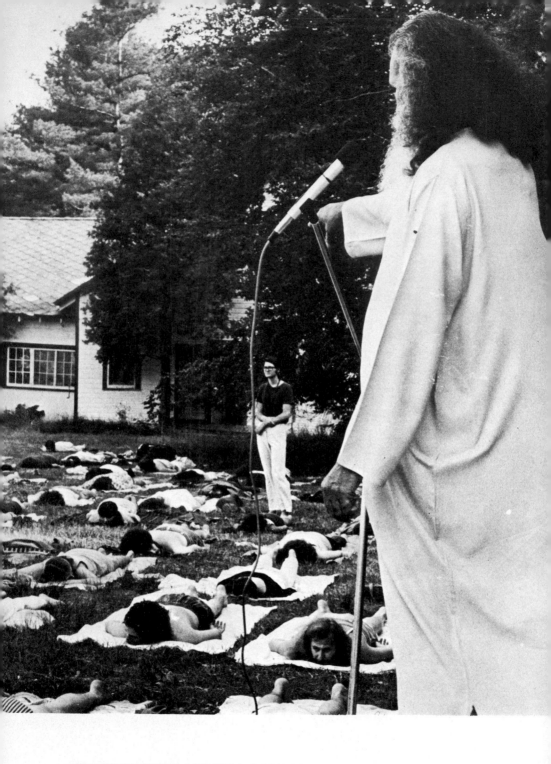

SWAMI SATCHIDANANDA CONDUCTING A HATHA YOGA CLASS

Seventh Day

Practical Advice on Meditation

Swami Nirmalananda

In his previous talks, Swami Nirmalananda dealt primarily with basic questions: the true nature of the individual and of reality and how Yoga is the path to recover that true nature; the significance of the mantram or sound vibration as a path inward to that essential nature; and the universality of that inner nature, that inner light, whatever tradition or path may be followed to find it. In doing so, he dispelled many misunderstandings about the "mysteriousness" of Yoga, emphasized its simplicity and its naturalness, and gave much practical advice as to how to approach the practices. Here in this final talk it is this practical aspect which he takes as his major topic. He talks at length about some of the nuts and bolts of Yoga practice, giving advice of inestimable value to the person who sincerely wishes to take up these practices on a regular, day-to-day basis; to the person who wishes to incorporate the practices of the retreat into his daily life.

This is our last session, so we should try to talk a little bit on *sadhana*, the really practical side. Philosophy in the long run does very little for a person. Of course, sadhana is meditation: everything else is a preparation and an aid. Some people put all of their attention and all of their time on the aids. It is something like a person who puts all his money into building a beautiful house but never lives in it. A lot of people spend a long time getting ready and then never start out. Of course, we should think about the getting ready part of it a little also, but mostly we should think about the doing. Doing, of course, is meditation, that inner investigation. The whole idea of the asanas and the breathing is to get the body and pranas flowing in such a manner that the mind will go inward with the least amount of resistance. Many of you have been meditating for years and some of you have just begun here at the retreat. So, I'd like to talk a little bit about hints and suggestions on your own individual meditation.

WHEN

The first thing you must have is a regular time for meditation. You should set a time and never violate it. This regularity is important for two reasons: First, if you set an exact time, then when that time comes you'll

166

have the idea, "Well, now is the time for meditation." If, instead, you think that sometime today you will meditate, you get up in the morning and there will be something you'll have to do right then. When you do it, then you'll remember another thing you need to do as well. "Well, I'll do it now, I'll meditate after I do that stuff." While you're in the middle of that, somebody calls you on the phone, talks to you for a while, and while talking on the phone you are asked to go to a certain place or you find out that something is happening in a certain place, so you say, "All right." Before, you were saying, "When the telephone conversation is finished, then I'll meditate." Then you discover that you have to go someplace to get something. So you say, "I'll go there and bring it home. I will meditate then." You go there and see another place to stop – you know what I mean; I don't have to go through it all. That's just normal life. Life just goes from one thing to another; that's the way we live. So if we know, "This particular time is when I meditate," then we'll make sure we don't keep on kidding ourselves.

Even great masters have this problem. Yogananda at the age of two and three years was in *samadhi*. He used to go to an old Siva temple. There was a big crack in the floor, and when he crawled through the crack, he would find that there was a tunnel that dated from even before the building of that temple. He would go into this dark place and find a little hollow in the wall of this tunnel, and he'd sit there for hours in samadhi. And yet, when he got older, when he was around thirteen or fourteen years old and he didn't have so much time, he'd always say, "I'm going to have a really long meditation." Time went by. About four years passed by, and that really long meditation never happened. Think of him, a perfected person in Yoga! And he realized how time had slipped by. You see, he loved to play football – their version of football, the British version – and he was always doing football plays in his mind, both morning and evening. He realized he had not done anything about God, but had thought about a lot of very good plays for football.

So that's us too. I knew a disciple of Swami Sivananda who isn't living anymore. She was an extraordinary woman who finally, after years of very steady practice, had come to the point where even during a very special social function, when she closed her eyes, she was *in*, she was *there*. And no matter what was going on, just the closing of the eyes turned the mind right there. She thought, "Well now, that's good. Thank heaven, I've reached that spot. I won't have to be so incredibly scrupulous." She said this because she had been inflexible in her schedule of meditation.

You might be interested to know that she married into a family that didn't like spiritual life. They sometimes kept her locked up with no food or water for as long as two or three weeks, trying to break her will so that she would quit her spiritual practices. You know, it's not right for people to say, "Oh, materialistic America and spiritual India." It is true that the spiritual current predominates in India. But you are mistaken in thinking that everything goes well there. Even if some of you have trouble from your parents, I doubt if they would lock you up for nearly a month and try to starve you to death to get you to give up Yoga. I know every person runs into some snags, but you can't imagine the incredible push towards materialism that Indian young people receive from their parents. They all want their children to get Masters degrees. They all want them to be engineers. So when you go to the ashrams today, there are very few young people. I mentioned to Swamiji that you wouldn't find 500 young people in India at a gathering like this. We shouldn't feel that this isn't India and that things would be much better if we were over there.

So they had done this to this woman, persecuted her horribly. But she persevered despite it all and got to the state of mind where she could just close her eyes and she was there. She realized this one day at a social function. Throughout the whole dinner, no matter what she was doing, when she closed her eyes — boom — there goes the mind. "Good," she said. Next morning she received a letter from Rishikesh from Swami Sivananda. It said, "Beloved child, be sure you're very strict in keeping your schedule of daily meditation." Before it happens, the great Masters know, not after the fact. Before it even happens. So she remained very faithful that way and kept it up. That's important. That way we won't skip.

Then there's another important reason for regularity. The mind is a creature of habit. We know that about eating. You're used to eating at a certain time of the day. When that time comes, you feel hungry. That's just the way we train the body. If we're used to sleeping at a certain time of day, when that time comes, we feel sleepy. We've conditioned it. So if you get the mind used to thinking that at such and such a time it will go in, you will find that the mind will go in much, much easier. It's just our way. We are definitely creatures of habit. So if we get the mind in the habit, then at that time every day we will find that it's much easier to put the mind in.

That's the most important idea behind this regularity. And please be sure that you are able to have two sittings a day for meditation, so that you keep the wheel in momentum. You know, it's like striking a wheel. You're all too young to remember old coffee grinders, but I do. If you get the wheel going well, then you just need to hit it once in a while and it will keep moving. You get the momentum going in the morning, then about 12 hours later you give it another shove and hopefully you can get to the point where the momentum carries on around the clock. That's a very important thing: two sittings at a regular time.

WHERE

Next is where to sit for meditation. It is really very, very essential to have a spot which is yours for meditation, because you imbue that spot with those very vibrations, with that consciousness. On the subtle level, you will magnetize that spot; and on the mental level, again, your mind is used to that spot. "When he sets me here, I go in." So the mind will go in. Now, it doesn't matter if you can't have a separate meditation room. It doesn't even matter if you're living with parents or friends where you can't take a spot and say, "All right, I'll fix it up." Make it that way in your mind. Pick a corner of the room and say, "That corner is my meditation corner." Just let it be in your mind. And just kind of make sure no chair is ever there and no wastebasket is ever there. It's just as simple as that. It doesn't matter if you can't put a permanent thing like an altar with pictures of holy people there. No. Just keep a picture in your drawer. Then just take it out, put it in front of you and sit there. That's all right.

Again, it's the conditioning of the mind. Why are we running here and there? Because of conditioning. Now we have to condition ourselves to stop it. So you do that. One spot. When you meditate, the burning of incense is very good, because it gives a pleasant kind of sensation. The smell of the incense, soothing and resting the mind, helps it to go in. Then again, it's sort of like Pavlov's dog. When Pavlov rang the bell, the dog salivated. You finally get so used to it that when incense is there, "Oh, meditation time." You know, the mind is a little baby. You just don't hit a baby and say, walk. You make it easy. You make it conducive. It's wonderful to see the spiritual training of children in India. I've seen it done. The mothers work with the children and they make it a game. They don't tell them, "You must or else you'll be lost forever." They just say, "Hey, let's see if you can do it (meditate) as long as I can." There's one kind of puja one family was doing where they would pour water in offering. The mother would say, "Now I'll get the water and I'll go out one door, you go out the other, and let's see who gets there first." So the little girl would run to try to get there first. The mother would rush to get there first. Then there were no complaints, "I don't want to do it." We have to play with this baby. We have to placate it sometimes and say, "Yes, baby, I know, don't worry," to get it to go where we want.

So it's important to have this place and try to get this atmosphere for meditation. The best, of course, is a closet or a separate room. But if you can't, it's all right.

Zen monks often meditate facing a wall, which is really a good practice. Because your skin is sensitive to space; if you feel a solid area in front of you, you feel like you're closed off, even though you're in a huge room. One of the best times I ever had for meditation was in the Soto Zen Mission in Los Angeles. It was really a wonderful atmosphere for meditation. Part of that was due not only to the other people – they were very good in meditation – but also to this facing the wall, which gave a feeling of isolation. So if you want to face a wall or face right into a corner, that helps too.

WHAT YOU WEAR

Regarding clothes to wear for meditation: It's a good idea if you can have some loose fitting clothes. And if you can, have something you wear only for meditation. Then you can get up in the morning, take a bath, put those on, meditate, and then take them off. Hang them somewhere. If you do that, they'll also get that vibration. If that is not possible, it's okay. It's also good to take a bath because that tends to equalize the pranas in the body. Water is very absorbent. That's why, in every religion, in rituals, you always find the idea of holy water or consecrated water. Some objects pick up vibration very quickly. Water is one of the most receptive. So, if you have certain magnetisms, if you are worried and your mind is kind of jittery, the water really will take it away. That's why, in India, you have to take a bath before entering many temples. This is not only because people may have gotten dirty from walking in the dust and so on, but also to get rid of the particular states of mind that they may be emitting at that time. If you can't do that, though, you should wash the face, the hands, and the feet. That's very good.

WHAT YOU SIT ON

Next is what you sit on. You should have a special blanket or a piece of cloth on which you sit for meditation, exclusively. Again, the idea is the vibration there. Wool insulates you from the subtle earth currents that tend to pull the subtle flow down rather than up toward the higher centers of awareness; but wool is getting more and more expensive. You might just want to get an ordinary kind of cheap blanket and then a piece of wool cloth that you can put over it. It's good to have some soft thing. You can even buy a square piece of foam rubber and over that you can place a wool cloth. Sit on that facing the North or the East. There is a subtle magnetic flow from East to West which is connected with the way the earth is moving. The earth is turning and it's creating a subtle magnetic field by it's turning. By facing the East there is a flow coming in. Or it can be North. In India, because of the Himalayas, but also because of the magnetic pull of the North. When we are facing that way, the various magnetic points of the body are affected. So that direction is also conducive to meditation. Now, obviously, you don't have to carry around a compass and meditate only in that direction. But those two directions are definitely the best, whichever one you prefer. You will see the difference yourself if you try it for a few days. So you face there. You have some picture and some incense, and so on, or no picture if you like. Put a candle there if you want to think of light, or just put nothing there.

POSTURE

So you sit there and you're seated upright. People ask, "Why do we have to sit up straight, why can't we lie down?" Because when you lie down, the prana currents tend to disperse throughout the body, to equalize and bring sleep. When you sit upright, and the concentration is either here (*pointing to the heart*) or here (*pointing to the center of the forehead*), and especially when you face North or East, the currents tend to pull back into the spine and up toward the higher centres. That's just the way it works. If you sit slumped, then the next thing you know, you're out. Also, you pinch certain nerves and that brings sleepiness — just as your leg goes to sleep when the blood doesn't circulate well. If you don't keep the nerves open so that the subtle currents flow well, there's also the sleepiness of the inner man. So that is important.

The position of the head is also very important. If it's down, automatically you will start to get what we call the "bobs." And if it's up too much, you can start to go strange ways. If the chin is about parallel to the ground it's in the right place and you'll neither bend forward nor backward nor sideways. And sometimes, after sitting for a while, the eyes may open up halfway. But never try to make them be halfway. It should be what is really natural. And the best thing is not to turn the eyes up. Unless you've been initiated into a system where they have told you to — in which case of course you do. But usually, the best thing is just to let the eyes be unfocused and closed. Then, whatever happens will be exactly what the subtle life force knows ought to happen.

As I said before, the idea is to be in a posture in which you can relax every muscle and still be completely upright and steady. Asana, Patanjali says, is any position that is steady and pleasant and that is also good for meditation. That's implied, because when you're asleep, it's steady and pleasant. So you can sit in a chair if you like. There shouldn't be a fetish made out of a special posture or cross-legged position. Those people who feel stiff should consider themselves completely free to sit in a chair and keep their legs out, or sit on the edge of a bed and then when your legs get a little asleep, just, with your eyes still closed, put the feet down, let the legs come back to normal and bring them up again. Always use good sense. That's what a Yogi is supposed to be: a sensible person. Absolutely, to the highest degree, sensible.

So we have to use good sense at all times. And never, never any pushing, and never, never any strain. And for your meditation time, be sensible. If you live with somebody who is antagonistic to your meditation, then meditate whenever they are not around or when they are asleep. That's only sensible. Why have somebody beaming vibrations at you when you're trying to meditate? Why have them downstairs thinking what an idiot you are? And why should you make a nuisance of yourself to them? That's important also.

CHAKRAS

So you're sitting and you're relaxing. Your awareness is here. (*He points between the eyebrows.*) Do you know what all of this means? There are chakras, psychic centers in the human body. Just as there are nerve centers in the brain — speech centers, sight centers, centers which control blood pressure, centers which control the heart beat — there are certain centers of awareness located in the central nervous system, in the spine, and by concentrating there our attention pulls the subtle life force there. As I'm talking to you, I'm not particularly feeling the bottoms of my feet, yet if I start to speak of what's there I find that I become aware of them. That's not only because I have connected those wires in the head, figuratively speaking, to be aware of that, but also there has been an increase of the flow of prana there which gives the messages back to the brain. So this (*pointing to the forehead*) is the center of intuition. All intuitive knowledge is functioning at this point. Physically you talk about the pineal gland, but actually we're thinking of the mental level, the mind-body, the mind structure. It is approximately the same, but far subtler. The subtle bodies are interwoven with the gross bodies. So here on the subtle level at this spot there is that center from which intuition is coming. Just as sight is coming from one center, hearing is coming from another, so intuition is coming from here. And this is also the master center; it is the controller of all the other chakras, all the other centers. If we concentrate on one of the other chakras, we can activate it and get the experience of it, but that one alone. But from the eyebrow center, all the centers are controlled.

Sometimes we concentrate here in the heart because this is where feeling — not just excited emotion but real feeling — is evoked. Those who prefer the path of Bhakti Yoga, of love, of openness toward God, and ultimately toward the whole of creation, meditate here. And when they do japa, they feel as though the mantram is vibrating at this center. Right there in the middle of the chest. Sometimes they make a distinction; they say Jnana Yoga here (*pointing to the head*) and Bhakti Yoga here (*pointing to the heart*). That isn't too good an idea, because the truth is you will find as you meditate that sometimes you'll be aware here, sometimes there, sometimes halfway in between — because there aren't just seven chakras, there are more than a thousand chakras in the spine. Your awareness will automatically go where it should, so never force it to be at one or the other. Sometimes it'll go clear to here (*points to top of head*). The best way is to start out being aware of one or the other. But then let the awareness go where it wants to. Never try to force it. Because the inner power is intelligent. Your inner life force knows exactly where it belongs; it knows exactly where to go. So, always be open to this when you sit for meditation.

So you sit and you put your awareness on the heart or eyebrow center. And if you know any particular saint — of course, if you have a guru, it's the guru — or some form of God, think of him; or, if you want to, think of light. First of all, feel that you are saluting that and, if you want, think of it as your own Self. Think of it as, "I am saluting that Spirit within may I have Your blessing, may I have Your grace, may Your light come now in meditation."

Sit there; just sit in silence, not thinking of anything. Just sit there in complete silence, the mind suspended in awareness, and then gently and easily let the japa of some mantram begin and let it go on easily and naturally at any rate you like, fast sometimes, slow sometimes, that's all right. If you haven't been initiated into a mantram, say any mantram you like. You might try two or three at the beginning, but then you should fix on one and stay with that. You might want to do japa in rhythm with your breathing: as you breathe in, you say the mantram once, as you breathe out you say the mantram once. You kind of keep it according to the breath. Or with the heartbeat, if you become aware of the heartbeat;

that also is good. Whichever will help you to become relaxed and absorbed in that, that's what to do. It's simple. And then again, at the end, whoever you saluted first, salute again and say, "Here, it's Yours, take it." For those who have a guru, this is a very good idea. Say, "All right, guru, I have meditated, now it's all Yours, take it." This is actually a very subtle point. Then you get up and go and try to keep that japa going throughout the day. Did I leave anything out? No.

That's how it is. Yes. Do what comes naturally.

Questions and Answers on Meditation

Swami Nirmalananda

Why do we offer up our meditation to the guru?

It helps us to realize that "I am not the doer." In other words, "I'm giving it to you because it's really yours." Otherwise, we'll have the feeling, "Oh, I racked up so many hours of meditation this week." It's good to have the idea, "I've given it away, it's not mine."

Actually when you have a guru, that force will go literally to him because of the connection between you and him. In a sense, the force will be stored up. See, sometimes people meditate well, and then they blow the whole effect of meditation by some mistake. So it's a good idea to subtly give this energy and power over to another person, who will hold it in store until the right moment comes; and then boom, you'll get it at the right time, when you're most receptive. Sometimes gurus keep it until the end of your life, so that at the moment of death you can get the full effect.

So there is both the devotional idea, the idea that it isn't mine, all of it is God's, and this other reason. In this way you have the feeling, "I've given it away." Even the idea, "I am doing sadhana, I am doing Yoga," has to be gotten rid of. There should be the feeling, "I am not doing anything. The body is moving, the mind is moving, according to its karma, according to God's command. So it's happening." That's how it should be.

What is the difference between the Ajna *chakra (the third eye) and the chakra on the top of the head?*

The Ajna chakra is the intuitive one; this (*pointing to the top of the head*) is the *Sahasrara*, the thousand-petaled lotus, in which the Shakti becomes united with Siva. This is the master center of all. But for beginning people, it is sometimes difficult to catch. Whereas, once you get here (*pointing to the third eye*), you automatically go here (*pointing to the top of the head*). Also, the Sahasrara sometimes produces certain psychic experiences which can distract a person. So that is the difference. Of course, the

175

Sahasrara is the Supreme One, but the Ajna is the one which is the most graspable, to which we can go.

Isn't the guru within you? Why should you offer your meditation to him?

If you've been initiated by somebody, they're really inside, and only delusion tells you they're outside. Still, you ought to say, "Well, guru, I'm giving it to you." It makes a total difference in meditation. There've been times when my meditation was, hm, just so-so. I thought, "What's wrong today?" And then I would remember I had not done my *pranam* (salutation) before meditation. It's not just a little devotional thing. In one sense, in Yoga, we don't really have Bhakti. That may sound surprising. But everything we do is to change the mind. People think of worship: "Well, it's just 'Oh, God, you're so nice, and I have pretty flowers, and I'm giving them to you because I like you.' " No. Real puja, real worship, is what we call a *changing act*. When you do it, it will change your consciousness. Actually, in our whole system we don't do a single thing just because it's beautiful, or just because it's nice, or because it's devotional. Every single thing we do is to change us. Take kirtan! Why do we sing mantrams and kirtan? To change the consciousness. Not really to glorify God. In one way, a bhakti is the most selfish. Everything he does is going to accrue back to his benefit. So worship, kirtan, all this has got a real effect on the mind, to pull it up toward the goal. So all of these things should never be dismissed as just devotion. They're real. They're buttons you push to get the right effect from the inner man.

What is the significance of the colours orange and yellow? Why do you and Swamiji (Swami Satchidananda) wear orange?

Ah — orange is the colour given off astrally by any object when it completely dissolves, when the energies are dispersed totally. That's one of the reasons fire has an orangish rather than a red colour. When we see atoms breaking apart, dissolving into their fundamental energies and becoming dispersed, that's orange. Swamis wear orange because it's the colour of fire. When a person takes Sannyas, he considers that he has burned up his old ways, his old life. He is cremated. In fact, part of the ritual is to perform a cremation ceremony for yourself. Cut off your hair. Burn it in the fire. Certain other objects — a horoscope, if you had a horoscope written out for you — burn that up. Because you say, "Well, that was another birth." All these things relating intimately, you burn up.

Then you do a memorial service for yourself, for the welfare of your own soul.

You also do another interesting thing. A Swami has to do a special sacrifice, where he sacrifices to the grass, to the trees, to the birds, to the insects. Every class of being is mentioned, saying, "May you be satisfied; may you be satisfied!" It is the understanding, "All right. I do owe you a debt. I owe a debt to every living being. But now, I am going to finish that and go for the highest Self alone. May you be propitiated. May I have no more obligations to you. May I have satisfied you. May I have paid my debt to you. If there's something left unpaid, then, please forgive me. Please release me from that."

Yellow is worn, especially by the Buddhists, because when the soul is going out of the body at death, the aura will give out a yellow color. In other words, it is the color of the separation of the spirit from the matter. So that's why they wear it. And Brahmacharis wear it. It means that they are dissociating their consciousness from the gross and putting it into the spiritual world. Whereas Swamis wear orange because they are trying to get away even from the spiritual world. To become a Sannyasi, you say, "I renounce everything of the earth. I renounce everything of the heavens. I renounce the subtle astral worlds. I renounce everything of the causal worlds. I don't want any of it. I want what's beyond it, what is really manifesting as all of it." That's why Swamis wear orange, and the Brahmacharis wear yellow.

Also, in meditation if you see different colors it's because each chakra has its principle which is rising up at that moment in your mind and you are seeing its color. That is why even though Yoga isn't formally practiced in the West, through intuition the Virgin Mary is always pictured in blue. She is the very embodiment of love, mercy and compassion. This is what she is.

When I meditate, sometimes I have beautiful experiences, but other times nothing happens. What's wrong?

When you meditate and you have what you consider a good meditation it's a mistake to get attached to that. Don't make the mistake of always hoping your future meditations will be that way. It's a very difficult thing, I know. It's a habit that I had to break in the beginning of practicing meditation: saying, "Wow, yesterday's meditation was great; how am I going to get that back?" But it's a mistake. You should just go on. If you have a meditation one day that seems very joyful and the next day it seems absolutely dead and it's like you're on the verge of unconsciousness, don't be discouraged. That's just the next step beyond; don't feel you've gone backwards. You should never feel that way. In fact, after a while, I got so that after I meditated and it was a struggle all the way, at the end I was satisfied because I thought, "Well, I've taken my little machete and I've hacked through the forest today. I've told this mind that it will sit there and go through it. So I dug a new channel." When you go down a canal in a boat you just sit there and you just move and it's wonderful, but if you decide to dig a new channel, you sweat a lot and you get a lot of aching muscles out of it.

No, meditation should not be a strain or cause tension; that isn't what I mean. But we should understand that when the mind just doesn't seem to be responding, it's because we're just drilling, drilling, drilling down deep to try to get that real water. When you dig a well, sometimes you have a soft layer and everything moves fine and the drill goes fine. Then suddenly, clunk, it hits the rock, sparks fly and slowly, slowly it drills. We say, "I don't know why. I made fast progress, now I seem to be making hardly any." Well, that's because you've gotten to one of those real tough layers of the mind and you're really working. Now you're really getting somewhere. This is the thing.

As Yogis, we should never get discouraged. As Mother Anandamayi has said, "Discouragement is the only evil for a Yogi. Anything else he may do, even a breaking of discipline; even though it's deflecting and it's retarding to him, it won't destroy him. But despair and discouragement, saying 'I give up,' that will destroy him. He's finished." So the only real evil is this feeling of discouragement or futility. We shouldn't ever feel that way. Sometimes people go through weeks like that, but we should remember that even the fact that it came, means that it has to go. Subconsciously, we know we are eternal beings. If only we could understand that. No matter what situation we're in, inwardly we know our nature is to be unchanging. We project it on our outside situation. If we're in an elevator and somebody steps on our toe, we just go wild — as though they're going to stand on our toe for eternity — and we say, "Hey, get off," and we give them a shove. Right? We overreact because we know our nature is to not change and suddenly we have this fear. We have a combination of fear and ignorance. "My God, he'll be on my toe forever." Or we meditate and we get in a really slumpy, dead period and we say, "Oh, what'll I do now," because we're thinking we'll always be that way. It's a projection of that subconscious knowledge. When you're sick you feel like you never were well. And when you're well, you feel like you never were sick. So, in Yoga, we must understand that we're going to go through many, many states. In fact, if you're not going through states, up and down and up and down, nothing is happening. Do you follow?

There's a practice in some parts of India which I would like to do today, since it's the last time I may get a chance to be with you. It's a custom of giving the *Brahma spota* — you could call it the God dot, maybe — and it is done usually by older brothers and sisters as a sign of love and prayer for the welfare of the other members of the family. It's the putting of a red mark here at the spiritual eye, and it is a prayer that the grace of God will be with that person. It is a prayer in action, so that the grace of God will be with them and then they will attain the opening and the fullness of this intuitive life; that they will get the vision of God. That is the prayer for them. It's not so much of a big ritual like what is done in temples; it's done by ordinary people. It's something done between family members to show their hope for each other's spiritual life. It shouldn't be considered a religious ceremony as such, or as a very formal thing, nor should it be considered even as belonging to one specific religion. So what I would like is someone who is good in leading kirtan to lead us. And then, whoever wants, just come up and I'll put this Brahma spota on your forehead. That way I'll get a good look at you and see who the members of all our family are.

The Mother and Her Children

Swami Satchidananda

Swamiji begins this evening's satsang with the chant, "SAMBASADA SIVA, SAMBASIVOHAM." Afterwards he explains the meaning, which in turn leads into the topic for the evening's discussion: The Lord and His expression as Mother Nature, as the entire world. Previously we heard about the Vedantic truth of the Absolute One and tonight we learn how that One expresses Itself through the Nature, and how to worship the Lord by knowing that we are His expressions.

The retreat has had a strong Bhakti, or devotional quality and some of Swamiji's talks have reflected this, but tonight especially. We come to feel that though he has realized his identity with the Supreme One and has no need to worship as a specific practice towards some goal, on the personality level he is a most humble worshiper of the Divine Mother, that is, of the Lord in all His forms. Fittingly, in the question/answer section of the program, he focusses on practical questions regarding women's role, family life, and married life vs. single or monastic life.

(*Chanting*) Sambasada Siva, Sambasada Siva, Sambasada Siva, Sambasivoham.

The meaning of it is: "Saha" means "with," "Amba" means "the Goddess." So "Saha-amba" becomes "Samba." Siva with the Goddess. We always place Siva with Goddess. And Siva means God. Without the Goddess, God is just a "shava." Shava means a dead body. Siva, without Goddess, without energy, without power, without Kali, is shava. Kali is portrayed as dancing above the body of Siva. Siva is just lying down. What does it mean? Without energy, He's lifeless. Without the expression, the Absolute is just useless. A dynamo is useless if it doesn't rotate. Every electrician knows that. A static dynamo is not even dangerous. Children can go, play, sit on it; they can put their fingers into it. It is dangerless and useless too. But the minute it begins to rotate, it produces thousands of watts of current. And then you have to put a fence around: "Danger, don't go near." Only the proper electrician can go, with good protection, with insulated clothes. Because only the electrician knows how to handle the running dynamo, not everybody. You may say, "Oh, the electrician is just a human being like me, why not I?" But if you touch, you may burn to death.

180

So Shakti is the moving dynamo, Siva is the motionless dynamo. Which do you want? Which is great, hm? Both. Without *sat*, there is no *chit*, and without *chit*, there is no *sat*, no use of that *sat*. God is everywhere, but what is the use if He is just everywhere. He must manifest in action. Current is everywhere, but what is the use? Tell me a place where there is no electricity? If you know the basic principles of electricity, you know there is no place where there is no electricity. Everywhere, even in space, you have electricity. Wherever you have atoms, you have electricity. The positive-negative force, electrons running around protons, hm? It's a dynamo by itself. An atom itself is a dynamo. So electricity is everywhere. Then why can't we just use it? Take a bulb and hold it in the air. Will you get light? No. It doesn't seem to work. Does this remind you of Sant Keshavadas's example? He quotes Ramakrishna: "Milk is all throughout the body of the cow, but you can't just pull its ear. Only at the udder will you get the milk."

It's the same with electricity. It is everywhere but you can't get it directly. You have to get it through a generating station. When the dynamo moves, it gathers, it collects the electricity and passes it to you through cables. If electricity doesn't express itself through a dynamo it is of no use to us. It is just there; it IS, but almost like it is not. So the manifestation is necessary. The expression is necessary. Mere being is not enough and that is the difference between Vedanta and Bhakti. In Vedanta you ARE. What is the good of you? You are, hm? So what can I do with you? Nothing. Express yourself! Current is everywhere. Can you just take a cup of it and pour and swallow it? Can you just go and hold the current and say, "I am getting light?" Or just touch the wire and get the music? You'll get a different type of music, no doubt: A shock.

So again, to use the electricity, you should have the right gadgets. It depends on what type of use you want to put that current to. If you want to get music out of it, connect a radio. If you want light out of it, connect a light bulb. If you want food out of it, connect an oven. If you want to cool yourself, get an air conditioner. If you want to get into motion, put a motor. So what is the function of electricity then? What is its quality? Cool, hot, vibrating, moving, running, musical? Can you pinpoint the quality of electricity? No. By itself it seems to be free of any quality. There is no quality. But according to the gadgets you connect, it expresses various qualities. So the difference is in the gadgets, not in the electricity. If somebody comes and says, "In our house the electricity always sings," another person will say, "No, no, in our home the electricity cooks."

"Fool, how can electricity cook? It can only sing, nothing else."

A third person may say, "It neither sings nor cooks, it is only to give light."

Who is right? Who is wrong? One is right in saying that the electricity cooks, but he is wrong in saying that electricity can *only* cook. The "only" makes the trouble. But the electrical engineer knows everything. He knows the electricity cannot do anything without the gadgets.

So the difference is in the gadgets, not in the spirit behind, the life behind, the force behind. You are all the gadgets. The same current runs through you all. One sings, the other swings, one steals, the other catches, hm? The difference is in gadgets, that's all. So the power that motivates the policeman and the power that motivates the robber is the same. Difference in gadgets. And certain gadgets do not function. Sometimes, when you plug in a lamp, you don't get light. You see all the connections, the wire is there, the holder is there, but you don't get the light. What does it mean? Everything is O.K., the switch is on, the electricity is on. So what is wrong? The bulb. The bulb looks right — beautiful, colored, good-looking. You don't see anything wrong with the bulb. But there inside the bulb, which you do not see easily in a frosted bulb, is a filament. The filament is a tiny little thing. When that gets fused, in all outward appearance it will look similar to any other bulb. But it won't give any light.

You can see many bulbs like that running around. No filament. They never shed the light. They go and "connect" — pray, sit, meditate, do everything, take all the retreats possible — but no light. And certain bulbs give light, but less than others. The voltage is the same, but they give less light. What is the difference? Coloring? No, same color. Quality? No, quality is the same. It's the *quantity* of the filament. In a 100 Watt bulb, you have a longer filament inside. In a 60 Watt less filament. The area that is allowed to glow is less. That means, if you have a longer filament, you get a better glow, you get more light. That also you see. Some have twinkling lights, a little tiny light — they have a little, little filament. It is not fused, it is there, but it is very little, very narrow. But the more you expand the filament the more you shed light.

What is the filament here? The heart. The mind expands it. If you are a very narrow-minded person you get only a very little current. If you expand your mind more and more, you get more current. You shed more light. The size of the bulb remains the same, 40 Watt, 60 Watt, or 100 Watt bulb. The size, shape, and everything seems to be the same. That's why you should open up your heart, don't be narrow. Then you get the current. The current is the same everywhere. It is the cosmic current. There is only one generating station. It sends light, wireless. We are all different gadgets. Some are built as a radio and they sing beautifully. You need not be jealous of that singer; he is built as a radio, so let him sing. You do your work; if everyone becomes a radio, we will be singing in darkness. Some should be bulbs also, and some fans, air-conditioners. We need everything. A nice vibrating chair, an air-conditioned room, nice soft light, then the music will be nice. So don't think that all must become singers, or all must become *one* thing. We need variety. Each contributes to the other. So who is great and who is small? None. All are equal.

Take a wrist watch. How many wheels are there? There are so many. Say roughly about fifteen or twenty. Are they all the same size? No. Are they all rotating in the same direction? No. Are they all rotating at the same speed? Big wheel, small wheel, slow wheel, fast wheel, rotating counter-clockwise, clockwise; each one is different from the other. The main wheel connected to the main spring is the slowest wheel. That should rotate, should it not? But you cannot even notice the movement, whereas the other end, the small wheel, will be running so fast. So the big wheel looks at the small wheel, and says, "Hey, you crazy little fellow. Why are you running like that? Can't you go gently like me? See me and turn like that, gently, softly."

The small wheel says, "Well, you laugh at me but at least I'm running in one direction. Look at that other fellow, he doesn't seem to have any direction. He goes this way, changes his mind, that way, again changes the mind, this way." Hm? Like a seeker running about here and there. Goes there, no, comes here, no, goes there. Doesn't seem to have any direction.

So the little wheel looks at the big wheel and says, "See, am I not better than that one who does not have any particular direction? You laugh at me. Why don't you laugh at him instead?"

The little balance wheel listens to this. "Ah, I see. So you both make me a fool? I see. O.K., well, in that case let me not move. Strike!" When you insult a worker, instead of arguing, he can say, "Okay, I'll sit and strike. I don't want to move. Why should I?" He just sits and "meditates." After awhile he slowly opens his eyes and looks at what the others are doing. They all seem to be sitting and "meditating." And the balance wheel asks, "Well, what happened to you? You all seem to be quiet, not moving. What is the matter?" And they say, "That's what we are wondering." So they call for an emergency meeting. They say, "What is this, are you moving, big brother?"

"No."

"How about you, the middle brother?"

"No!"

"You, small fellow?"

"No. We all seem to be stationary now."

Then the balance wheel laughs at them. "Ha, you fellows; you teased me. Now you know the truth! We are all interconnected. We have equal responsibilities. If anyone of us stops, we all have to stop. We have been assigned certain duties, certain speed. Everything is being controlled by the main spring. And that in its turn is controlled by the man who winds the watch. We don't have any purpose of our own here. Don't you know that? Why am I rotating like this? Why do you rotate like that — slowly? Do you have any purpose of your own? Who knows the purpose? He, the one who winds us. What is the purpose? To show the time to Him."

So they all have a common purpose — to show the time to the owner. So there is no inferiority or superiority. We're all needed. Every tiny little screw, bolt and nut is needed for the mechanism. Even if one is missing, the whole mechanism will be faulty. We are all like that: the different parts of the Universal Mechanism. Each one is a screw, a bolt or a nut. Keep yourself tight. Don't get loosened. Perform your duty. Wherever you are, just do your duty. Don't try to copy the other man. The only thing that we should have in common is to know that we are all moving because of the Mover. If you want to know why you are moving, ask the Mover. Or, maybe, one of us might know. "Hey, why am I moving? Why are you moving?"

"Well, I am being moved."

"Oh, then, is it the same case for me also?"

"Yes, we are all moving because of that unseen Hand. If ever He stops moving us, we'll be dead."

So one person is placed here to tell you that. You are placed there to learn it. He put me here to be a Swami and He put you there to sit and listen. If you don't listen, I have no purpose here. If I don't talk, you have no purpose there. Who is great? Both. The minute we see that, you will have to search for your ego; it will have gone long before. There is no need to drive it away or crush it or control it; just know this truth. The poor ego will have said goodbye long ago; it won't deceive you anymore. Let us know that: that one Cosmic Consciousness you call God runs through every atom in this world. Everything in this world has a purpose — from a blade of grass to a mighty king. Whoever it is, we are all equal. Nobody should think that he is inferior or superior.

This reminds me of a saint who once answered the question, "How did you become a big saint like this?"

"Oh, that is a big story," he said.

"Oh, what is that story?"

Then he said, "You know, years before, one fine morning, the Creator, Brahma, came to His court and He called His subordinates. They all assembled there and as soon as He walked into the court the subordinates said, 'Sir, all the components are ready. What should we make today?' Creation. All the components are ready, just like in a Detroit factory. 'Should we make an LTD today or a Thunderbird or a Mustang?' So the subordinates asked the Boss. And certainly Brahma asked His chief assistant,

'What is the program; what is pending? We seem to have created many things, almost everything is done. Is there anything pending?'

'Well, today's program shows that You have a choice, Sir. You can make either a pig or a saint.'

'Well, all right, make a saint.'

"And that is why I am here. Casually, He decided to make a saint. And that is why I am here. If He had decided the other way, I would be squealing in the mud with all my little ones."

Swami Nirmalananda probably didn't tell you the story of Devendra, the king of the devas, the celestial beings. Devendra asked the Lord, "Can You explain the force, the power of maya? Will it delude everybody? Is there anybody who can escape from that?"

"Well, Devendra, it is very difficult to explain what it is. It could be understood only by experience. If you want, just take a walk, probably you might have a chance to see. Go down to the Earth, walk around, and see what's happening."

So he came down to the Earth and as he was walking, he saw a number of piglets. They were running around here and there, crying, "Mama, Mama, Mama." He saw that and wondered, "Why are they crying like that?" Then he slowly walked around and he saw a few others who were jumping around the body of a mother pig. The pig was dead. The mother was dead and the young ones were really in a terrible state, crying for the mother, hungry, running around. Well, he just took pity. "Oh, poor little ones. How can I see this and go away?" Even Siva once saw this situation and He became the mother pig, to feed those young ones. So when Devendra saw this, he said, "Oh no, I can't just leave them and go. Let me transform myself into a mother pig." So he transformed himself into a mother pig and started feeding the little ones. Once he got into that form, and once he saw the young ones playing, he became so happy, he totally forgot about his true identity.

Years passed. He had a whole family there. The celestial beings were getting worried. They asked, "What has happened to him?" So they went to the Lord and said, "Lord, where is he?"

"I don't know; you better go down and see what's happening."

So they sent a few people to look around and when they came down, they could recognize him, but unfortunately, Devendra couldn't recognize them. He was just so happy. They came and said, "Hey, what are you doing? You are Devendra." He replied, "Huh?" He had totally forgotten.

"You are Devendra."

"I don't know anything about that. Look at all my little pigs; see how beautiful they are. Would you like to take one home? Here is my first child and my second child, and my grandchild, and my great-grandchild," and he started praising the family and talking about his family tree. He was so happy, he didn't even want to come out of that form. He didn't want to believe them. Nobody could make him realize.

Ultimately, one of them came up to him and said, "All right. I am going to do something." She just borrowed the sword from Kali — Whessst — and cut off his head. The soul came out yelling. As it came out of the body, there stood Devendra. They released him out of his body and looked at him. "Devendra? What were you doing here?"

"My Lord. Do you really mean that I was there? No, no, it can't be!" He didn't even want to believe that. That is the play of maya. It can easily deceive you. That's why, who is the greatest among all? The one who knows his true nature, the true Self.

Self-knowledge, or to know that you are the instrument — either way — is fine. As the great devotee Hanuman once said to Rama, "Rama, this is my realization: whenever I treat myself as the body, let me be Your servant. When I feel that I'm the Atman, then I'm You." When you think you are the body, it doesn't matter; we don't need to knock the body. Don't worry about it. Take yourself to be the body, but become a good body. "Yes, I'm the body. You're the master. You are the electricity flowing through this body; without You I can't even move. Thy will be done. I'm the tool in Your hand. I've been given the awareness just to know that I'm the tool." That is why the free will is given, not to go and do all kinds of things.

We should just know that, but instead we want to know everything else. I can very well prove that without that cosmic force of God we cannot even move. We're all interested in living, is it not so? Nobody wants to die. What is the most important thing that is necessary to live? Even without bread we can live, without water we can live, but not without the breath. How many times do we breathe in a given minute? The average amount is fifteen breaths in and out. When you say you are breathing, it seems that the air comes in and goes out, does it not? It goes in fifteen times and comes out fifteen times. If it doesn't go in, will you live? Fifteen times a minute it goes out of you, is it not? That means you are almost dying. Does it say, when it goes out, "I'm just going out, I'll come back soon?" Does it tell you? Are you aware of it? Many people are not even aware that they're breathing. Do you consciously do that? No. Whether you remember it or not, whether you know it or not, the breath goes in and comes out. If you are interested in living, and if you know that the breath is the most important thing for your life, you should get scared every time it goes out, is it not? It's going; will it come back? We don't even worry about it. But it comes back. How? Nothing moves without a force behind it. There must be a command, a consciousness behind, that controls everything, that moves everything. So what is it that sends back the air when you yourself are not interested in getting it back? Nature or God or some force, some cosmic force which takes care of everybody. And that cosmic force wants you to live even if you forget it.

So somebody seems to be sending you air. When the air comes out, "Hey, better go back." The air even revolts, "Oh, what is this, you push me in again and again; everytime I go, he kills me, murders me, burns me." Aren't we doing that? Every time that air with the life, the prana, comes in, what do we do? We burn the poor thing. Every time it comes in, we murder it. And what little is left over runs away, "Oh, I don't want to be with that fellow, he burns me." It jumps out, runs away, "Oh, I don't want to be with that fellow, he burns me." It jumps out as carbon dioxide. But God says, "No, it doesn't matter, go back."

Do you agree that you are not living because you want to live? Call it God, cosmic consciousness, Nature, anything. The name doesn't matter, but you're not living by yourself, that's all I want to tell you. Call it any name. Somebody is causing you to live, somebody who is interested in your living.

Who will take care of my glasses? Every time I take them off, I put them in the case, clean them, put them away. Why am I interested in treating them so carefully? Hm? Because I am using them. If I don't use them, will I carry them? No. If they are of no more use to me, I will just discard them. As long as I use them, they don't demand, "Oh clean me, put me in the case, take care of me." I need their service so I take care of them. Now, somebody is taking care of *you*. Why? He needs your service, so he keeps the instrument clean, alive, well-sharpened. If you take care of your car, it's not because the car asks you to. It's because you use it.

What does it mean? We're all instruments. He has created the instruments. He made different instruments for different purposes. And again, all the instruments need not be the same. If you are going to a workshop, you see a chisel, a saw, a knife, a file, screwdriver, pliers, a hammer, all kinds of tools, is it not so? They're not the same size or shape. And the workman knows what to use and when. When he needs the hammer, he will use the hammer. The pliers should not be jealous of the hammer. "Oh what is this, I am just lying here since yesterday and you seem to be using only the hammer, why not me? Hm? You seem to be favoring him. You should be impartial, you must use all of us equally." When he wants to use the pliers, he will use them. When he wants to use the file, he will use it. Until then, their duty is just to be in place. And that's why we are all built in different ways. He will use everybody.

And if anybody is useless, if He doesn't need any instrument, then you know where He will put it. Some instruments He will put in an expensive box, because sometimes when you have been using a nice tool for a long time, you say, "Oh, I have been using this pen, this is the pen my father used. Put it there in the showcase." But some people say, "Oh, a tool is a tool, why keep a space for that? Burn it. Dust goes to dust." Some people think that way and probably that is the best way of disposal. It saves a lot of economic problems also. The best way is to put the body somewhere, buy a cup of gasoline, pour it, shhh, finish it. If you are rich enough, buy sandalwood, and then burn it. The Hindus do that. They don't worry about burying. It came from the dust and it should go back to the dust. So He knows how to dispose of us. When the tool is of no more service, junk it. That clearly shows that we're all nothing but instruments. Saint Ramalingam sings to the Lord, "Lord, You are feeding me, so I am fed. You are putting me to sleep, so I am sleeping. You are showing me things so I am seeing them. You are making me happy, so I am happy. You are pulling me, so I am shaking. Not only me, the entire universe is like that, I know. Therefore, what do You want me to say to You? All I want to tell You is this: that I noticed, that's all. If You want me to praise You, make me praise You. If You want me to worship You, make me worship You. You get things done. All I can say is, I know that and I'm ready. I'm prepared, like wood is carved or stone sculptured."

With this attitude, where is the room for egotism? Where is there room to say, "I did it, I built it, I'm going to rescue that man, I'm going to save that man." There's no "I" at all then. Because almost every one of us is functioning on the body-mind level. All this taking, all this doing, is within the body and mind. The Self doesn't do anything, neither myself nor yourself. As Self, I don't need to preach to your Self. The Self is just there. Silent. All this preaching comes from the mind that gained a little knowledge. It's a little pill for ego, that's all. Don't think that the guru is egoless, talking to you. If he is egoless, he won't be of any use to you. Even to come here, sit up and talk to you, there must be an ego. The only difference is there is no greed, that's all. But the Self need not and cannot say anything. It's just there. As Self you don't need any instruction. So it is on this ego level, intellectual level, emotional level, physical level, that we are communicating.

How? It's something like if one knife is blunt, you use another knife to sharpen it. Don't you do that? In the same way, a tempered knife tempers the other knives, when they are losing their tempers! Do you know how to temper steel? Heat it, then suddenly cool it. To raise the temper of steel is to heat it well, then all of a sudden cool it. So, to temper you, just burn you a little and then cool you suddenly — ups and downs. It's not necessary that I should do it or some other guru; Nature itself does it. The Nature is the bigger guru. She is the Mother. Sometimes she makes you a little high, excites you; you get all warm. All of a sudden, freeze. By that way you get tempered. Scientifically, what is tempering? Crude iron is mixed with carbon. Every time you heat and cool, some of its impurities are burnt away; it gets cleaned. When it gets cleaned well it becomes steel, and it is tempered. So this crude iron is being treated to be tempered.

When the treatment is complete, you are a tool, an instrument — you just know that. That is what you call knowledge. We seem to have forgotten it. When we know the truth, the Master is so happy. "Wonderful instrument, I can handle him any way I want." But some are possessed with the egoistic devil. So any time He wants to use them in some way, they twist another way. He says "What is this, I have to fight with this tool." Something like a loosened car, if you steer it this way it goes that way. So keep yourself in good shape so He can use you well. Don't allow your ego to come in between. Let Him handle. That is what you call renunciation or surrendering. You don't even need to choose what to do. He'll decide what to do with you.

But our ego is terrible. Even in surrender you say, "Oh, I let Him do everything, but don't you think I should do something? God helps those who help themselves!" That is also a type of Bhakti, a type of devotion, no doubt. But unfortunately, even in surrendering, a little ego slips in. So one group of devotees says, "You have to surrender. You have to depend on Him; but still you have to hold him."

Have you ever seen the mother monkey jumping around with the baby monkey? Go to the jungle some day and see these things. When you really go to the jungle and learn from the Nature, you'll learn many, many beautiful things. Everything will teach you a lesson. I'm really sorry for this so-called civilized country, city people, city dwellers. Gentle nature can teach you many things. I will tell you. The baby monkey catches the stomach of the mother. It holds with the fore paws and the legs. It will hold the entire body, hanging underneath. The mother monkey will not even worry about the baby. She will just jump from branch to branch; it's the baby's duty to cling on to the mother. Whenever the baby wants to go somewhere, all it has to do is take hold of the mother and then the mother will jump. When the mother jumps from branch to branch, who will have the fear of falling down? The baby. The baby is depending upon its mother, no doubt, but it still depends on its own strength. "God, I won't leave you, I'm holding on tight."

There is another animal whose baby also depends on the mother for its movement. The kitten. That probably you've all seen. Whenever the kitten wants to move, all it has to do is meow. The mother will come, pick it up by the back of the neck and jump here and there. When the mother jumps with the baby, who will have the fear of dropping the baby? The mother. Both monkey and kitten depend upon their mothers for their movement, but in the first case the anxiety and the fear is in the heart of the baby monkey, whereas here the anxiety is with the mother. The kitten is totally free. "It's none of my business — you take me wherever you want. I don't know anything. All I know is to meow."

So there are two different schools of thought, even in surrendering. One group says, "You must be like a little monkey and hold and then He will take you." The other group says, "Even to hold, where could I get the strength if He is not to give me that? So, why should I worry? I am His child."

You know, these two schools of thought created so much difference, they became totally separate cliques and enemies. If you go to South India you will see it. Do you know the mark here (*indicating his forehead*)? Probably the Hare Krishna people do that. Do they just put a "U" or do they put a little mark here (*indicating the bridge of his nose*) also? A "U" and a little here, hm? In South India we have the two types of Vaishnavites (worshippers of Lord Vishnu) — the ones who follow the monkey and the others who follow the kitten. And they have to show that they belong to one group or the other, so they have the difference in the mark. One is just "U" without the extra mark. So we call them the U-mark people and the others are the Y-mark people. And they get into terrible fights.

They even kill each other, yes, and they go to the courts and because of them, sometimes the temples are locked and the keys are kept with the official attorney until the dispute is over. It's all a kind of religious ego. Ego in the name of God.

Actually, who could escape from this? The poor, childlike, ignorant, illiterate people. That's why all the great saints have said, "Forget all you have read, go back to the childhood." Children are the kingdom of heaven. Become a child again, you are saved. Just say, "I don't know anything." If you know even a little you are in trouble. If at all you want to know something, know that you don't know anything. The real knower is somebody within you. It doesn't matter, wherever you are, whatever station of life, stay totally free from this egoism. That is the only thing that is necessary. You may be a Sannyasi, you may be a householder, you may be single, you may be illiterate, literate, rich, poor, whatever it be. That is the best form of liberation.

So where did all this begin? Siva and Shakti, the Absolute and His expressions, hm? So, that is what the *Shakti Purana* says, "Without the Shakti, neither Siva nor Brahma nor Vishnu can do anything. Even the three functions — creation, preservation and destruction or dissolution — cannot be done without the Shakti." That is why they always keep their Shaktis with them, all the three. It's all beautiful, beautiful, scientific, if you go into the esoteric meaning of it.

Brahma creates the whole world, not with any components, just by the words, "May it be so." That's all, and it is created. That's why "In the beginning was the Word." Brahma used the word to create: "Be it so." To produce a word, to produce a sound, you need a tongue, is it not? So the power must be in the tongue. That is why Brahma's consort, His power, as Saraswati, resides on his tongue. Saraswati lives on the tongue of Brahma.

Vishnu is protecting everything, taking good care of it. To protect everybody and everything you should have a heart, is it not so? A compassionate heart. That's why Lakshmi resides in the heart of Vishnu. See? And now, one created, the other is protecting, so the third one should excel both these. To dissolve he must have much more strength. So that is why he has one half of his body as the Shakti. Parvati takes one half of Siva. The left half. That is why he is called Ardhanadeshwari: Ardha is half, nadi — woman, Ishwara — God. So half woman, fifty-fifty. Hm? To dispose of everything, no one-sided decision, hm? When you want to dispose of something from the house, he consults you. "Honey, how is it? You need it?" "No, you can dispose of it." "Okay." That's why Parvati is one half.

So whatever it be, the power is there. Anything that moves is the expression of power, and that is the reason why you say Mother Parvati, Mother Nature — not Father Nature. So let us know the greatness of Mother. Let us know that She is functioning within us. She is taking good care of us. We are always Her children, whether we are good or naughty. She still loves us. Just love Her. Allow Her to take care of you. And that is the reason, even great Vedantins like Shankara, who said that God is without name, without form, Absolute, used to sit for hours and hours and worship the Goddess as Saraswati. He was a great Vedanta exponent but he was a great devotee too. He established great temples for the Goddess. At the same time, he says, "God is nameless, formless, don't even worship images — you are that Brahman." Vedanta philosophy, hm? If you ask him, "Well, that is the Truth, but the Truth is of no use by itself." Like wheat, it should be cooked into bread to be useful. Only Mama can do that. You can't eat it as it is. All the great Vedantins were Mother worshipers. Look at the great Ramakrishna — Mother worshiper. Vivekananda, a great worshiper of Siva and Amba. They're all great bhaktas. So let that Bhakti be with us. Let your heart melt. Be devoted. Recognize that highest power that functions through you. Then we'll all be saved. That is the only way to be at ease and peace with everybody. Don't just listen to me and go away. Think well. Think of the greatness of Mother. Put aside all of your intellectual gymnastics. We're not going to gain anything with all of these intellectual fights. The world is seeing enough troubles with all our so-called intelligence. Let us learn to use the heart.

Questions and Answers
on Women, Family Life and Monkhood

Swami Satchidananda

With all due respect, your view of women as weak, submissive and incapable of independence — which you have given in some of your answers — seems to be a limited and limiting stereotype. Did I understand you correctly?

Did I say it that way? No. I never said that she is weak. She is Shakti. How can Shakti be weak? As I said, she is more tolerant, more patient. Only a strong person could be patient. Tolerant. She is the power, the Goddess, she is the Mother Earth. If we really want to compare man and woman, she is stronger. I'm not talking about the physical strength, but the mental strength. They have more patience. They have the greater capacity to make or break. If you go into history — I'm not a historian, but, of the little I know, most of the wars are caused by women. At the same time, most of the great kingdoms were built by women. They can make or break. In the *Mahabharata*, Draupadi caused the war. In the *Ramayana*, Sita was the cause. Great kingdoms depend on the capacity of women. That means they are really stronger. Even in the house, the girl can make her husband a slave if she wants, if she knows how to handle him. Hm? Just a tear is enough if you know when to shed it. They don't use brutal physical strength. A smile is enough to make him a slave. Yes. If there is a capable wife there is nothing wanting in the house. There is everything. She can bring all the wealth there. Please, if I have given a little room for you to think that way, I humbly withdraw whatever I said. I am a worshiper of the great Mother. How can I say that She is weak or incapable of independence? No, she is the giver of independence. She can bind or free. If I say that they are generally the weaker sex, it is physically I mean. Physically, they are weaker. If they want to make themselves stronger, they can. But in general, by nature, physically they are weaker. They are tender, creeper-like. But if they want to show that they are men, okay, do it. You can show yourself to be a man but still you are a woman. You can never grow a mustache and beard like me. That is the gift of God to you. Who said one is weaker

193

than the other? The positive, the negative. Without one, the other won't function.

In one and the same body, you have both feminine and masculine. In one and the same atom, we have positive and negative charges. Electron and proton. Electron runs around the proton, is it not? It is the electron that runs around the neutron and the proton, because they can't stay away from that. That's the very nature. Affinity. They are the ones in whom love predominates. That's it. The secret is that. Love and devotion and bhakti is the feminine aspect. That's why even if a man is a devotee, he treats himself as a woman. God is the Lord; all the devotees are feminine, are the electrons that run around that nucleus. So the entire nature is like that. It is charming, being like that. I really don't know why the women should show themselves to be men. There's a beautiful charm in women. There's no need to imitate a man. It's a really sad thing to hear people say that or even feel that way. I don't even understand why this "Women's Lib." Who binds you? Nobody binds you. If you give room, naturally anybody will bind you. So we should lead our own lives. Nobody can bind us.

What is marriage?

Well, should we talk about marrying somebody? Are you interested in it? We're all married. Purusha (the Self) is the only husband. His wives are all the egos, hm? One saint said, "My wife is desirelessness." A high-class wife. Her name is *Narosi*, that means desirelessness. Dispassion is my wife. So we live together. We have a child and the name of the child is peace, Shanthi. "My wife is dispassion, our son is Shanthi." Why can't we have that wedding? That's the best marriage. Never divorce that one.

We're all sent with a companion. We're already wedded. And that wedding has been performed already, in the heaven. What is it that you are wedded to? Your own peace. Never divorce it. Let nothing separate you from your peace. You are born with that. That's your husband or wife, or whatever you want to call it. And she will never go to the courts to divorce you as long as you don't want a divorce.

Isn't sex a part of the Divine Plan? I think some people use mysticism and religion as a cop-out.

That means a kind of escape? Well, that is probably *your* feeling. But what do they want, people who use mysticism and religion? They are also aiming for satisfaction. But *permanent* satisfaction, not temporary — that is the difference. With sensual satisfaction, you get something, you are satisfied; you don't get it, you are dissatisfied. And if you are satisfied when you get it, you have to keep on getting it. If sex is going to satisfy you, the more you do, the more you should be satisfied. Come on, let me see how much you can do. If it is going to satisfy you, the more you do, the more you should be happy, isn't it so?

That means satisfaction is not something which can come from outside; that something can bring you. It is always inside. You forget that. You just ignore that, you don't even know that it is within, and you get a glimpse of it reflected from outside. Something ... you just want something, and then when you get that want fulfilled, in the fulfilment your satisfaction is reflected. And it is only a temporary reflection, and then again you don't see it. It is something like walking around, close to the wall. Wherever there is a clean mirror you see your face. So, "Ha!" you say, "I've got my face." You walk further: "I lost my face." Then again you see another mirror: "Aha, I got my face again." So if you want your face always, you feel you should stand in front of a mirror always. Because every time you walk away you miss the face. But to have the satisfaction of having a face, should you constantly stand in front of a mirror? That's not a clever thing to do. Instead, know that you are the face. Whether you see it or not, you have it. Even that reflection cannot be seen if you close your eyes. And that is how we get satisfactions. Wherever things are a little clean and nice, your own satisfaction is reflected.

So anything that comes from outside is nothing but your own reflection. And if you depend on the reflection, you have to keep on waiting for it. Instead, these religious people, they want to really know why it comes and goes, why it seems to escape. Where is the source? "If it is there, it should be permanent. So where is the permanent satisfaction?" After having tried everything and found that nothing satisfies them permanently, they want to know the source. Then they find that the satisfaction is always there. You don't need to go out and do anything. That is why they are not interested in that. Not that they abandoned anything or "copped out." They are no longer interested because they don't see satisfaction through that.

Until you realize that, go and experience things. And then one day you'll know that this is not the thing that can give you satisfaction and you can leave it. We only say that you cannot get *permanent* satisfaction through that; nobody insists that you not do that. In fact, no teacher will say you should not do it. He will not command you; he will not tell you, he will not say, "This is not the right thing; this won't help you." He will say that only when you come and ask him. He will not go out of the way to your house and say, "Don't do this and don't do that." No. That's why, "Ask, and it shall be given." We are not missionaries, remember that. We don't go from door to door, saying, "Oh, you sinner, don't do this, don't do that; do this, you will get high." A real teacher will not do this. He will wait until you are ready, until you want it. Either you know what you want, or you do not know what you want. If you come and say, "I want something but I don't know how to get it," then he will tell you, "This is the way to get it. If you like, try it." "Oh, that's too much, I can't." "Okay, go, when you are really ready, come back again." He won't hold you. So don't think scriptures or any teachers will ask you not to do this. If you come and ask, they will tell you, "That's not the right thing to do, you won't get the right thing there. It's just a trifling thing." If you don't know, ask him; if you don't care to ask him, don't worry about it. All the scriptures simply advise you: "If you want a natural, permanent satisfaction, this is not the way."

But if you have a reason for it, not just for your satisfaction, but some other reason, then go and do it. That is the natural way. The natural purpose for sex is reproduction, not just for your satisfaction. If you depend on that for your satisfaction, you will always miss it. So don't just use flowery words and say this is the natural way for satisfaction, and this and that. If you mean what you are saying, then you will know the truth.

I am convinced of the benefit of observing celibacy or Brahmacharya *but I find it difficult. The body seems to have it's own will. I would like to know how to overcome this.*

To overcome this you have to educate the mind, because this urge doesn't come from the body, it comes from the mind. It's the thought that kindles up certain glands. If you take care of the thinking it won't affect the body. So we have to analyze, what is this desire? Should I have it; if so, how, how much, when, where? It should not control you. Instead, you can control it. It's not bad to have this urge; it is just normal. It's a part of your nature. But here we are trying to win over the natural tendency. The natural tendency of the river is to flow. You arrest it, build up the energy, channel it, and bring illumination to the cities. You harness the natural flow, use it for some greater purpose. That is another reason why I say, "Don't waste all your energy in that. You can use it for a better purpose. Harness it." Just to say to someone, "I love you," you don't need to waste all your energy; you can show your love in many other ways, without wasting your energy. If you are going to waste your energy every time, to show you love somebody, you'll totally run down. You can't even start the car again. Then you have to go to somebody to jump it.

So if you are interested in something more, you can even ignore it. You can use that energy for something higher. Or you can experience that in a reasonable way. But that should not control you and come to the surface whenever it wants. Instead, you should control it. That is to be achieved only by concentrating on it, pondering, meditating on it. Analyze it, try to sublimate it. Another way is to occupy the mind in something else, something more useful. Then you won't even have time to think of it.

To be more plain: imagine a couple. They desire to have that physical relationship one evening and they are all ready. All of a sudden they get a telegram that somebody very dear to them is in a serious state, or has passed away. Will they still be ready to satisfy their physical urge? Immediately all the urge goes away as if it is quenched by a bucket of water. Because the mind is taken somewhere else, all this goes away. Why? Because it is the mind that has created it. All of a sudden the mind is pulled out, the main switch goes off. If you have a two-fold switch and you put it one way, one light goes on. If you put it the other way, the other light goes on. One cannot function simultaneously with two things. So engage your mind in something more useful. More elevating. And you won't be bothered by this. So try both the ways.

Would you please talk about Tantra Yoga?

Some people unfortunately think of it in terms of a physical relationship. The masculine and feminine that Tantra Yoga talks about are within yourself. Siva and Shakti are within you, you have both the polarities. The *prana* and the *apana* are to be united. As I said before, the feminine force, or in other words, the creative force, is locked up in you. The Siva and the Shakti are to be united and that is done by awareness, deep meditation, and by the application of the entire mind. You can do it by your own thinking, because wherever the mind goes the prana follows and vice-versa. You can send the prana or the vital force with your own thought. If you look at your thumb and keep saying that it is going to become warmer and warmer, ultimately it will become red hot. If your thought is really powerful it will really happen there; even a blister could appear. By your own thought you are driving the vitality there, you are increasing the circulation. You can command all the cells of the body. Wherever the mind goes, the prana goes, and wherever the prana goes the mind goes. That is why when you want to control the mind it is good to do a little pranayama to begin with. Pranayama calms the mind quickly and helps to bring the mind to one place. Then the mind takes over the concentration. That is why when the mind is agitated, you breathe heavily. When the agitation of the mind is calmed, the breath will be calmed.

You can use your thought, in connection with the prana, to awaken certain psychic forces or whatever you want. According to Tantra Yoga there are fifty-one important psychic centers in the trunk, the petals of the different chakras. Each lotus has certain number of petals and each petal corresponds to one particular aspect of the cosmic power. According to the *Tantra Shastras*, a deity resides on each petal and the vibration of the deity is the vibration of a particular syllable. In Sanskrit there are fifty-one syllables and each syllable corresponds to a particular deity. The sound of the syllable itself is the deity; each has its own power. You can pinpoint one, whichever you want to develop, and focus your mind there. You can awaken that. If you have that feeling of devotion, then you say, "That Divine Force is in me." You feel, "Come and bless me, help me, give me all this." So more of a feeling is there. And to help that, you do some outside pujas, which will ultimately lead into *antar puja*, or the inner worship.

That is what you call Tantra. If you worship the God as Siva, that is called Siva Tantra; if you call it Shakti, it's called Shakti Tantra. Otherwise, if you just bring that to an ordinary physical level, it's nothing but mere Tantra! Tantra has another meaning, also — trick!

Recently when you talk I feel that you are saying, "Marriage is okay if you have to, but monkhood is much better."

Did I say that? It's not that you have to. If you find a good partner, marriage is good, no doubt. But it's seldom you find that. That's the trouble. Certainly you would all agree with me. If you find somebody you are the luckiest person in the world, I should say. There are huge temples built in the name of chaste ladies, in India. They were able to control even the nature, even the gods. What more penance should one do than to just be a wife? (*laughter*).

I'll give you an example. There was a couple and the husband became a leper. He was the worst fellow. Even in his leprosy he wanted to go out having dates, though he was married. So he used to say, "Now I can't walk, I can't go by myself, but I have to meet that girl today."

So his wife said, "Don't worry. If that is your desire, I'll help you." She used to put him on a chair and carry him on her head to the prostitute's house. "If that is your will, go ahead, do it. I give myself to you, to your service. I'm happy in making you happy. It doesn't matter. I'll do that."

And she did that. One day when they returned it was very late. They were passing through a place where the public executions were performed. In those days the executions were not by hanging. At least in India it was by torture. They used to have a long spike planted on the ground like a thin needle and they take the person and then from the anus it passes through the whole body. They don't die for a number of days, just like crucifixion. (*There are groans from the audience*) You say, "Oh, oh, oh." What is crucifixion then? It's another form of crucifixion. Instead of so many nails, there's just one nail. and once a saintly person was caught in some trouble and he was punished that way. There is another story behind it. I'll come to that story later on, hm?

So when the lady was bringing her husband like that on the chair, this saint was on that pole. And by mistake, the chair touched one of the parts of his body and it gave him a good jerk and you know how agonizing it is. So he goes, "Ahhh." And somehow momentarily he lost his peace, his presence of mind. And he cursed. "Whoever touched me, they should die before the sun dawns." That was the curse. And he was a man of penance, a man of powers, a *siddha*. If you meditate, you attain certain powers; your words will come true. You can bless somebody, you can curse somebody. So during the momentary weakness he said that. And she heard that and immediately she realized that it would come true. She said, "Yes, my husband touched him, but I did it; but it's not even my mistake, I didn't do it purposely. He should have inquired before he cursed. So what am I to do? God, I have been living as a chaste wife; I took this life as a penance, as a spiritual practice; I accepted whoever came into my life as a husband and treated him as God, and served him with all faith and loyalty and devotion. If the divine law approves that, I say, let not there be a dawn!"

Even to say that one should have courage, is it not? He said, "You will die before the dawn." She said, "Let there be no dawn." And it did happen. The sun didn't rise. Hours passed, all the sages and saints who used to get up early in the morning to do their practices, they woke up to see it still dark, dark, dark. "What is this?" They started praying, "What is this? Something is happening." They appealed to the gods. All the gods appealed to the superior gods — Brahma, Vishnu, Siva. They all called for an emergency meeting.

"What's this? What's happening? Sun, what's happening?"

"I don't know. This is a command from a chaste lady."

"Don't you know that we ordered you to go through this function daily."

"Well, sir, you did. I was obeying all these days. But here there is a higher command that seems to be more powerful than you all. I can't break that. I can't do anything."

"Okay, that's your right." they said. The superior gods went on, "Let us all go to that girl. Only she can help us out of this situation." So they all came down and begged her, "Please, he made a mistake. We request you to withdraw your order."

"Well, that's all right. You are requesting me, but if I take away my word, the sun will dawn and my husband will die. I can't afford to lose him. What are you going to do about that?"

Then they all turned to the saint. "You have to do something."

"All right, then, I withdraw my curse." So he withdrew the curse, and she withdrew, and the sun dawned. Who is more powerful than the gods? A chaste lady. Why? You may call it just a story. But there is a scientific reason for this. The reason is, all alone I can be a good devotee. To worship a god is easy. Even to worship a master is easy, because at least you see him as a Swami, he talks nice: God, Yoga, this and that. He looks like a spiritual presence, hm? You can easily bow at his feet. And it's even a little more easy to bow at the feet of a statue, because it is always sitting there quietly. It doesn't grumble at you and if you look at it with a smiling feeling, you see the smile coming back. You know it's there. You can bring fresh fruit, take it back! You can bring decayed fruit, take it back; isn't that right? He doesn't ask, "What are you doing? Why are you bringing me this fruit?" You can sit and meditate in front of him. The statue will just be there. If you sit and sleep, still the statue will be there. It's not going to question you. It is you who are worshipping. According to your feeling, you get the result.

So image worship is easier than the worship of a living person. And it is still more difficult to worship an ordinary man who comes as your husband. You don't see a spiritual guru in him. Just a husband. How can he be a guru? So to treat an ordinary equal or even a little less than your equal, as a guru, means you should have tremendous capacity. That is why the wife who could see that leper, a fellow who runs after prostitutes, a terrible sinner, as a god — what more penance do you need? What more control of mind do you need? You're the God of gods. The entire nature will obey you. That is the reason why a loyal chaste lady is respected, adored and worshiped. She is doing something that cannot be done easily by anybody and everybody.

Does it make sense? It is not just a story. Not everybody could do that. Even in those ages, *Satya Yuga*, the age of virtuousness, there were only about seven of them. Because it is rare. So you see how difficult it is to be a householder? But if you could follow that, you are even greater than a monk. If not, take an easier path. It is more simple; just let go.

I want to become a householder but it creates a kind of guilt in my mind that I am doing something second-best. Why aren't both paths the same?

It was really good somebody asked this question. I want to assure again and again and again, please don't think it is a second-class thing. It is the first-class thing if you can get the first-class compartment. You know, in the train we have first-class compartments. So you can make it first class if you have the right person. Or, even if you have the wrong person, if you have the courage like that lady. If you don't mind whether he is a drunkard or an ordinary person or a vicious person, "I'll take him as my husband or as my wife. I don't worry. This is my part, let me perform my duty well. You have your freedom. Go, come, go, come. I have certain duties to perform, I'll do it." And that is the best way to bring him around. He can never go like that constantly, continuously. One day or the other his conscience will tell him, "What kind of thing am I doing? Look, there is an angel, there is a goddess in my home. And I am going here and there, doing all these things." One day he will come and fall at your feet. We have stories like that also. Yes. Not, "Okay, if you go that way, I'll go this way." Who is going to teach whom then? It is not a competition. At least one should be a saint. Then you are freed. Like a Sannyasi. When someone takes this vow, he sticks to that. He is an individual. So as an individual he can still be a householder.

I understand that you are going to give a marriage ceremony. How will it be different from an ordinary wedding? What special qualities do you expect of the householder?

You should have an understanding partner who will have the same goal in life. If you will be like the two eyes seeing one thing, then you can always be a householder. But let not the house hold you. You hold the house. That is something really great — much greater even than monkhood.

Yes, that's why even Siva has *Parvati*, Vishnu has *Lakshmi*, Rama has *Sita*. That's why, you know, all the gods are married, according to the Hindu philosophy. And not only that. You know how they address the gods? It's not like here. *You* lose your name to become Mrs. Jacobson but there the lady comes first. Sita-Rama, not Rama-Sita. Sita-Rama, Lakshmi-Narayana, Parvati's Pati (Parvati's husband). Who is he? Parvati's husband. You see? Because of Parvati, He is respected. Because of Lakshmi, Narayana is great. Because of Sita, Rama is glorified. Almost all the gods are addressed that way.

That means, as I said, there are two eyes. Can two eyes see two things at the same time? If you ever try, whoever sees you at that time will take you to the asylum immediately! We have two eyes but we see one. The eyes cooperate. There's no divison. There's no right and left. They're two halves of the one whole. Just like two wings of the bird, two oars of a boat. If a householder can be like that, that is something celestial, heavenly. The monks will salute them. There are many, many great householder saints. For example, Janakan. Janakan was a king, a householder, the father of Sita. That's why her name is Janaki. Janakan's daughter is Janaki. All the monks went to him. Many of them went to him for initiation. Know that. We don't need to go into those older days. Even in our present days, Ramakrishna and Sharada. They were a married couple. You saw Sant Keshavadas. He's a married man. In what way is he different from me? In a way, he is a better Sannyasi, I should say. Having a wife and child, he's still doing so much. Why? Because of the beautiful, beautiful girl, Rama, his wife. She's an angel. Anyone could lead a householder's life with an angel like that. Because they both have the same interest in service.

If you marry somebody, and you're interested in spiritual life, and you want to go to the retreat, she must be the first one to say, "Come on, come on, it's getting late." Not, "You're going to the retreat? I planned to go to Miami." That is enough to make you a monk. A householder's life is harder than a monk's life, no doubt. You learn a lot as a householder. I say that those who want to become monks, if they have even the slightest doubt about their resolution, better be a householder for some time. That's a good place to learn many things. The Hindu steps are like that: first brahmacharin (celibate student), then a householder's life, and after that if they are both tired of all these fun and games, "We've enjoyed enough, let's get into some Yoga, no more husband and wife. Let the children take care of the house, maybe go into seclusion or do meditation." Then for some reason if they want to separate further, they become monks, or if one dies, the other becomes a monk, a totally free Sannyasi. If your wife is not going to stop you from serving, why not have her? She'll be a wonderful secretary for you, she'll be a good road manager, same way for a girl.

So what comes first? God and his creation. Your station of life should help you to reach that. Whether it is as a monk or as a householder, doesn't matter, if it is going to help you serve God and humanity. I say God and humanity because God never needs your service; the expression of God, the expressed God, humanity, the entire nature, needs your service. God in the form of nature includes your house also then. The house is part of the nature, so then you can be a good householder.

So it's something really great. The only thing is, it's a bit hard to find a companion like this nowadays. We always seem to be independent. It's very difficult for the egos to go together. Even a couple of renunciates living together have their own egos. How can there be this freedom or understanding between two ordinary individuals? Each one would want something for himself or herself. They don't marry as renunciates. But the purpose should be that they both come as renunciates. "I renounce myself in your hands, you renounce yourself in me." That means, "I am for you, you are for me, and we are both for the world at large." That is a vow you make when you marry. "I've dedicated everything of mine for your sake, for your help, for your safety. Your comfort comes first." That's what the couple should say to each other. Then they both should say, "Our comfort comes after the comfort of the world." Imagine a couple like that. Is there any need for them to take monkhood? No. They're already monks. Married monks. If you can't find a partner like that, better be alone. Then you are a single monk.

You asked about a marriage ceremony. Yes, I am going to conduct a marriage ceremony for a dozen couples, and the next week I'll be performing a monkhood ceremony for another dozen people. That means it's all the same. I was a householder myself. Now I am a big householder. The world is my house, all are my children. Who said I am not a householder?

Eighth Day

A Great Morning

Rabbi Shlomo Carlebach

Today the retreatants are treated to Rabbi Shlomo Carlebach. Like Rabbi Gelberman who spoke two days before, Shlomo (as he is commonly called) is both a representative of the Jewish tradition and a teacher for people of all faiths. He too incorporates many aspects of the Jewish tradition, chief among them the Hassidic. But perhaps it would be more accurate to say that he embodies that tradition, because — like the Hassidim of Europe — his presence is vital, exuberant, physical and heart-felt. His talking is mostly story telling, and singing and dancing are as much his way of teaching as is talking. Many of the songs he sings are of his own composition, and all of them come from the heart. Many people said that he was a Jewish Santji, as both he and Sant Keshavadas radiated the same Bhakti approach, alternating their spoken words with songs in which everyone would join, and bringing their listeners to a state of tremendous exuberance and feeling. In fact, there was a great deal of concern on the part of the staff of the retreat that the wooden structure of the satsang hall (though solid) might not withstand (literally) the rhythmic jumping and dancing that Shlomo induces in his audiences. But it did survive quite well, and everyone shared in a time of spontaneous group feeling and expression that was unique.

Shalom, Shalom. Good morning. You know, we have three fathers: Abraham, Isaac and Jacob. Abraham taught us how to say good morning, Isaac taught us how to say good afternoon, and Jacob taught us how to say good night. So we have three prayers to say — in the morning to say, "Good morning, God"; with afternoon we say, "Good afternoon, God"; at night we say, "Good night, God." But the people who really pray don't only say good morning to God, they say good morning to the whole world.

One of our holy masters, before he would go to the synagogue in the morning, the first thing, he would run to the houses of poor children who didn't have any parents. Because when do children feel most that they have no parents? When they wake up in the morning and nobody says, "Good morning." What a sad morning. So he'd run and he'd knock on the door of all those children with no parents. "Poor sad little babes." He'd knock on their window. "Hey, good morning." He would give them so much strength for the whole day. Then he would knock on the windows of all those women who were widows, because when does a woman feel most lonesome? In the morning, when nobody says good morning to her. What a sad thing. He would knock at the windows of all those women who had no husbands and he would say, "Good morning." You never know when you meet somebody on the street and you say good morning, what you are doing for them. You never know. Maybe you gave them a whole day, and maybe a whole life. Maybe you gave them back the world, and maybe you gave them back their own soul.

So, "Good morning" to you, friends. Good morning to the lake. It's a beautiful lake. Good morning to the trees. (*He sings: La la la la la la la la*) What happened to all the tambourines you had? Why don't you join me? Does anyone have a guitar? Play anything you have. Ahhh. Listen, if the holy Swami says that I should stand here, I should stand here, right? (*Swami Satchidananda has just come in and suggested that Rabbi Carlebach stand on a higher platform so that everybody could see him*). You know what a good friend is? A good friend is somebody who tells you your place. (*La la la la la — more singing.*)

Let me tell you something very strong. What is the whole idea of dancing? I'm not talking about ballroom dancing, I'm talking about real dancing. I have nothing against ballroom dancing, but that's not what I mean. What's the whole idea of dancing? Let me tell you. The Earth has something very strong about it, a tremendous gravity, right? Very strong. If you have to eat, it's pulling you. When you have to pray, the gravity isn't that strong, right? If you have to go to the bank before three, wow, do you have gravity! That means that there is something very special about the Earth — gravity. Heaven is very holy but it has no gravity, right? So it's very simple. You realize, "I have to get out of this gravity," you got to get out of here. So you tell the Earth, "Thank you very much, you know. I love you. You're sweet and cute and everything. It's just that I'm not so turned on to your gravity." Right? So, you tell the Earth, "I'm taking off!" So you jump a little bit, give a little jumpela. But while you give this little jumpcla, y'know, the Earth is practically laughing in your face, because the Earth says, "You crazy? I know you'll be back." So this is crazy. So you have tears in your eyes, you want to get out of the gravity, and the Earth is laughing. So you come back. You say, "Earth, I'm not finished, I'm going back again." Each time the Earth laughs a little bit less and finally the Earth sees you continue to do that, y'know, you're just getting out of the gravity, you're reaching for Heaven. You come back but it's okay, you're getting out of it. So the Earth asks, "How about taking me with you to Heaven?" And then the strangest thing happens; each time you put your feet on the ground, the

Earth doesn't pull you down but gives you a little push up. The more you dance – you can feel it physically – the more you dance, the Earth doesn't pull you down. On the contrary, the moment you touch the ground, tssst. Earth says, "Please give my regards to Heaven; get there fast."

(*Chanting*)

Tell you what, maybe sit down for a few minutes. I'd like to tell you a good story. I want to share a few things with you. I see that you are strong into the holiness of silence, the holiness of words. You know, there are two kinds of words. Sometimes, I tell you something because how else will you know what I mean, right? But imagine, if you would know exactly what I want to tell you, I wouldn't have to talk to you. Right? But then, there are some real holy words. It's not that I want to tell you something which you don't know. When someone comes up to you and says, "I love you," the words are so holy. They're not spoken just because I want you to know what I think; the words themselves are heavy words, heavy words. I want you to know something very deep. Words which are only uttered to make you know what I think, after you know what I think, you don't remember the words. But the words which I speak which are real, these words stay with you. They walk with you. Can you imagine if people would communicate on that holy level of holy words, real words? You see, when I utter holy words to you, and you utter holy words back to me, then we are always together. You can be at the end of the world and I can be somewhere else, but these words tie us together. When God spoke to us on Mount Sinai, He said, "I'm God." Do you say, "Listen, God, I knew this before. Couldn't You just tell me something new. You know? Tell me something that has importance." I knew God is there before, but when God told me, "I'm God," what holy words. Right? And we answered back, you know, we answered back, "We are your people." What holy words.

Anyway, I'd just like to wish that you, and myself, all of us together and the whole world, should begin again to utter holy words, real words. I'll tell you something very deep; when someone calls your name, it's a word, but you feel it. When someone doesn't love you and just wants to get your attention for something, they utter your name, it's meaningless. When someone really loves you, they say the deepest words there are: they call your name. Ahhh, you called my name. What a deep thing it is, what a deep thing. I don't know if this is true according to medicine, but according to our Kabbalistic beliefs, if a person is dying, God forbid, and if a true friend would stand there at that very moment, when he wants to die, and call out his name, he'll stay alive. But it has to be on that level, you know? You must have a friend who really can call your name. Can you imagine how many people are dying, and how many people would not die, if they would have one good friend who would call them by their name?

The second thing I want to tell you, which is very, very deep, is what gives you most strength. There are spiritual vitamin pills, right? What gives you the most strength? There are two, three things which give you strength. Whenever you do something good, it's not only for that moment you do something good, it really gives you strength to do more good, or to do less evil. If you don't do something wrong, it gives you a tremendous amount of strength. "I didn't do it." It gives you strength. I mean, reading books and knowing all the laws is very sweet, but it doesn't give you one ounce of strength, believe me. Not one ounce. Maybe it even confuses you sometimes. What gives you strength is doing and not doing, that's strongest.

I want to share with you and tell you a little story. I don't know if some of you are turned on to the Psalms. Then again I have to tell you the sad thing that the Psalms, the way they're translated into English, makes it such a sad book, y'know? I can't even recommend it, the way it is. But if you would know a little bit in Hebrew with the commentaries, it's not just a book of prayers. It's a book . . . really giving you holy advice, how to serve God, in the deepest sense. There's a very beautiful passage that says, "I am hiding your words in my heart. It will give me the strength not to sin." Do you know what David Melech Tov (The Good King David) says? That "the strongest, strongest thing is, stronger than doing or not doing, is if you want to say something and you don't." That gives you the greatest strength. Inner strength, you know? I want to say something, but I don't. But then, Hassidim, holy Hassidim, puts a little sugar on it, and they say like this. Sometimes you have to talk, right? It's a very holy gift, God gave us the gift of talking. But the question is, where are those words coming from, a shallow place? So they say, "Words are uttered, but before I uttered them, I was hiding them in my soul." Those are very holy words, secret words. When you utter those words, or when someone else hears those words, they really purify you. Nothing holier than words. You know, one of the holy masters says, "Don't tell what you do good," because imagine I do something very good and I walk around telling everybody. This good deed would not give me any strength. It would give me publicity but not strength. One of the holy masters said, "If you do something good and somebody knows about it, it's a punishment from Heaven." You know, the whole thing is, God is so secret and so deep and so holy, how can you serve him unless it's also a secret, very deep and holy? Idol worship doesn't need secrets.

I want to share this little story with you. I don't know why I'm telling you this story. I'm telling it all over the world, so I might as well tell it to you too. You know, friends, in Krakow (*in a singing tone*), in Krakow, a city in Poland, we little Yidalach (*little Jews*) lived there for many hundreds of years. We were driven out, we came back. We had nowhere else to go, so we came back. My great great great great grandparents came from that city. So the story is, somewhere, somewhere, in the old cemetery in Krakow, there's a grave hidden away by the gate, and there is a little tombstone. And on the tombstone it says, "Here lies Yosaleh, the Holy Miser." So join me softly.

(*Rabbi Carlebach sings, "Yosaleh, Yosaleh . . ."*)

In the sixteenth century, everbody was so poor. But there was once a rich man in the ghetto, his name was Yosaleh. But Yosaleh never gave one penny to a poor man. You know, he knew every part, he knew where his nose was, where his feet were, but he didn't know where his pocket was. Couldn't find it. You know, he tried to, but gave up. Can you imagine? Not one time in his whole life did one person see him giving one penny. But you know, friends, even misers have to die, right? The only thing is, when a non-miser dies, you think that maybe he'll come back one day; but when a miser dies, you know he'll never come back, because who needs a miser, right? I want to share something deep with you – in Kabbala, Jewish mysticism, which is very deep, a sinner is not an anti-God; he's just not living up to God's will. A miser is an anti-God, because God is giving, and he's only taking. Anyway, Yosaleh's dying, so the people in charge of the cemetery – you know, in those days, it was so hard, Jews had to pay so many taxes even to be buried; not only when they wanted to live did they have to pay, even when they wanted to die they had to pay. So they come to him and they say, "You never gave a single penny to the poor; you're dying now, buy yourself a grave and give a thousand rubles to the poor." Leave it up to Yosaleh, he chisels them down to fifty. So they get very angry and they say, "Yosaleh, if you don't give us a thousand rubles, you have to bury yourself." Leave it up to Yosaleh; he says, "Okay."

So, his trip was coming to an end, and you know, before you die you say, "Hear, O Isreal, the Lord our God, the Lord is One." So Yosaleh said, "God is One," and he took off. Which is even more disgusting than the rest, right, because which God is he talking about? (Can you imagine what a low creature? The last minute of his life, he only thinks of rubles, which he can't even take with him. And suddenly, you know, he says,

"God is One," and he goes.) The whole city would have nothing to do with him. This was Monday night that he died. Tuesday night, because Yosaleh had a wife and children, someone felt compassion toward them, and late at night took a little wagon, put Yosaleh in the wagon, and took him to the cemetery, but he wouldn't dare bury him where all the people were buried. He dug a little grave at the gate, threw Yosaleh in, and covered Yosaleh with the earth. This was Tuesday night. Thursday night, someone knocks at the door of the chief Rabbi of Krakow, Rabbi Kalmin, and says, "Rabbi Kalmin, please help me, I have no money to buy food for Sabbath." Rabbi Kalmin says, "You? How did you live all these years?" He says, "I didn't have a job in ten years, but I don't know, every Thursday morning there was money under my door. But not this Thursday morning." Two minutes later somebody else knocks on the door and says the same thing. "Thursday morning . . . but not this Thursday morning."

(Sings: "Yosaleh, Yosaleh . . . What a holy miser. Yosaleh, Yosaleh . . .")

That night all the poor people of the ghetto came, and everybody told the same story: "I don't know what to do this Sabbath because I didn't find any money under my door this Thursday morning." Y'know, friends, it's strange how few people really see another person. People look at you, but do they see you? Suddenly it all came back to them and they realized that maybe they had looked at Yosaleh but they had never seen him, because you know Yosaleh was a strange character.

When someone would come up to Yosaleh and ask him a favor, he would shine in a million ways. He was no miser, stark and bitter; he would say, "Oh, I'm so glad you're asking me a favor. What's your name?" He'd get out a piece of paper and write down his name and ask him, "Where do you live?" Write down his address. He'd say, "You have a wife and children?" "Yes, I have a wife and children." Then, Yosaleh would say, "What can I do for you?" He'd write down every word the other person's saying. But the craziest thing happened – after the person finished telling Yosaleh what he needed, Yosaleh suddenly changed his voice and said, "Are you crazy? Do you think I'd give you my precious money!?" Then he would laugh, throw him out, and walk away. But Thursday morning, Thursday morning, there was that money under the door. But naturally they didn't think that it was Yosaleh.

(Sings: "Yosaleh, Yosaleh . . . Yosaleh, Yosaleh . . .")

So Rabbi Kalmin said, we have to make a fasting and on Sunday the whole congregation has to be in the synagogue and ask Yosaleh for forgiveness. The whole city came, and all day long they were reading the Psalms, and they were asking Yosaleh, "Please forgive us, we didn't even bury you." Well, just about sunset, Rabbi Kalmin was so heartbroken because he felt he hadn't really asked Yosaleh for forgiveness, such a holy person, a really holy person, a real servant of God. So he opened the holy ark and he said, "Yosaleh, please forgive us." At that moment, Rabbi Kalmin suddenly felt very weak, he had to sit down. He fell asleep, and in his dream he saw Yosaleh. Join me.

(*Singing: "Yosaleh, Yosaleh."*)

Yosaleh was shining like ... not like the sun or the moon ... much, much deeper than that. And Yosaleh was smiling and he says, "Rabbi Kalmin, please, tell all my brothers and sisters to stop asking me for forgiveness. This is the way I wanted it. On the contrary, I thank them, I thank them that I was able to do a little bit of good without anybody knowing." He says, "Please tell them I'm here in Heaven, it's very beautiful here, but it doesn't compare to what I felt when I put money under broken doors." So Kalmim says, "Yosaleh, just permit me one more question. Weren't you lonesome when you were buried there all by yourself?" So Yosaleh says, "Believe me, I was not alone. Our Father Abraham, our Father Isaac, our Father Jacob, Moses our Teacher, they carried me, Elijah the Prophet with a candle in his hand ... he showed me the way, and King David with his holy harp was singing a song till I found my place."

(*Sings: "Yosaleh, Yosaleh ... What a holy Yosaleh." Singing, clapping, joyously.*)

I have to tell you one thing, very very important. You know, there's two lights, there's the inner light, which we are vessels for, and then there's a surrounding light, which is so high it has no vessels. You know, sometimes you meet people and they have a little light inside. Some people really have a surrounding light. It's something. They don't say one word to you, but something happens, right? This surrounding light is coming from the secret good deeds. When you do something good, you know it, someone else knows it, it's an inner light, it doesn't surround you. The surrounding light comes from holy secrets. Imagine two people. Nobody knows, just those two, so a great light surrounds them, and puts them together. So I'd like to wish you surrounding lights, deep lights, holy lights, a lot of secret and holy words, and holy deeds. What a beautiful thing to do something for somebody, without anybody knowing. How beautiful to save somebody's life when the other person didn't even know he was in danger.

Friends, could we *Mamish*, get together very close? Let's get together. I can't come down to you so you'll have to come up to me. Let's get very close. Let's just say "Good morning" to each other very strong. Maybe I could ask my holy Swami to join me. It would be so beautiful.

There is a story, that two holy masters hadn't seen each other for a long time and they were so happy to see each other. The story is that one kept talking, so the other one said to him, "Listen, Holy One, I have to go to sleep." So the first holy master said, "I want you to know that you're very sweet." So the other one said, "Holy one, I want you to know you're also very sweet." But then, listen to this one . . . The first one said, "Holy friend, tell me what you do at night?" So the other says, "At night I correct yesterdays." Did you hear that? "Every night, every night, I correct my yesterdays." This is what he did. Then the first one says to the other one, "What do you do at night?" And this is what the other said: "I prepare myself for the morning." Did you hear this? This is so deep. So, Shalom, Shalom.

You know, my darling friends, let me tell you something. A lot of people teach us how to correct the yesterdays, but we need holy, holy teachers to teach us to prepare ourselves for the Great Morning. So I would like to bless my holy friend and Master, the holy Swami, that he should find holy pupils to teach them how to prepare themselves for the Great Morning. Because this is what the world needs, a Great Morning. Everybody talks about what we did wrong yesterday, but so few people tell us how we can do better tomorrow. So, Shalom, Shalom, Shalom.

And maybe some of you know that the textbook of Jewish mysticism says one thing very beautiful. "Some people ask what, and some people ask who." Some walk up to you and ask, what are you? And some ask you, who are you? The person who asks you what you are hates you, but the person who asks you who you are loves you. But also, some people ask God, what are you? And God doesn't answer. But if someone asks God, who are you? He always answers. Shalom, Shalom, Shalom.

(Swamiji requests a strong song. Rabbi Carlebach sings with joy and liveliness.)

I want to say something very deep. I think I told some of you that the world needs a face, right? People need faces. The world needs a face so badly. The world has no face any more. And the name of that face is peace, right? And we think people are peaceful, they have a face, right? People have no peace, they just have a nose, something sticking out there in the middle. You don't know what it is. And something sticking out here, but not even ears, just little fleshy pieces. Ideas need faces, right? An idea, if it doesn't have peace in it, has no face. Everything needs a face; friendships need faces. If you are friends with somebody, would you always fight or sometimes fight? It's a sweet friendship but it has no face. I want you to know one more very deep thing. When I honor somebody, I don't honor them to their back. I have to bow down to their face, right?

Do you know what peace is? Peace is that I love you so much, that I give you back your face. So when I give you back your face, I can honour you and then there is peace between us. You know, a lot of people love each other but they don't honor each other, give each other faces. So the world needs desperately people who have a face.

Do you know what the saddest thing in the world is? Children, when they're born, they have faces, the most beautiful faces in the world. We don't know how long it takes to unface them, but we're doing a good job, y'know? Especially schools. You can look at a child who's already in first grade, if it still has a face. Look at kids in high school. Oy Veh! "No face" is written all over their faces. A *nebuch* (nothing). It's heartbreaking. When you go to college, you're not even human any more. Not only you don't have a face, you don't have a heart any more. You don't have a head. They're defaced. Oy Gevalt, Gevalt. You know what a person who has a face does to you? It depends how close you are to them. Sometimes they give you back your face or sometimes at least you feel, "I wish I would have a face." That's also very deep. "I wish I would be peaceful." That's also a little bit of peace. Not only peace is holy, the prayers for peace are also holy. And even if the person is not on the level yet to pray for peace, but he would love to pray for peace, he can pray to God, "Please help me to pray for peace." It's also holy. And even if a person is not on that level, he's just praying that he should pray that he should pray for peace . . . that's also holy. I don't know if you know — sometimes you wonder how come Nature is cruel, y'know, animals eat each other. I want you to know something very strong. According to our Kabbalistic tradition, at the very moment when Cain killed Abel, the vibrations touched the animals. But if man would never have killed, the animals would never have thought of killing. It never occurred to any animal — killing. But the sad difference between animals and man is that even if the vibrations of killing touched animals, they never kill their own kind. But man is so low, he can kill his own brother.

I want to share something with you; it's just a consolation. Do you know that Cain didn't want to kill Abel? Because he didn't know that you *could* kill. He just hit him over the head, and suddenly Abel fell to the ground. He didn't move. So Cain was crying. He says, "Please forgive me, I'm so sorry. I was only angry with you. Please open your eyes." And the Talmud says something so beautiful. I don't know if you know this, Abel had a little dog. Abel was very strong with animals, he was very close. Cain was working in the fields, but Abel was only with animals all the time and he was close to animals. So he had a dog and this dog was also crying, barking away, "Please, open your eyes." And then all the animals of the world came and they were begging, begging Abel, the first human being who was killed, they were begging him, "Please don't do this to us, don't do this to us. Don't be killed." And the Talmud says that for three days, they were all sitting around Abel, crying and crying. But do you know what will happen on the Great Day? On the Great Day, God will take all the Cains and put them next to all the Abels, and all the Cains will say, "Brother, I didn't want to kill you, believe me, I didn't. I was just angry. Please come back." And a great miracle will happen, that Abel will come back. Shalom, Shalom, Shalom, Shalom.

Can you imagine, Cain and Abel will do a little dance, what a dance, what a holy dance. Then all the animals will dance. All the hills and all the valleys, and you know what we will do? We'll tell the sun, "Sun, have you ever seen the moon?" Sun will say, "No, what's the moon about?" So we will tell the sun, "You're very beautiful because when you shine, there is no darkness. But do you know there is a little moon, so holy and deep, shining even in the darkest night. It's a very deep light." Then the sun will begin to shiver, and the sun will say, "My light is beautiful, but it doesn't compare to the deep light of the moon." So the sun will not move and will wait after sunset for the moon and the sun and the moon will meet. What a dance. The sun and the moon will dance together, and then we'll ask them both a question. We will ask them, "Holy sun, holy moon, have you ever seen a candle?" They will ask us, "What is a candle?" And this is what we will say: "When the sun is shining there is no darkness, when the moon is shining it drives the darkness a little bit away, but the candle leaves the darkness as it is; it's just shining." What a deep light. It doesn't even disturb the darkness. It's just shining. And then the sun and the moon will ask, "Who brought such a great peacefulness to the world?" And we will say, "One candle." Because it takes a light which is really a lot to bring light to the world, but it takes only one candle to bring peace. Shalom, Shalom, Shalom, Shalom, Shalom.

I wish you to be little candles, friends. Holy candles. Do you know how beautiful the darkness is? Darkness is also beautiful. But it's only beautiful if there's a candle. The candle is so deep, it tells the darkness, "Do you know why you're dark? Because you think you're nothing. I'll show you something. You're beautiful. You're deep." That's what the candle does. Some of us have friends like the sun, like the moon. We need a friend like a candle, that doesn't change us; it just tells us, y'know, "You're so deep." Because how do you know that only light is light? Maybe darkness is light also. On the Great Day, the little candles will know, "I have so much light. Why am I not shining?" Then there'll be peace in the world. And people will see each other. People will walk around as little candles and look at each other. And they will say, "I'm so sad I never saw you before. I saw the electric light, I saw the sun and the moon, but I didn't see you." Everything in the world can be seen with light. But the face, only by the light of a little holy candle. So, walk around as candles, the secret candles, and put faces on everybody. Tell the world, it's time.

Shalom.

(*Swamiji says, "He's come all the way from Europe, just to be here." Rabbi answers, "I just want to tell you, because Holy Swamiji says I've come from Europe. Believe me, I would have come from the other world just to be with you. Thank you.*)

Satsang with Swami Satchidananda's Devotees

On this Friday evening the retreat is exactly one week old. By now, everyone is fully into the spirit of the retreat and it is building towards its climax on the weekend.

This evening, for the only time during the ten days, Swamiji is not giving satsang. Instead, he is giving mantra initiation to more than 100 of the retreatants. So, in his place, the evening program consists of shorter talks by several of Swamiji's senior students and disciples. These are not talks about Yoga, as such — instead, each student talks about himself and how he or she became involved with Yoga and with Swamiji. These are very personal talks, and are very much appreciated by the retreatants. It gives them an opportunity to get to know some of the staff that have been serving them, and to see that the staff — like themselves — are persons who are still seeking and working on the spiritual path.

Hari, the coordinator of the retreat, serves as MC and introduces each of the speakers.

The first disciple to speak is Amma, one of Swamiji's personal secretaries. She has been with Swamiji for about five years and is looked to by many of Swamiji's "children" as a mother figure because of her constant, helpful counsel and love for all. After leading a short prayer, she begins:

I'm the last person who should be speaking here, because I really don't know much about Yoga. I am just beginning to learn how to be a Yogi. What do you want me to tell you?

Question from audience: Can you tell us how you met Swamiji and how you got to be his secretary?

I don't know. I still wonder sometimes, when I write a letter or do something for him. I still wonder how he signs it. Or when I do a little something for him, I think, "Swamiji really put on something I ironed." I still can't believe it yet. It's something almost all the followers of Swamiji desire, because we always have the idea that being physically close to the guru means much more bliss, much more love, much more attention and all the things we're always trying to have in life. When we find the guru, all our emotions are geared towards him and even intensified. Even the negative, the ego, we transfer to him: "I want him to approve of me. I want to do this nicely so that Swamiji knows I'm serving him well."

217

Before I became Swamiji's secretary, I had a very intense life. I had everything under the sun; I was pampered by life. And I have suffered also a great deal. But still I would say, "Oh, Divine Mother" — because I am a great devotee of the Mother — "I know there must be some real greatness in this world of Yours. Please, before I die, let me meet that greatness face to face." Ah! Because nothing used to impress me.

But I remember the first time I had an appointment with Swamiji. I walked in and saw just some wooden benches. It was so simple. But as soon as I walked in I felt that finally for the first time in my life, I was walking into the palace of an emperor. He wasn't even there waiting for me. I had to wait for him. Anyway, it has all developed and finally, by the grace of God, I am working with him in a personal, close capacity.

I would like to tell you something else about this also: I've worked a lot in my life and I've been pretty successful in what I did. So when I came to Swamiji I was sort of confident. At least I would not make so many mistakes in certain areas of life. Like answering the phone, for instance. Well, when I began working for him, I realized that I didn't know how to do anything — not even picking up the phone and answering it.

That's how it is when one starts working closely with the guru. It's funny, people look at those who are closer to Swamiji, who walk close to him and hand him the glasses and do this and that and they might think that we are sort of privileged. Well, with whom does the doctor spend more time in a hospital? Hm? You tell me. With those patients that are getting better? Or those that are very, very sick? He spends time with those who are very sick and less time with those who are getting better. And those who go out of the hospital, he might just see once in a while. They might just come in for a check-up once a month. And that's the truth with the guru also.

In my association with Swamiji, I have found, as hard as it is, that the ego has to die. This is what Swami Nirmalananda has been telling us all these days. And this death, this agony, seems to be eternal. It's a hard process sometimes, but it all depends on what one wants.

All through my life, ever since I was little, I didn't know exactly what I wanted to do or be but I did know that I wanted to meet greatness face to face. I knew it must exist and I wanted to experience it. I wanted to love it. To love until I died. I was always dreaming of this great love. And I've always wanted to be free.

I had already started practicing Yoga before I met Swamiji but when one encounters one's own guru there is no doubt whatsoever. That's it. And through his teachings, and through all that he is purging out of me,

I'm, beginning to have a glimpse of this true greatness. I am beginning to find love. And I'm finding that love is not something we can *do*. It is just being. It is just loving. It is just being totally possessed by that love. And that love that possesses you completely is the only way to be free. That's the only thing I know.

Probably it is an easy way, because this love which is all-consuming does its own thing in you. As in the practice of all religions, the practice of Yoga ultimately is to calm and purify the mind so that it can become the reflection of the true Self. But, believe me, if I tried to just analyze my mind or purify it in my own little way, I just couldn't do it. For instance, if I see Swamiji scolding someone, my first instinct is to go to the defense of that person. I don't even know why he is being scolded, but that's where my heart goes. So sometimes, my mind might say, "Oh, my God, Swamiji is being unfair to him. How can that be?" But then immediately my love for Swamiji races up like a fire and just burns out the thought. Then only my love for him exists. So it's easy. It does it by itself. And ah, it's a pretty wonderful thing, when sometimes in the midst of tears, I realize, "Oh – how wonderful. It is one little step more towards freedom."

And, you must have seen by his talks that Swamiji is no abstract guru. It is by working, by doing, by participating in every little detail of life, that he teaches us. One thing I have learned through him is that there is nothing else for me but *now*. I have no past, because even if I think of what is past, I'm thinking of it now. And even if I'm planning something for the future, I'm planning it now. So the future doesn't really exist. It is now that exists. And this conviction, this complete realization of the "Now," is very freeing. Swamiji is really a free man.

As I have told you, I have been very pampered in my life, so money has gone through these hands sometimes just like they had holes in them. I never even had any consciousness of saving anything. And I am a Catholic, so I grew up with all these ideas of sacrifice and rebelled against it. And you know how Swamiji speaks about renunciation very often. Well, with love, there's no renunciation at all. It's just a taking over. One doesn't renounce anything. One only becomes free. Simple. For instance, when I go to buy something now, it is a beautiful experience for me. "Here, this costs so much. In two months, it'll cost two dollars less. Fine, I'm going to go and buy it when it costs two dollars less." That means I'm two dollars freer. It's a wonderful feeling. Or when I'm walking in the street and I say, "Oh, I have to take a taxi." Then I think, "No, why should I? I'd better take a bus; it's only that distance." Then, "Why take a bus? I might as well walk. It's good exercise." That means that I am one taxi and one bus freer. So that is renunciation. That's the way I see it. It's just becoming free. Slowly it happens. So these are all the things that I'm beginning to glimpse by the grace of God.

What is your normal day with Swamiji like?

The sure thing about a day with Swamiji is that it is totally unpredictable. But it is very full of work. We rise at 5:30 and do our sadhana. And around 9:00 he calls us and we usually go to him and have darshan and report the business of the day. This brings to mind another thing I've learned through Swamiji. I had been used to working like this: "From 9 I'm going to do this, at 10 I'm going to do that." So when I began working for Swamiji, I used to say to myself, "I have so many letters to read. I'll finish them by 11; by lunch I'll be free of that and in the afternoon I can give him all these things. He will be happy."

But it never works like that. You never know what's going to happen. It used to make me very nervous at the beginning, because I used to think, "Oh, I'm never going to get the work done this way. How can one work like that? This is a little bit crazy!" So that is something I'm learning too — to be elastic. The mind has to become elastic, not to be nervous, to be calm whatever happens and be ready. Like sometimes, he might say, "All right, I'm going shopping now. Get the checkbook ready. And I have some things to pick up." Where is he going shopping? What is he going to pick up? Nobody knows. You just have to be ready and go and see what happens. So that's how a normal day is.

What does Swamiji eat and how many hours does he sleep?

He normally eats just once a day, when he's not fasting. He eats at noon, usually sauteed or steamed vegetables and some grain or dhal (lentils), something like that. Then in the evening, he eats a fruit. In the morning, he has a warm beverage. I don't know how many hours he sleeps. I really don't know what he does at night — whether he works or meditates; I couldn't really tell you but I suspect that he sleeps very little.

Well, that seems to be all. Thank you very much. Om Shanthi.

After Amma, the retreatants hear from Sister Hamsa, one of Swamiji's newly initiated pre-monastic students from California. Her warmth and wonderful sense of humor about herself keeps the audience in almost constant laughter. She helps many who might have felt they were the only ones who face obstacles to see that even those who have practiced for a few years have many trials, but that they are all nothing in the face of sincere dedication and a sense of humor.

Hari OM. Can you hear how fast my heart is beating? I'm awfully scared to be up here. Anyway, I'd like to tell you a few experiences I've had which brought me to what I'm doing now. When I first started going to the Integral Yoga Institute in San Francisco, I would just come in off the street all filled with anxiety and confusion and just mixed up. I would come inside and get filled with this peace and calm. I'd never had that experience before. And I came to know that it was Swamiji. I could just see it in his photograph. I just wanted to be like that. For a long time I never talked to anyone very much 'cause you'd come in the door and see everyone in white clothes and they'd go, "Om Shanthi," and I thought, "Wow!" They all looked so pure. (*Laughter and applause from many retreatants.*) It was wonderful but I just didn't dare speak to anybody for months. So I just kept coming to Hatha classes and Family Days every Sunday and I would just feel this peace and calm. But then, I'd go out and be three feet out the door and have all the anxiety again. The peace didn't last very long, though I felt it was something so deep inside. Who understood it? But that's what I wanted *all* the time. So I just kept coming and coming. And I would see Swamiji at satsangs and lectures and different things. I was blessed in that way many times. And I used to meditate for five or ten minutes at a time. That was as long as I could sit up straight. At one point, I heard that Swamiji would be giving mantra initiation. All I knew was that it was an aid to meditation. And I really needed an aid! It was going to be given at a five-day retreat like this one. Well, I only signed up for the weekend because I didn't think I could make it for five days!

I'd been to one other retreat and it was horrible! We had two bananas for dinner one night and one and a half cantaloupe another night! I just thought I'd starve to death. The night we had one and a half cantaloupe, we were sitting there in the hot sun. There was dust everywere. You couldn't even sit on *grass*. It was just dust. And we were observing silence. And I was experiencing a lot of mental pain because it was just very heavy with all the discipline. I'd never done anything like that before. So we were sitting there in a circle and everyone's silently eating their cantaloupe. And you're so miserable you think you're going to die! And I was eating it and eating it. And all of a sudden the person next to me scoops out a piece of his cantaloupe with his plastic spoon – and you know how slippery it is – a piece just went "shwoot" and fell in the dust. Well you can imagine how it is when you have half a cantaloupe and one bit goes in the dust — and that's all you're getting for dinner! It was terrible! (*Laughter*) Well, not only that — it happened to the guy twice. I just looked at him. And he looked at me. It was so ghastly. So we just sat there laughing, 'cause it was so ghastly. But you know what? They say that karma means that your every thought, word and deed comes back to you. And mine came back. The next thing I know I'm sitting there, and mine goes in the dust. It wasn't so funny then. Well, anyway — that's enough about cantaloupe!

So that's why I just signed up for three days! I figured three was all I could handle. But anyway, at that retreat I received the initiation. We were taken in groups. I felt like I had rigor mortis. I was so scared I would forget my mantram, I didn't know what to do. Well, it turned out you get them on written cards, so you see, you never need to have anxiety. But who knew? So we sat there for six hours because there were so many people to get initiated. And it was just terrible, you know, because I couldn't sit there with my back straight, and I just wanted to go home and lie down and go to sleep and get some food. And I started thinking about cheeseburgers and french fries.

Of course, that's just one side of it. You know, I really didn't know what I was getting into. I didn't know at all. And look at me now! (*pointing to her yellow renunciate clothes and cropped hair. Laughter from the audience.*) I started out telling a funny story but instead it's a beautiful story. When I went to bed that night after initiation, I lay there and I had a mantram! I didn't even know what I had. But I just knew then that I had never had a blessing like that in my life. It was so fantastic.

What happened next was that I went home to my boyfriend and in two weeks he left me. He said to me, "Well, I'm splitting." I was crying and crying; I didn't know what to do. I just didn't know which way to turn. I thought I needed him. That's what I thought, that all I needed was someone to love me and someone to love. That's all I'd ever thought. So I didn't know what to do. I thought, "Well, I'll sit down and meditate; I'll say japa." But I sat there and just cried and cried and couldn't stop. I just had to go to bed. But I couldn't go to sleep so I just took Swamiji's photograph and I held it to my heart. And I just said, "Swamiji . . ." and I was just crying "Please help me. I don't know what to do, where to turn." And I think the crying stopped, because I did go to sleep that night. And I had a beautiful dream about Swamiji. I just couldn't believe it, it made me so happy. I had just been as low as I had ever been and the next day I was so happy. I didn't know what to do except dance around. A friend told me to meditate on the dream. I had never even thought of that. So I did and it came to me what the dream meant. It meant that

Swamiji was saying, "Give all the love that you were giving your boyfriend, all that affection, all the energy and devotion, to me. If you give it to me, I will *never* let you down. I will always love you. You will never be disappointed." that was it. I just couldn't believe it.

And I knew then what my life should be. All I had to do was give everything to Swamiji. I knew what the answer was and it was so incredible. At the initiation, Swamiji had said, "Some people will feel the effects right away. And some people won't feel it for a long time." Well, every time I would think of the boy who left me, I'd say my mantram. And just like that (*snapping her fingers*), it would go. I never again had a moment's anxiety over him *ever*. And from that moment on, Swamiji just pulled me in. I guess he does that with all of us. You know, I don't know exactly what's happening, but I know *that's* what's happening. So that's the story.

Question from audience: Would you talk about life at the Institute?

Well, it's phenomenal in many ways. When you move in, your spiritual growth is speeded up a lot. That's what happens immediately. And another thing, when you walk in the door to move in, you feel like you've come home. That's what it is. You're home. And there's that peace all the time. What I mean is, you always feel that refuge whenever you walk in the door of the Ashram or the Institute. It's fantastic to have such a supportive environment. The people are all doing just the same thing as you. They all love Swamiji. They are all having difficulty with all these things. They all want the peace that they see in Swamiji. And you always have someone to help you, someone to give you love. So that's very wonderful.

The schedule is: we get up for 4:30 meditation (*each Institute decides what time, some meditate at 5 or 6*). We sit until 6 am; then we do our Hatha Yoga by ourselves in the meditation room. Then there's some time to do whatever you like: your personal study or sometimes going back to sleep! (*laughter*). At 9 o'clock the business day begins. In San Francisco the Institute is mostly a teaching center. One person is in charge and she also happens to the housemother who cooks for us. And there's a secretary and treasurer. We work really hard all day long. And what's fantastic is that you get up and say, "Well, today I'm going to do this." But all day long, people hit you with things that "must" be done. So you never know what you're really going to be doing. You think you're going to do a certain thing, but someone comes and asks for your help. That's the thing. You always have to help people. That's what we're there to do, but most of the time you *want* to do what you want to do. That's what's fantastic, because you think, "If one person asks me one more question, I'm going to ring his neck." But people are *always* asking you for your help and you always have to serve, serve. We hear that word "serve" so much. When it seems hard, I think, "Look at Swamiji. He never stops serving for an instant. Why can't I do that?"

Then we have our main meal in the middle of the day. We eat quite a bit (*laughter*). I think that's because we're giving up a lot of other things and so we just cling to that one pleasure. Did you see that fantastic sign in the retreat dining room? It says, "Brothers and sisters, if you overeat, maybe you're hungry for something that food can't satisfy." That must be it.

So, after the main meal we do work the rest of the day, have a light fruit supper and then there's meditation from 9 to 10 at night. It seems that we sit there and say, "Wow, I wish I could go sit in a cave somewhere and just meditate all day and get really high and have a beautiful smile all the time." But Swamiji's way in the ashrams is to do Karma Yoga — to just work as hard as you can. And that's what makes us happy really — to be as busy as you can be, to do things for others and not for yourself, to eventually get out of thinking about yourself. That's when you'll be happy.

How did you come to take the pre-sannyas initiation?

Well, once in a family meeting of all the Institute people on the West Coast, Swamiji just slipped in a little sentence which said, "When you are ready for Brahmacharya Diksha (pre-monastic initiation), I will let you know." And I thought, "Well, that's wonderful." But I didn't even know what it was and I didn't ask. But I felt that when I was ready, he'd let me know. So some time went by and then he told us that if you wanted to progress faster, this was a way to do that. It was very exciting — we all want to go faster. And here was a way we could do it with our practices. Then the bomb came, which was that he was going to be giving Brahmacharya Diksha in one week. We're just standing in the Institute kitchen and everyone was asking everyone, "Oh, should we take it? Are you going to take it? What is it?" (*laughter*). And no one was quite sure what it was, except that you received a new mantram and it was going to help you be a renunciate. Who could ask for more? (*Laughter*) I mean, if that's what you want! (*more laughter*)

Well, anyway, the first thing they told me was that you had to wear yellow all the time — yellow for the rest of my life! It *was* my favorite color — but that's a bit much! So there I am, thinking maybe I won't do it cause how can I wear yellow for the rest of my life? I didn't even have to talk to anybody. I just knew that this was what I'd been born to do. I had been born to give my life to God and to Swamiji. I didn't know anything else, but I knew that. I didn't know what was coming next and I couldn't believe the whole thing — it was like watching someone else, 'cause it all came so fast. I didn't know what it was but I *did* know. And there was nothing else. It was no big thing either. That's the funny thing. It was perfectly natural. But people had a lot of silly questions about what it was all about and what we'd wear, etc., but Swamiji wouldn't even answer them. He said, "I'm not even going to read this list. If you have one question, if you have one doubt, then you aren't ready." And he said, "You should be so hungry for it, that even if I said, 'No, you can't have it,' you'd make me give it to you. And that's the thing. We just knew. You didn't know what you were getting into, but you knew it was right.

So that's what it is — something to help you become a renunciate. But we're sort of like little babies. We're just like everybody else — except we have a fire in our hearts that might be a little stronger right at this time. So, we took the initiation. We received the Gayatri mantram, which we say along with our personal mantram. And, Swamiji's taking care of us now. He's just helping us all the way. We don't know what's coming next but it doesn't matter.

Why is your hair all cut off?

This "crew cut", — Well, we all had to cut our hair. In India the women never cut their hair, I understand, except when they take Sannyas and have their heads shaved. Again, it's Swamiji's way to help us, because he said, "You're going to have doubts. You're going to lose sight of what you're doing." You see, the maya will come in. It will come again and again. But every time I wake up in the morning, every time I touch my head, every time I look in the mirror, I'm reminded of what I'm striving for. And he also blessed us with these orange scarves. We're to wear them always. This reminds us because it is the color of renunciation like Swamiji wears. This is what we are striving for.

What exactly do you mean by renunciation?

I think it means giving up all worldly desires and attachments. Isn't that it? (*great gales of laughter from the audience*) I think an even better way to put it is giving up everything you want to do that's tying you down.

Swamiji says that whenever you're unhappy, whenever you're depressed, whenever you're disappointed, look at what is causing it. Do you know what it is? It's because you wanted something for yourself, and you didn't get it. That's always the way. The only way you can be happy is to get rid of that, get rid of trying to get things for yourself.

Do you feel free?

In a way, I know I'm caught, if you know what I mean. I feel as if I have no choice. I don't mean it in a bad sense. I have no choice — God is drawing me like a magnet. It's a fantastic feeling. I feel like I have a little secret inside, which is that I know a way to be happy all the time. Do you know? I can't say I am happy all the time — it goes up and down, up and down, a million times every day, but I know how I can get out of going up and down — I just have to continue my practices.

Couldn't a person choose to be a householder and still be holy?

Oh, yes. Both ways are holy. It's just that I've been drawn this way. I don't understand how, because all my life I wanted to be married. In fact, I think marriage would be fantastic. That's the part I can't understand. How phenomenal to have a partner who you could have that fantastic union with — to have the closeness, to have someone to share with.

But the thing is, as you get closer to God, you feel God more in your heart and you feel fulfilled in your heart. But I think being married is fantastic. I think both ways are fantastic. They're both miracles.

What are all these Sanskrit names about? Where do you get them?

People who have Sanskrit names have been blessed by Swamiji with them. The names seem to be something that you grow into. I'm not sure how it happens, but I know Swamiji picks it just for you. It's something that you will turn into. And they're so beautiful. When we break silence, you should even go to some of the staff members and ask them what their names are and what they mean.

How did you come to move to the Institute?

I'd been going there for a year and a half and I always really knew I'd like to live there. But there was so much I had to give up before I could move in. I had to give up boyfriends; I had to give up smoking dope. I knew someday that I would, but there was stuff I had to work out first. Then one day I was lying in my room. I was on unemployment and the sun was shining. It was a beautiful day. I had plenty of food in the icebox. I was as happy as a clam. I had slept late; I was well-rested. I was in perfect health. There was nothing more I wanted. It was fantastic. If I had been offered a trip to Hawaii, it wouldn't have made me happier. I woke up and I knew that there was nothing more in life I wanted to do. I couldn't wait to move to the Institute.

Thank you for listening to me. I hope you are all blessed with peace and joy. Om Shanthi.

Next the retreatants hear from Madhava, the Executive Secretary of the New York branch of the Integral Yoga Institute. As were Amma and Hamsa, he is introduced by Hari. By way of introduction, Hari says, "Executive Secretary means simply that he is director of the daily affairs and oversees what happens at the Institute."

Did you say I was director of the affairs at the Institute? What we seem to learn in Yoga is that we're not directing anything — we just watch. I'm thinking now how wonderful it is to have a sister like Hamsa. It's really great to have people of your own age who are understanding and learning and giving. It's really an inspiration to see.

How fortunate we all are to have all of this incredible energy flying around. Maybe you think that people who live close to the Institute or close to Swamiji are always in this incredible state of glowing. But I must tell you, it's really not quite that way (*laughter*). So it's nice for the people who live and work at the Yoga Institutes to come here and let go too.

Is there any question anybody has or should I just talk about whatever comes to mind?

What are your duties as the Executive Director of the IYI?

I think my duty is to let go. That's really my latest inspiration. New York is a very hustle-bustle place and naturally I get into this "*my* Institute, *my* classes, so many Hatha Yoga classes, and *I've* got to organize all this," you know? In other words, I'm saying that I pick up the vibration that all of New York City has. It's like all of us have slowly, slowly picked up a completely different vibration here. You're not the same as when you walked in five or six days ago. Everybody now is really glowing and energized. Well, in New York, it's easy to get lost in the New York kind of vibration. In fact, it's almost impossible not to. It takes a strong person, a developed person, not to. So I'm sure you've seen us running around like New York, too — you know, "Do this, rush, do that, storm into the chanting," etc.

The unfortunate thing is that it makes you very unhappy to be like that. Swamiji accepts us, whatever we are. He accepts our craziness. He says, whatever you do is okay; just do it in the name of Yoga. Do it for other people. So if Hari is a great real-estate dealer, he becomes a great real-estate dealer in the name of Yoga and finds us the Yogaville Ashram. Sure! Do you think buying the Ashram was done overnight? Or the New York City Institute building? No. So all of this is going on and Swamiji watches over all of it.

I was a great mechanic, oh a really good mechanic! So I became the Institute mechanic. And it's fine just as long as I don't carry that weight of "I am the mechanic with my heavy bag of tools and my sexy tool belt and my 300 lbs of mechanical knowledge, which nobody else has except me and which makes me so valuable as a person . . . " You know what I mean? It's fine to have all of those things, but probably I'm learning that the best way to be miserable is to carry around the weight of being the mechanic or the Executive Secretary or the real-estate man or whatever the weight is that you carry.

Amma was talking about heart — that she wanted to love something all her life. That's something I think we all really have in common. In my first meeting with Swamiji, I was very shy and withdrawn and found it really difficult to even say anything. I was like that with others too because I was worried about how I looked, how successful I was. "Does this person really dig on me? Am I really coming over all right? What's the impression I'm making?" And you're really blocked up when you're like that. It's really something to experience. And naturally I'm still carrying a lot of that around.

Anyway, at the first meeting I had with Swamiji I told him that I seemed to be able to do all kinds of things — "I can write papers on French literature, I can do theatre, I can be a mechanic . . . I can do anything. But somehow I don't seem to feel anything in my heart." That was what I told him three years ago. I told him how in relating to girls I always seemed to try and grab onto them and own them, you know? And it made me miserable. But I didn't know what to do about it. It was almost at the point where I could actually feel a physical pain in the heart sometimes from emptiness.

He just said, "It's okay."

And I said, "I would really like to work at the Institute." I wanted to be like the people there — they really impressed me a lot. They were so cool and calm and pure and collected, you know? Actually, it was like a game of one-upmanship: who could be the coolest and calmest and wear the whitest whites (*laughter*). I didn't know then that they were all lunatics! Yes, they're all lunatics. I know that now, but then I wanted to be like them.

Swamiji said, "What can you do?"

"Anything, I suppose."

So he said, "Fine, just be there. There's one thing I believe in — natural growth. The Institute should grow to the point where it needs you and you should grow to the point where you need the Institute."

Well the first part was completely obvious. If there's a job open, there's a job open. The second part didn't strike me until about eight months later. You know how you're walking down the street and suddenly — "Dong!" — you understand something. What he was trying to tell me was that I should come to the point where I would feel that the Institute was really a field where I could work out everything I needed to work out — to have that faith. And there was even a time when I told myself, "If you're really going to be consistent about this, you have to assume that everything you need is going to come from the Institute. Everything — if you need a wife, it's going to come from the Institute; if you need money — whatever your desires are — somehow it's all going to come through this relationship with the Institute." And I would hang on to that faith, at least mentally, just to hold myself back, when my mind wanted to pull me away.

So, back to the heart and letting go. Three years later, I'm still the same except that being at the Institute has given me a little more capacity to be as loving as I want to be. That's really my only desire.

Do you accept new people to live in the Institutes? How does it happen?

Yes. You know, it's important that we hold hands in the cities. If we don't make that little effort to smile, to be nice, to put our effort into Yoga, to give whatever we can give, we'll have to wait another six months for the next Yoga retreat! Remember that.

Sometimes people say that the people in the New York Institute are cold, you know, like business people. And it's true to a certain degree, but don't think that they're happy being like that. They don't know any better. But we learn by doing. By really being in pain, you learn where you don't want to be. So sometimes people come to the Institute and see one of the staff's a little bit uptight because he's just taught three or four classes or he's just dealt with so many business people over at the Building

Department or this, that and the other. Somehow he's lost sight of himself, he's become unconscious. He see's you sitting there on the couch and he just says "Hi" and zips right on past you. And you go home and say, "Oh, that's terrible; there's no warmth in the New York IYI." It may be true. But, you know, you have a lot to offer. You yourself. I'll give you an example.

There's a girl named Day. She came to the Institute and just about bowled us over because she'd come and bring us lemonade. And we'd say, "Lemonade? Day, are you all right?" because normally you got up to the kitchen, grab your own and go back to work. So, that softness taught everybody. She came without even asking. She busted the doors down. She's still doing it and it's a wonderful experience. So, don't think you don't have a lot to teach us. Don't think we don't all have a lot to share together.

So, people who are interested in practicing the disciplines and who want a kind of shelter to do that with other people can come and live at the Institute. We're not saints; we have pizza — it's the whole thing. We practice and try to understand and love Swamiji. And serve other people — which sometimes is difficult and sometimes is beautiful. And we're learning that every time we're unhappy, it's because we didn't get something that we wanted. We're learning about that and about what we really want, what works and what doesn't work. And hopefully we're opening up our hearts.

Does Swamiji visit you at the Institutes?

Swamiji gets pulled here and there by our interest. But I would say, don't always wanting him to make you high; become happy by yourself serving. Our trouble is, even if we are happy, we can't believe it. Even if he tells you you are divine, you really don't have any faith. A part of you says, "What a wonderful experience I just had. I feel so light, so even," and another part says, "What's this? I can't wait to blow it apart." You know? Unconsciously, you'll say, "Oh, no, it's impossible, I must be unhappy somehow." Because our conditioning in that direction is so incredibly strong. We have to let go of that feeling, "Well, I must be unhappy; I must be dissatisfied somehow." I think it's a lifelong process almost.

What helps most along the way to developing an attitude of selfless service?

I would say, just doing it. Everybody starts from their own place. And that's why Swamiji more or less accepts wherever we start from. You have to want it. That's really the main prerequisite. Want it. You may not know how it's going to happen. It doesn't even matter. But you want the change — you want to be more happy. And things come out of that. You have to have faith in that.

Did you know immediately when you saw Swamiji that he was your guru?

No, that was the one part of Sister Hamsa's talk which I couldn't personally relate to. I experienced intense doubt. People always used to say, "Isn't Swamiji great? Don't you feel all the love pouring out of him?" And I would feel embarrassed because I wasn't feeling a lot of love at all, much less from Swamiji. So, I would have to hide a little bit from those people. I felt, "Leave me alone. Don't bug me with this. I'll develop at my own rate."

At my first retreat, I remember thinking, "Is he or isn't he? What is he? Who is he? Do I feel it? No, I don't seem to feel it — it isn't there — but I want it — this must be it!" You know, up and down, up and down. One of the most beautiful parts of my experience in Yoga is my relationship with Swamiji — how it has gradaully and slowly opened me up. It took me three years to be able to say, "I love you," to him, to let go that much. So we all come from different places.

Do people who live in the Institute have jobs outside?

Yes, they may, because that's how they pay rent.

Is it required that you practice celibacy while living there?

Yes.

How to visit the Ashram?

Phone ahead; give them some notice. There's even guest applications which explain the routine there. You know, it used to be people would just pop in and flop somewhere. It's not that way any more. It's like a mini-retreat.

Isn't it more spontaneous the other way?

Well, you can be spontaneous, but the minute someone lets you know that they're coming, there's a certain graciousness involved in that. Anybody can just drop in, it's easy. But there's a certain graciousness to say, "Hey, I'd like to come." It's something that I've learned here. Don't forget that everybody is serving everybody else, so you serve them by telling them you're coming and then they can serve you by giving you what you want – in all ease and harmony and peace. That's it.

Thank you all. Om Shanthi.

MC becomes lecturer as Hari takes the speaker's platform himself.

Now it's my turn to introduce myself. My name is Hari and I'm staying at Satchidananda Ashram-Yogaville as the President. Swamiji has somehow managed over the years to provide me and all his other disciples with all kinds of nice "toys" – positions, jobs, titles, experiences, relationships, material things – everything that somehow it was in our karmic arrangement to come in contact with. As indicated by some of the other disciples who just spoke, the things that come to us seem to be the things which are necessary for us so we can undergo certain experiences.

You see, people think that "renunciation" means you're going to come to an Ashram and give up everything you had before. But renunciation is basically a state of mind. You might be renouncing your job with some Wall Street firm and find yourself working twice as hard on the Ashram's books! The only difference is that you begin to understand that the job you are doing is sadhana or spiritual practice. You're not just grinding out another job to get your pay check at the end of the week, so that you can have fun on the weekend and dread the coming of Monday morning when you have to start the miserable cycle again. Instead, you become more conscious of what you're doing while you're doing it. The work itself becomes a meditation.

You may wonder why I'm speaking about work. Well, everybody has their particular orientation and when I came to the Institute, the thing I got most immediately and directly involved with was Karma Yoga, or work. You see, Karma Yoga involves the body and the mind in a very obvious, I'll use the word "gross," way, in the sense that it's very apparent that you are *doing* something. In a more subtle practice like meditation, it may not be so apparent that you've fallen asleep (mentally), but if you're supposed to be sweeping the floor or cleaning the toilet, you can't fall asleep. It's very obvious that you're either doing it or not doing it. So for those of us who have grosser minds, it's necessary to have grosser forms of sadhana. Consequently I found myself getting involved more in the service aspect and it seemed to suit my personality. I would spend more and more time doing Karma Yoga as a way to meditate and at the same time to thin out the ego a little bit. It purifies the mind and makes it a little more subtle so it can appreciate the subtleties and the greatness of meditation, which is several degrees harder to comprehend than something like service.

I remember the first time I did some service at the Institute. The place just glowed because it had Swamiji's presence in it everywhere. It was like the place itself expanded in my consciousness to the point where I was more conscious of every little detail there. One Saturday I got a call from the Executive Secretary. I was accustomed to sleeping till ten or eleven o'clock but I had signed up to do some Karma Yoga. "Do you think that you could come down here and mop the floors and clean the toilets?" I was so excited. "My goodness, the *Yoga* Institute – I'm going there and I'm going to clean!" (*laughter*) Then a thought struck me – I'd better not tell my mother exactly what I was doing. She'd feel terrible because there I was, 19 or 20 years old, and I hadn't cleaned a toilet in my life. And here I was, on my one day off from school, going down to the Yoga Institute to clean. She'd definitely think I was nuts.

But not half as nuts as the proprietor of the hardware store, when I went there to buy some implements – a towel rack and a garbage can – which the Institute had asked me to get for the new dressing room. Oh, I was so excited – you may think I'm just putting you on, but I really had this experience – "Oh, I'm not only going to clean – I'm going to buy something; it's actually going to be there in the dressing room and the students are going to come and use it. This is great! This is fantastic!" So I went to the hardware store and I was really excited at the prospect of actually succeeding in this divine mission! (*Hari is laughing as he tells the story and the entire audience with him*). I said to the man, "Do you have a towel rack?"

"Why, there's a whole rack of them."

"You *have* them! You have garbage cans too?"

I was literally beside myself. I even dropped the dollar bills out of my pocket, I was so excited. That poor man in the hardware store couldn't figure out why this poor guy was so excited about a garbage can and towel rack. And I didn't try to explain. I just ran out of the store and got to the Institute and put the garbage can in the right spot, the perfect spot. I thought about it for ten minutes. Then I put the towel rack into the wall, right under the mirror – lined up – just so and later on I even got to put up a dixie cup dispenser! Oh, the service was just intoxicating!

Of course, sometimes I'd look at myself and say, "You're really pretty weird; what's happening to you?" But through some kind of inspiration it seemed to be that way from then on. Every possible opportunity, I wanted to serve at the Institute. It wasn't even that I thought of it that way; it was just that where there was a vacumn, where something was needed, I found myself drawn in.

And within a few months, people would say, "Oh, you're Swamiji's secretary now — you write letters for him, teach classes, he asks you to do this and that for him — how did you do it? What did you swing?" And the funny thing is, the important thing, as I can understand it, is that I didn't really do anything except have the keen desire to put myself there and wait for an opportunity to do something. And just that keenness and enthusiasm created an energy field which had to attract something. I wanted to serve; I wanted to do something, so along came the necessary opportunities.

How did you first come in contact with Integral Yoga and Swamiji?

Well, the beginning that sticks out in my mind is December 1, 1966. A few weeks before that, I had seen Swamiji's picture in the newspaper, saying he was giving a lecture and Allen Ginsberg was going to introduce him. (You know that picture of Swamiji with his beautiful face and all the love coming from him?) And I had just about gotten to the point where I was thinking. "Well, you know Larry, as really together as you are when you go to school and drive and meditate and take your 100 acid trips — still it seems that, as masterful as you're becoming, these 100 acid trips don't seem to be doing the thing for you. Maybe you should consult someone who might know a bit more than you, eh?" Just about this time I saw that announcement in the paper, and even in the face of scathing criticism from my friends ("What are all these Swamis coming here; Swami — what's a Swami?") I decided, "Well, I'm just going to go and see what this is all about."

So the week before the lecture, my friends and I were taking one of our traditional, ritual weekend acid trips (*laughter*), and suddenly a funny thing happened. I decided to recollect a long lost memory of some Yoga postures I'd learned somewhere when I was thirteen. So I started doing them all night in this kind of acid frenzy. Then the sunrise came and it was time for the next part of our usual ritual. We went trooping out to Central Park and began our "sunrise service," which this particular morning consisted of jumping around in the trees! So there we were, jumping from branch to branch — really carrying on and having a good time. All of a sudden, I landed on one branch without the usual safeguard of being ready to grab another one – because I was getting a little confident. So, suddenly I heard this very disconcerting sound – "snap" – and I landed about forty feet down.

As a result, I was hobbling around for about a week. And this is right before Swamiji's lecture. That would normally have been enough to discourage me from doing anything. And the night of Swamiji's lecture, none of my friends with their cars were around. Should I go on the SUBWAY? I *never* went down to the subway. So first of all, you have to have a friend with you when you're making a new scene, right? But there was nobody into going with me. Then second, I had to go down on the train, and third, my leg was really hurting. But somehow I had just decided that I was going to do it. And I did it.

I hadn't even met Swamiji yet, and already, somehow, he had made me overcome my usual *tamas*, my usual laziness, to get down there to at least see him. Then I had a very interesting experience at this talk. First, I was amazed at Allen Ginsberg's introduction. Since I was 19 years old and a hippie from the Bronx, and trying to leave behind the cultural trappings of the bourgeoisie, Allen Ginsberg was naturally one of my folk heros. I couldn't believe the reverance he had for Swamiji.

Finally, Swamiji spoke, and the one point that I still remember from that talk was that we tend to see everything according to what we have in our own minds. We project what is in our minds onto the outside world and then say, "Um hum, I know what *this* is." Then we start calling the shots. "This is this. And this is that." That's a common psychological principle; a lot of people may have known of that. But it really impressed me. Particularly when I walked outside and some friend from my college sees me and says. "Look; come here, I want to let you in on something." His attitude seemed to be that he had found out what was behind this whole scene. And he showed me this photo of Swamiji which was given out at the lecture and the tiny print at the bottom of this beautiful photo said, "Sponsored by the Integral Yoga Institute." See, this fellow happened to be an advertising executive. He said to me, "This whole lecture was just promotion for the Integral Yoga Institute!" and waited for my response, as if he had just unveiled the big secret to me. I said, "Didn't you hear what the Swami just said – that we tend to see things according to . . . " and as I was saying it I knew he wouldn't get the point. But that imprinted the point on me all the more.

One final experience about that night. You know how after one of Swamiji's talks or after any great saint speaks, the vibrations around the room are so nice that you don't immediately feel like leaving? That's the way it was around that church. So I was just waiting around outside.

Now, I had no contact with religion; no respect or knowledge or feeling to talk to anybody like a clergyman; I didn't know what they were all about. I couldn't relate to them at all, because I saw them as clergymen and I didn't know anything about their religion, so what was I going to say? But these two priests came by with their collars and they looked around, wondering, "What are all these people? What's going on?" So I just gravitated over to them — and I'm not the type that goes around talking to strangers — and started explaining to them, "Well, this was a talk on Yoga. It was given by Swami Satchidananda. He's with the Integral Yoga Institute and Yoga is . . . " And I just started repeating the things that Swamiji had said. And I was watching myself, "Hey, what's going on here?" I hadn't even met him yet nor had he met me and all of these things were happening.

So from that day forth, I just started coming down to the Yoga Institute every day, and having those other exciting experiences with the garbage can and the towel holder that I told you about — and then becoming a Hatha Yoga teacher. And little by little, I moved in, then became a full-time worker and had the job of Executive Secretary which Madhava has now. (But I think it was easier then!)

Some of you might be curious about the organization of these retreats. The foundation of it all is Swamiji's teachings of Integral Yoga as manifested in Integral Yoga Institutes and this new thing — the Satchidananda Ashram-Yogaville. The practices of Integral Yoga are taught in the Institute branches. More people are concentrated in a small space, so if you want to serve people, that's where they are. Then there's the country center — the Ashram, which is removed from the city vibrations. In other words, the Ashram can be a complete yogic environment much more easily than in the city. But it's also being done in the cities. And the people from the Institutes can come and get rejuvenated and spend some time in retreat at Yogaville and the people from the Ashram can go into the city centers to serve, being refreshed, having moved forward in their spiritual practices. So together they make a complete spiritual community. Both are equally important — and both serve as places which are open for anybody to come.

That reminds me of what I experienced when I first came to the IYI. You know how you felt when you started this retreat — hopefully not any more — or when you first came to the Institute, "Oh, it's a new thing and I'm just coming. They're the inside people, the people that are close to Swamiji. They are the teachers, the staff, and the whole thing is set, locked in place. And here I am, an outsider. I only rate second in this game, because these other people have been here longer." So what happened when I went to the Institute was one of the teachers there came up to me and said, "Don't forget that this place is yours, as much yours as it is mine. It's here for you. We're here for you. Swamiji and these teachings are here for you." Those weren't actually his words, but it was coming so much from his heart that the feeling got conveyed in just a few words. That was it. And I really felt it. From that time on, I really made it my own. The whole thing is here for people. The only reason that all these staff people are here at this retreat is because you're here. If the retreatants weren't here to give the staff an opportunity to do their sadhana or service in the form of Karma Yoga, then nothing would be happening. And of course there would be no retreat for the retreatants. We're doing this dance together.

There's just one more little story I would like to share with you about the guru. Once we were riding in the car with Swamiji. You know the expression, "Chip off the old block"? It's a very American expression, right? Somebody in the car used it. So Swamiji asked, "Oh, what's that?" So I explained in my formal way, you know, because you don't want to waste his time and attention: "Swamiji, you see, 'chip off the old block' refers to someone who is very much like their father. If a young boy is like his father, instead of saying he takes after him, they say, 'Oh, he's a chip off the old block.' "

Swamiji's mind is very quick. He looked at the three of us in the car and said, "Oh, then the three of you must all be chip-monks!" (*The crowd roars with laughter*). Think about it for awhile. It really gets to you. You may remember it later, right before you're about to go to sleep and you'll crack up again. He's so quick — he just came back with that immediately. The walls and roof of the cab nearly exploded because the three of us just couldn't believe he said that. And he laughed even harder than all of us.

Tell us about your first personal interview with Swamiji.

Well, it was beautiful. He received me so graciously, like a long lost friend or son. He took me into his room so graciously; that's his style. You know, he's pure grace. He just ushered me in. I had sent him a letter in Ceylon a few months before but he had never met me. I had sent him this letter, saying, "Swamiji, if you return to this country . . . " So when I sat down, he said, "Thank you for your wonderful letter." I said to myself, "How could he remember that that was me?" I had never been introduced to him and he got the letter on the other side of the world and he comes three months later and immediately says thank you for the letter!

Then I said, "Swamiji, when I was a young child, I always felt that I had some kind of calling that was something beyond ordinary things, something that was going to be completely fulfilling." When you were young, didn't you have the experience of thinking that your personal salvation or great satisfaction in life was going to be that you were going to become something, you were going to become a doctor or a teacher or something? So I told him that and also that I'd explored the usual channels — school and relationships, etc. — and I was beginning to feel that this was not really where my satisfaction was going to be. And he said, "Well, a lot must be the impressions that you have in your mind, the past experiences that are preparing you for the spiritual life." And as I was walking out the door, he put his hand on my shoulder and said, "Everybody in this world gets married, raises a family, has children, lives and dies, but one in millions renounces that and lives a completely selflfess life." That's what he said the first time I met him.

But don't feel that it's too austere, because here I am $6\frac{1}{2}$ years later and I'm very far from selfless.

Well, I've enjoyed talking to you, because you've made me remember things that are nice. Thank you so much. Om Shanthi.

Ninth Day

Honoring Siva

Ram Dass

So far on the retreat there have been, among the guest speakers, a Hindu singer and saint, who is also a married man; an American who, though raised a Christian, has become a Hindu and a renunciate; a Rabbi with a background in pshychotherapy, and another Rabbi u hose songs and stories come directly from the heart. It has been not only a mixture of different traditions and temperaments; each of the speakers himself has had a unique blend of unexpected features.

The same is true of the present speaker: Ram Dass. Certainly he has a background none of the other speakers have, and one which many retreatants identify with. Probably it would be best to say, not that he represents a religious tradition, but rather a secular tradition, a background independent of all the faiths represented here. And this too was part of the ecumenism of the retreat — that spiritual life is truly universal, embracing not only all faiths, but also those who do not identify with any particular faith.

Ram Dass of course used to be Dr. Richard Alpert. He had been an academician and a psychologist, a colleague of Dr. Timothy Leary at Havard University. That period of his life could be called his first "incarnation." The second came when, along with Leary, he began experimenting with hallucinogenic drugs, first within the academic context and then (when expelled by Harvard) independently. This period is interwoven with the whole period of the 1960's, a period of massive experimentation, mostly (but not entirely) on the part of youth, with drugs of all kinds — but particularly with drugs which seemed to promise to open up new areas and levels of consciousness.

For many, this experimentation was really a search for spiritual reality, and like many Ram Dass became more and more aware that this was the real quest. He himself has written about his own odyssey in his book Be Here Now, *in which he came to his third (and present) incarnation as the result of a trip to India. It was there that he met Maharaji, who became his spiritual teacher or guru, and upon his return to the West he himself became a transmitter of those teachings.*

Ram Dass (as he is now called) has been teaching in America off and on since his return from India in 1970. He still has much of the appearance that one associates with the 1960's: long hair, colorful clothing, and mellow vibes. He speaks in the language of the youth or counter culture, a language that is a mixture of words that come from East and West, a language that draws upon words from drug experience, Hindu mythology and philosophy, Western science and music. As a result of all this, many people find him an ideal conveyor of yogic teachings, spoken in a language they can understand and identify with, and with an unmistakably American point of view. For unlike Swami Nirmalananda, who became a Sannyasi and a renunciate, Ram Dass has returned to this country to develop a purely American brand of Eastern teaching. In both you see the mixture of East and West, in different ways and in different proportions; both seem to be providing a living synthesis between East and West, which is what ecumenism, on its largest scale, is all about.

In his talk, Ram Dass goes over much of the ground of his recent history, describing the evolution in his own attitude and understanding of Yoga and spirituality. In particular, he relates his own shift from a preoccupation with Raja and Jnana Yoga (the Yogas of meditation and analysis), which he had always assumed were the "higher" Yogas, to an appreciation and practice of Karma and Bhakti Yoga (the Yogas of selfless action and devotion). As many newcomers to Yoga share Ram Dass's earlier prejudices, his description of his change in attitude was really a valuable sharing by a man who considers himself to be more our "older brother" than a guru or "father."

Namaste. Just our being together here is such grace. So much blessing for one birth. Last evening, Hari described how, as Larry, despite a sore leg from a fall during a morning ritual under LSD, and despite the subway ride, and despite the fact that nobody would join him to go, he still found himself going to hear Swami Satchidananda in New York City, and he said, "He was already working on me — that he could overcome my tamasic nature to get me to go through all that to get to him." Certainly we cannot believe any less of this moment, that forces are afoot in every one of our lives that bring us here. It is not by chance that we happen to meet. It is interesting to examine that "chance occurrence," because it's certainly easy at the moment when it's all beautiful to say, "What grace, what a blessing. Certainly the guru is smiling upon me, to have allowed me to have satsang again." The reason it's worth examining is to see that the concept of an over-riding plan can become such a dominant theme in our consciousness, that when the drama changes, when the melodrama gets heavy, when you've just fallen from the tree, you can equally say, "What grace. Oh, thank you."

Swami Ramdas is reported to have said, when he had been thrown out of a temple one night and had to sleep by the riverbank where the mosquitos were particularly fierce and thus he couldn't sleep at all, "Thank you, Ram, for coming in the form of mosquitos to keep me awake so I could remember You." In the Ramayana, in the Tulsidas version, there are two places where Ram makes it very clear that unless one honors Siva one cannot come to Ram. Now Ram is an incarnation of Vishnu, generally connected with the preserving and maintaining and very loving and supportive forces of the world. Siva, on the other hand, is often associated with the chaotic or destructive or unpredictable or what are often called the malevolent forces in the world. Ram says, "Unless you honor Siva, you cannot come to Me."

There's a temple right at the very tip of India. It's where Ram did puja to Siva before going across to Ceylon, to Sri Lanka, to rescue Sita, His wife. It's interesting to reflect on what it means to honor Siva. It's so easy when you get high in a situation, whether it's satsang, meditation, or · whatever, and you say, "Oh, I feel the presence. I am being given grace." But what about when you're despairing and you don't feel the presence? Do you think that that's any less grace?

Last night Hari said one thing which I guess I disagree with, a sort of attitude which he reflected. He said he guessed he was doing Karma Yoga a lot because he was too gross to do any other form of Yoga. Now I must say that I shared that opinion about Karma Yoga. When I went to India the last time, in 1970, I went in order to meditate — in order to "get holy." I had been lecturing and teaching in America and doing whatever my hypocritical poor light would allow, and my own hypocrisy overwhelmed me and it drove me back to the feet of my guru. I was just drunk for satsang. I just needed it, I was hooked, I needed to get back to my connection. And my plan was to check in with him, get his blessing, and then go to a cave which he would bless me to do — this was my mind — and there I would sit and I would meet Babaji and I would meet Buddha and I would meet Christ and I would hang out with the astral team, and they would give me all the secrets and maybe I'd go north to the edge of Tibet and I would get some deep teachings from the Tibetans. And I would take deep meditation practices on various visualization exercises. I might even be walled into a building for three years, three months, three weeks, three days, three hours, three minutes and three seconds. I thought, "Now when I come to America the next time, boy is it going to be different. I'm not just going to be a phony Yogi, I'm going to be the real thing." And I went with the group that was together at that time. I went to Bodh Gaya, where Buddha got enlightened. It seemed like a good place to start because, you see, I couldn't find my guru — he was off being "irresponsible" somewhere, as he is wont to do!

So I went to Bodh Gaya and there was a meditation teacher there who was teaching Southern Buddhist meditation. So we all enrolled in these 10-day courses and we took a series of them. It was very intense and very austere. We learned how to cheat and how to cut corners but it still was pretty fierce. And there was no doubt that some headway was made in that meditation. But after about four of the courses I could see that the slippage was increasing considerably, and that the thing that was missing was that my heart was very dry in that situation. I couldn't open my heart. And just at that time I was invited to *Sivaratri* with *Swami Muktananda* in Delhi and I thought, "Wow, a good Siva festival. That will really get me moving again." But I didn't want to just walk out of the meditation, 'cause I felt, "Now that's kind of a cop-out. Here I came to meditate and I'm walking out to go dance and sing like any sloppy Bhakti would do." So I entered into an arrangement with the meditation teacher; I found out where he would be up in the mountains for the summer for the monsoons, and we went and made a survey. We went up there in advance and found another house that would hold three people and we rented it, fixed up the house, put a new roof on it, new water system, got the house all ready, and I arranged that when he went off for the summer, three of us would go and we would be with him, and we would get all this intense training in meditation. So I thought, "Well, as long as I organized for it and prepared for it, now I can go dance and sing. I can do my sort of sloppy stuff now, 'cause I'm really going to do the work later."

Well, on the way to Sivaratri it turned out that we met Maharaji, my guru, and in my puffed-up pride, I said to him – you know, like the good little boy reporting his work – I said, "I've arranged for this teacher, and this house, and I'm going to meditate," and I told him this whole story with a question mark at the end, like, "Aren't I good?" or "Isn't that wonderful?" or "Isn't this just what you want?" And his answer was, "If you desire it." (*laughter*) Well, that left me hanging. Cause what he was saying was, "If you want to go ego-tripping, go ego-trip." Now, I couldn't understand that. What self-respecting guru would say that meditating was ego-tripping?

That seemed like the height of profanity, yogic profanity. So I thought, "Well, he's just a silly old man, and he doesn't really understand, and maybe he's saying something much more profound that I'll understand only later, after I've meditated. So I'm going to do it anyway." I said, humbly. (*laughter*)

So when the time arrived, I went up there. I was so happy to get this place, because up until then, everywhere I had gone, there were always Westerners. After all, you don't go to India to hang out with Westerners, Western consciousness. And I was always hanging around Westerners, who were looking to me for something or other – which seemed absurd. I mean, they go to the well to drink, and then they're looking to polluted water they brought from the city. It's so bizarre. But there's a certain culture shock in India, and it's nice to have something to cling to, and I was sort of it. So, I went to the mountains, and I was so happy, I was finally away from all of "them," and that draggy feeling of having to be with them, and answer, and deal with that stuff all day. And I put away all the musical instruments, and all the Bhakti schmaltz, and I was going to settle down for serious business that was going to bring me to God.

Got the set of the mind?

Well, when I arrived there, within about two or three days, Westerners, other than the three people who had been invited, started to trickle in. First three, then five, eight, then eleven, till there were about twenty others. And I said, "What are you doing here?" because I thought we were hiding out, and we had kept it really secret, and they all said, "Well, Maharaji sent us. He said, 'Go be with Ram Dass.'" (*laughter*) So we took over a hotel in the town. But I stayed up in the house, with the group up there, and I wouldn't have anything to do with the people down there. I said, "Look, if you're in the town, that's up to you; I'll come down and visit every week but that's all. I don't want anything to do with any of you. I'm here for serious business." Well, then another week went by, and the teacher didn't show up. And a letter comes from him, saying, "Unfortunately, due to circumstances beyond my control, I will not be able to come this summer." Now I could see whose big hand was behind that! (*laughter*) There wasn't any doubt about that. So we arranged to take over the Gandhi Ashram in the town. We all moved in and we ended up having an ashram for the summer. We all disciplined ourselves. We read the Ramayana and fasted and meditated and lived in silence. We had a very profound, good summer together. It was a very beautiful, holy place.

And now the next component in that training program that is in answer to Hari's point last night, is that when I got to India this last time, when I was with my guru, he said, "Who'd you like to see while you're in India?"

"Well, I'd like to see Anandamayi Ma, the Mother. To have the darshan of the Mother, wow, wow."

He said, "That's good, who else?"

And I said, "I don't want to see anybody else, just you."

So he said to me, "See Lama Govinda."

"Lama Govinda?" I said. "I've already seen Lama Govinda. He's a very nice man. He's a good German scholar. He's a wonderful Lama, and that's lovely, but you know . . . "

But he said, "See Lama Govinda!"

So that was that. I kept stalling, but then I heard that Lama Govinda was going to be leaving for Dallas, so I went over to visit him.

Just to put a little flesh on the bones — just to give you a little feeling for the Divine Play in the whole dance — let me tell you the story in the rich way rather than the bare bones way. Because the means and the end are one. So there's no conclusion to anything I say. It's just like hamburger, it just keeps coming out. We had included a picture of my guru and Lama Govinda in *Be Here Now,* and also in the picture was Li Gotama, Lama Govinda's *shakti,* his wife. She had taken the picture on an automatic camera. And we had cut her off in the one we had used in the book, and since we were not acknowledging anybody's contributions in the book, we didn't acknowledge that she had taken the picture. And since all her pictures had stamped on the back of them — taken by Li Gotama — we knew she might have a slight investment in this matter. And I expected to get a little flack from her about this when I should see her. Now there was an additional matter — that Lama Govinda had written a letter to an editor of Newsweek in Chicago who had photostated it and sent it on to me, in which he said, "These Westerners go to India and they take the first guru that comes along, they're so hot to get a guru. Take Dick Alpert, he went and he got hooked up with the second-rate mind reader . . . " So now, I figured, if Li Gotama gives me any trouble about the picture I will discuss second-rate mind readers, but otherwise I won't do it.

So I'm not going to just start out. I have a little thing in storage. All loving, you understand. All yogic love — it's just the social dance. So the time came for taking pictures, which it does at most of Lama Govinda's scenes and I said, "Well, I'll stay inside, you go ahead." And Li Gotami says, "No, you've got to be in the picture too. I'm going to get back at you for . . . " And I thought, "Uh-oh, she just did it." So as we were standing, posing for the picture, Lama Govinda and I, with some other people, I turned to him and said, "Do you really think he's a second-rate mind reader?" That's all. And I just looked right at him. Well, he went through the change and realized that he had just been had. And he lit up and we looked at each other with total love. We had just broken through all the formalities and from then on our relationship was totally joyful.

So that evening the three of us sat together after the other guests had left and his mind was beautiful. It was like an exquisite crystal — like a beautiful jewel — very clear mind. He represented to me the kind of meditative Jnana Yoga — the intellect and meditation aspects of Yoga — which to me have always been the manly, tough forms of Yoga, as opposed to the Bhakti and Karma things which are what you do if you can't do anything else — if your mind is too gross to do anything else. So I said to him, "Lama Govinda, what is it you want me to do? Do you want to me go and study, do visualizations? What is it you'd like? Maharaji sent me to you. He must have sent me to you for a teaching. I now take you as my teacher. Tell me what to do next. I can go on with my Southern Buddhist meditation. Or go into Northern Buddhism. I've been very interested in the Ningma Pa. And I can go on with my Padma Sambhava mantram, or what do you suggest?" I sat as a seeker.

And he said, "No, you don't understand at all. I've looked at your book and all that. Your path is the path of the heart. Your heart is opening. It's all happening to you. You don't have to do anything."

He said that and I wouldn't hear it. I said, "Oh, I know all that, but tell me — what should I do?" Because you certainly couldn't assume that you don't do anything. You know?

And he said, "No, you don't understand. You're doing your path already."

Now, coming from him, it was incredible. It's one thing if a Bhakti says, "Oh, go be Bhakti." You say, sure, he's protecting his own investment. But when Lama Govinda says that, he's got to go against everything he ever talks about. So, in a way, it was incredible that Maharaji would send me to Lama Govinda to get him to tell me that my Yoga was Bhakti. So I began to reassess Bhakti Yoga. It took on a new dimension for me now. It was going to be made respectable.

So later, when I was sitting with Maharaji, I would say to him things like, "Um, Maharaji, um, how do you awaken *kundalini?*" I mean, just a question in the passing of the day. And he'd say, "Feed everybody." Feed everybody? I'm ready for *pranayama* and *bastrika*. Feed everybody? "Maharaji, how do . . . " "Love everyone." All he kept instructing me and all of us was, "Love, serve, remember . . . Love, serve, remember."

Now, I couldn't help but break up over the Cosmic Joke that I should go to India, to the deep, dark mysterious East, to learn the secrets that will bring man to final realization, to bring them back home to the primitive tribes in the outerlands, and I come back bearing the gift of three words, "Love, serve, remember," which have already been hanging around here years and years, as I seem to recall Christ reminding us. And in the two years I was in India, in total there were 14 days when I was not surrounded by Westerners, doing exactly the same thing I do in the United States. So what I was forced to do was what you could call a figure-ground reversal. I had seen hanging out and talking with people about God as what you do until you do the real thing. And now I had to flip it over and see that maybe that was the real thing and all the other things were support systems. Now, faced with the possibility that the rest of this incarnation my dharma was to do Karma Yoga and Bhakti Yoga, I started to examine the nature of these Yogas a little more carefully. And I must say I shared that little tone in the way Hari put it, that "I'm, you know, so gross, I just do Karma Yoga and Bhakti Yoga." It's sort of a very gentle path, we used to think, like going to church on Sundays. It's like, there were steep paths like Zen Buddhism where you just sit and think of nothing. But most people can't stand that because that's too steep. They need a support system like a God or something or a church or ritual to cling to. So there are these different steepnesses of paths and Karma Yoga has always been connected with doing good – grey ladies serving in hospitals – you know, a sort of nice, gentle way to come to God over the next 10,000 incarnations.

So I got into a deeper study of the Bhagavad Gita, which of course is the text for Karma Yoga, among other Yogas, and I entered full steam into Karma Yoga. I figured, "Well, if it's my Yoga, then I'll do it." Now, when I came back to America in '72, I was going to live not in time; I was going to live like my guru lives. He's just somewhere until he isn't there any more and then he goes somewhere else. You never know when he'll be there or when he won't. I figured I'd live outside of time – because time was really scaring me about the West. Schedules, like you're going to lecture Saturday morning at 9 o'clock. And many hundreds of people are going to expect your consciousness to get them off at 9 o'clock on Saturday. So everything you did Friday night, everything you did Thursday, you know if you had a lustful thought on Wednesday that was going to affect Saturday morning, so you had to watch it, you had to get so programmed. If you had two talks a week, you know, it wiped out the whole week. You had to just sort of sit in a straight-jacket to just stay together enough. So time was my enemy. I was always afraid to let go. So I thought, "Look, I'm not going to live in time, I'll just be where I am," and people would call me from New York to New Hampshire and they'd say, "Will you be there tomorrow afternoon? I want to come see you." Meaning, "Will you be holy tomorrow afternoon at two?" And I'd say, "I don't know." They'd say, "What do you mean, you don't know?" I'd say, "Well, I don't know where I'll be tomorrow afternoon at two." Meaning not only I don't know where I'll be geographically but I don't know where my consciousness will be. Because my consciousness – unlike Swamiji's – is not nice and even and smooth and together.

At this point, Swamiji sneaks up to the stage and takes Ram Dass's watch which was laying beside him on the stage and goes back to his chair in the audience. There is a lot of laughter.

My mind is a little bit like a roller coaster and it's not any roller coaster where you ride the same route each time. Each time it's a different route, so you can't tell. It's all pouring through you and everybody looks at you and they see the Highest Light, and you say, "Oh, boy. All I've got to do is keep cool and this is the way it's going to be. I can just be the transmitter." And so you make a plan for tomorrow at three. Tomorrow at three comes and somebody drives up the driveway and you think, "Oh, God. Do I have to see them? Oh, God. I want to see Perry Mason on television and I've got to see these people." Now I don't *want* to want to see Perry Mason, see? But because I want to see Perry Mason, I hate these people driving up the driveway. I don't want to hate them, because I'm a holy man. I want to love them. But I hate them. So I thought, "Okay, I'm going to change all that. I'm only going to be holy when I feel holy. If people come and I don't feel like seeing them, I'll say, "Go away," or I'll just disappear or whatever. I just won't be holy unless I feel like being holy, and when I'm holy, I'll be really holy." Because I was tired of being a phony holy man. You'd see they'd driven up from Ohio, and they'd come to see Ram Dass . . . so at the last moment you'd turn off the TV set and rush around, and light an incense and a candle and sit down and they'd come in and you'd say (*Ram Dass speaks in a hushed "holy" tone*), "Well come . . ." You know? Well, with that kind of hypocrisy you can live with yourself only so long; I mean, it's too ugly. It's just too horrible. And my guru had kept saying to me, "Tell the truth. Tell the truth, Ram Dass." He kept catching me not telling the truth, really little things.

I'll just give you a little quick example. I mention this in lectures. Once (I won't tell the whole story, just a little part of it), a judge, a high Supreme Court official came to have Maharaji's darshan and we — the Westerners — were sitting on the outer rim, and the Indians were in close; this alternated from day to day. Maharaji gave this high court official a tremendous build-up about what an important man I was in America, which he had never done, and I had never even thought that it was remotely relevant to anything he and I did together. He said, "Ex-professor from the University," you know, just full of lies, oh, incredible stuff and he snowed the official. Finally, the official — with great awe, really — turned around and said, "Well, I'm honored to meet you." I said, "How do you do." He says, "Perhaps you'd like to visit the high court." I come from a family of lawyers. I've been in courts, and I didn't go to India for that particular trip. So I said to him. "Well, that would be very nice." So he said, "Well, tomorrow at 10?" So I thought, Uh-oh. "Well, you'll have to ask my guru," figuring he'll get me off the hook.

So the judge says, "Maharaji, can Ram Dass visit the high court tomorrow at 10?" Maharaji says, "If he says it'll be very nice, it'll be very nice." So he's wagging his finger like this, "Watch it, baby, tell the truth." Just little ones, those little white ones, you know, the little ones that don't hurt anybody.

There was a woman with him one day, and he came up and he said, "Do you remember her?" and I said, "Oh, yes." And I didn't. And he said, "Yes, she's Dada's sister-in-law." And Dada's from Allahabad.

So I said, "Oh, yes. We met in Allahabad." She says, "No. We met right here." I said, "Oh." Maharaji went like that (*wagging his finger*). It's just those little ones. He was always getting me. It's like, "Tell the truth, baby. Come one, tell the truth. The truth gets you high." So I thought, when I come back to America I'll be straight. If I'm not feeling high I won't make believe I am. I was trying to get very, very straight.

Okay. So I just sort of floated around the country, just being wherever I was and when I felt really together and it was clear and I was calm and centered and loving and had something to offer, I was with people and it was beautiful and I could feel the guru's grace coming through to people and then when I wasn't I just went off and read and studied.

I had just done four or five lectures with Allen Ginsberg as benefits for Trunga Rinpoche — those were in time, the first things I'd done in time — and then I thought I'd go into a retreat for a month. So I rented a cabin in Tucson, Arizona, in the mountains, which has a kitchen, refrigerator, stove, beds. It was a bird sanctuary, so there were lots of bird lovers. Those were the only people there, me and bird lovers. So I was not relevant in their universe. It was a certain kind of privacy, even though there were other cabins.

I walked into the place and I found to my dismay that the one other thing that the cabin had was a television set. I had gone there to do a prayer. I was going to do a prayer for thirty days. Well, I spent the first eight days, roughly twelve hours a day, looking at television. Now, after I looked at television for the first day, I was so horrified that I might spend the next twenty-nine days doing it, that I took a screwdriver out of my car and I unwired the TV set and I put it in the closet, and I put a blanket over it, put it way behind my bag and everything and I closed the door and I sat down. And around 5:30 I thought, "Well, I could just look at the news." So I took the TV set out and I wired it up again and looked at the news and suddenly it was one in the morning, right? Three or four cans of beer later. Now it's very hard to think of that as sadhana. However, in that cabin, besides that television set, and all the food I had filled the refrigerator with, and the bed and bathtub that I could take frequent baths in, and all the different ways I could play in my sensual delights, there was also my consciousness, sitting in that cabin saying, "Far out! Imagine that. Are you going to tell anybody about this one?" I'm sitting there with the guy who said, "Gee, if I take the broccoli and put some of that spaghetti sauce over it and bake it, it'll be just like a pizza, and oh boy, if I can quick get that done I can watch Kung Fu and . . . " That guy was doing his thing and this other voice was saying, "Far out!" or Maharaji was saying "Tik, tik!" That's the way it is. There was the voice in me that was saying this and watching all this, just noticing it, witnessing it, watching with — at first — horror, because when you meet Siva in yourself, when you meet him anywhere, he's really scary. In the *Siva Stotram*, it says, "When Siva dances, the beings in all three worlds tremble." All three worlds tremble because his dance is so violent.

Now when I'm sitting there with the TV set, I get in this funny predicament. I get my food ready just as the program begins. This happened to me not long ago when the Watergate hearings started. See, watching Watergate has me even more than my orality. And I was sitting with the Watergate hearings just beginning, and I had the food, but I couldn't eat the food till I had consecrated it, but I couldn't stop watching Watergate long enough to consecrate it, and if I didn't consecrate it quick the food would get cold. And you can't just do it real fast, watching TV, it's just too shoddy. You're faced with these real dilemmas in doing sadhana and I think you should recognize that his is where it really hurts and this is where we live most of the time, unfortunately.

Well, the next week, I would just unplug the set and put a cloth over it and put it in the closet. And I found that I was getting a little bored so I would look at the television for only three or four hours a day and then I got into feeding birds and studying bird names and things like that. By the third week, I was sitting a little quieter and deepening a little bit and I could sit by the river for a few hours and I was starting to eat more simply and I was losing interest in television and by the fourth week, I was in a pretty calm, centered place and I was beginning to feel that energy again. I was getting to that place that you get when you've been here on retreat for nine days: that connectedness, that "Yeah, that's right, O, that's it . . . this is the real . . . " You all know, I'm sure. Well, while I was there, I looked at the whole scene and I thought, "You know, if I'm going to do Karma Yoga, I really should just go and do it, just get right into it."

So, I had a big folder of places that were inviting me to speak — I just kept them in a folder and wrote back and said, "I don't do that sort of thing, but if I ever do I'll let you know." Benefits and lectures and all kinds of stuff. So I said, Okay. I got the inner message 'cause I live totally intuitively now. And sometimes it's a reflection of a deeper voice. And I never know which one it is. Sometimes it tells me to do something and I start to do it and then it turns out to be just another ego trip and it falls away; I see its impurity. And sometimes I start doing it and it feels right on and I just stay right in this space as I'm doing it. I feel right. It's all a hunt and peck process of learning to hear that inner voice. Because you can't hang on to the coattails of the guru every minute and say, "Swami-ji, what do I do now? Should I sharpen this pencil now? Should I sit? What should I do now?"

When I was coming back to America, I said to Dada, Maharaji's devotee, "Dada, you're lucky, you hang around Maharaji; if you do something wrong he tells you. He says, 'Dada!'" He's always telling him, "Do this, do that." I said, "Look at me. I'm thousands of miles away and I can really go off the deep end. And I don't mind doing myself in, karmically, but I don't really like doing other people in. That's a heavy. And I can do that because I have a lot of lust and stuff left. I may manipulate the whole game just to make it with someone. I don't trust me at all." And he went to Maharaji and he told Maharaji this, and Maharaji sent back the message, "Ram Dass shouldn't worry; I wouldn't let him do anything wrong." Now, how does he not let you do anything wrong? Do you think, suddenly, a little angel comes fluttering in and says, "Stop!" like in fairy tales? No, it's the guy sitting in that cabin in Tucson, watching me, saying, "More Kung Fu? More beer? More baths? More, wow, right." It's that place in me that knows; it knows, and it's just letting me do what I need to do as I'm getting closer there. And it never lets me out of its sight.

To let you in on the secret of the game from where I'm sitting, the universe I live in has only two beings left in it. There's who I still *think* I am. And then there's Sam. You can call Sam God, or you can call Sam guru, or you can call Sam whatever you like. I call it guru. As far as I can understand it, my universe – the universe of the illusion of who I think I am – exists solely for the purpose of bringing me to the guru. That is, that everything that is happening to me, is a teaching being given to me as grace to bring me to the guru. Not just sitting in satsang, but tripping on the rock as you walk down the path. It's all the teaching, if you can flip it around and see it that way. Now under those conditions, Karma Yoga takes on quite a different aspect.

So, deciding to do this tour . . . I decided, "All right, I'm really going to do this to myself." I mean, if you're going to do Karma Yoga, really do it! Don't just screw around. So I took a big map, and I laid out all these lecture dates in terms of schedule and geography. And I got to the point where I had scheduled myself to lecture in a different city every night. For two months. And then on the third month I started to loosen up a little bit, so I was only doing, say, one on every three nights. So I started, and I went up the coast of California, to Seattle, and Portland, Olympia. Everywhere I went, either Swamiji had just been or was about to be, it turned out. I'd get to a place and they'd say, "You know who slept in this bed last night?" But the difference between us is he doesn't do it as Karma Yoga, he's just doin' it, 'cause he *is* it. That's what Karma Yoga is about. Not to say, "I am serving, "but to become the service.

Here's what happens, here's the routine. Every day you get up, have your morning beverage, which for me is coffee, sometimes a bagel. Okay. Then you go to the airport. You go through security, open your bags, go and get on the plane, sit on the plane for so many hours. The plane lands, you get off the plane, you walk down the runway, and you walk into the hall. And there are these beings saying, "Oh, Ram Dass, Ram Dass," and you say, "How do you do?" and they pick up your bags, they take you to where you're staying. You either do some press conferences or radio stuff or meet a group, and then at three o'clock I take a nap, 'cause I say to everybody, "I had hepatitis and I have to protect my liver," and I go nap for a few hours and when I get finished, there is dinner, which is usually some kind of gathering, some very beautiful pot-luck thing somewhere, and we all get together and it's all very lovely. Around 7:30 we move to the lecture hall, I sit down, tune up the tamboura or get the shruti box ready, whatever it is, work with musicians that have gathered to help me out. I start at 8; 11 or 12 I stop, I am delivered back to the hotel or motel or room, I take my peanut butter and crackers and my milk, drink that, look at the late news, go to bed, get up the next morning, meditate for a few minutes, have my coffee, go to the airport, go through security . . . It's no different than working at a lathe, see? You know?

Now, what happens is, I started to get sicker and sicker and sicker. First of all, because the schedule was grueling, and by the time I got to Vancouver, I didn't have any voice, which was funny. I mean, I was about to head for Anchorage, Alaska, and I didn't have any voice left, to speak. And I was sitting over a hot vaporizer, and doing the whole thing, mantram and everything, saying to Maharaji, "What have you got in mind now? It's pretty far out. How am I gonna speak without a voice?" And he had said to me in India, "There's gonna be a time when you're not gonna want to lecture any more." And I kept repeating that to myself, and I kept saying, "This must be the time," but I still wanted to do it, because quite honestly, what I'm working with is power and fame and all these worldly things which are connected with what happens when Swamiji says, "Who *doesn't* know Ram Dass?" And of course everybody applauds.

What am I supposed to go through then? If 40 people came to see me in a day on the farm in New Hampshire, I get stoned out of my head from the satsang and my father will walk in and say "Had a pretty good crowd today." Like he's counting cars, you see? I mean, that's the cultural background that I come out of. And I have to work with that all the time – that's my work. You have to understand what Karma Yoga really is. It's working with your desires right in the middle of the fire, right in the field. It's dying into the thing, it's dying into the service. I realized that the only reason I was getting fatigued and wiped out and physically run down was because I still wanted something. Like after a beautiful satsang I would be hardly in my body, I would just be floating around and we'd all be staying, nobody wanted to be going home – that place where nobody wants to leave. Somebody would say, "Hey, I've got a beautiful place just a few miles out of town and there will be like ten of us and we'll cook a beautiful thing. Why don't you come?"

It would be around 12 o'clock at night now; I know if I go it will be until at least 4 o'clock in the morning. Next morning there's the security and the airplane and the coffee   that's not going to change. So I'd say, "Oh, I wish I could go but I can't." That's what I had hated about time. Time kept making me turn off my desires." All I have to do is just desire to become the pure instrument of service. That's all. I'm going to become like one of the 747 planes. Not like the pilot but like one of the planes. Somebody gets into the plane and moves it from here to there. It doesn't say, "Oh boy, I'm flying to New York," it doesn't say, "Oh, I'll bet I'll be big in Denver." It's just an airplane. You move it from here to there and it does its thing. It goes Roaarrrr and it just flies. And I recognized that for me to understand the exquisiteness of Karma Yoga was going to mean that I was going to do this every single day until there was nobody doing it at all. It was just being done every day. Every day there was just the moving, the flying, and it was all sadhana. There wasn't one tiny bit that wasn't. You come up to the security guard and the guard sees you as a potential bomber, you know? That's Maharaji, that's my guru, who has gone to central casting and has come out as the guard and he's saying to you, "Well, see if you can see through me this time. Do you know I'm God in here, or do you think I'm a security guard?" Are you so paranoid that you are busy reacting? Saying, "I'm not the bomber, I'm not the bomber. I'm a nice guy." Everybody I meet every day is the guru in drag as far as I'm concerned. And the sickness and the fatigue and all of it is the grace. It's *all* the grace. There is nothing left in my life other than teachings that will bring me to God. It's the only game in town. Nothing else has any meaning. What else am I going to make meaningful?

Like I'm busy watching the Watergate. I can't wait for Dean to get on the stand. You know? And at the same moment, I am sitting inside, saying, "You can't wait for Dean to get on the stand." Because, let me tell you that once that thing has happened enough to bring you into this room, as far as I'm concerned it's all over. Now it's the mopping-up operation, which may take many lifetimes. It's all purification from here on out. It's just getting cleaned up. It's getting your body together, your heart opened, getting your mind calmed down and understanding that a conscious being recognizes that she or he has taken birth and that the function of an incarnation is to end suffering. Wherever it exists. On any plane it exists. And you recognize that the optimum thing you are to do to end suffering is to work on yourself and how you work on yourself depends on your dharma. What is your route through? For me, my work on myself is through doing what I am doing this minute. If I think *I* am doing this, I still have a way to go — until this is just being done, and I am just as much part of the audience as you are. Am I attached to being the speaker? Am I looking for the rush of your appreciation?

Now, the honoring of Siva . . . it's easy when you're just talking about Siva. You know, way over there in India. With his ashes and all his buddies he hangs out with that are so scary, and his wife Kali, whew! That's easy. Then you can bring it over here and say, "Look at pollution and look at lying and stealing in government, and look at murder and paranoia and rape and, oh boy, that's Siva." But get a little closer to home still, when you're ready, and realize that in you are all those forces as well.

The *Bhagavad Gita* is talking about an inner battle, the battle between that voice that says, "Kung Fu and broccoli with some sauce on it," and the guy that says, "I want to watch Kung Fu and I want to have the broccoli." That's that battle, those two guys. And that goes on and on and on and on in everything you do. People come to me and say, "Should I do this or that?" And I know, as a good Yogi, I'm supposed to say good yogic things, like "Do this" or "Stand on your head" or something like that. But I must honestly admit that what I mainly say to people is, "It doesn't matter." Because whatever you do, you'll do as consciously or unconsciously as you are. Do it all to bring yourself to God. Don't get caught in the form you're going to do it in, just do it. And as you come closer to God, you find out in fact that there are only certain things you can do because you can't do things which increase illusion. You can't do things which increase suffering. You just can't do them because they're just absurd. It's like taking needles and sticking them into your hands; why do it? If I screw you, I'm just screwing myself. Who am I hurting? It's only us; that's where I'm sitting.

I've got this economic story that's a fun image to play with. My father heard that we were putting out some records, very cheaply, and we were trying to lower prices of things and do everything very economically. And that I was not trying to collect or amass money. He says, "What's the matter — you against capitalism?" This is the ex-President of a railroad talking, right? So I said, "No, Dad, I'm not against capitalism; for you, I think it's great. It's just not my style." He says, "I don't understand you." I said, "Well, *that* I understand." It's interesting. We love each other incredibly, even though we are on different trips, because compassion doesn't mean you lay your trip on anybody else. It means you become it so perfectly that you become the light that draws. You don't go out and say, "Come on, Dad, wake up." But I said, "I'll try to share with you since you don't understand." Didn't you just try a case for Uncle Henry?" My father's a lawyer. He says, "Yeah" I said, "Did you win it?" He says, "Damn right, I did, and it was a tough case." I said, "Boy, you worked a lot on it." He says, "I sure did." I said, "I bet you charged him a big fee." He says, "Of course not, he's my brother-in-law." I said, "Well, that's my predicament. Everybody's my brother-in-law. Who am I going to rip off?" And he could hear that. He could hear that out of a Jewish middle-class background. Family, you do one thing with, and "them" out there you do something else with. And if his son is *mishugana* enough so the whole thing is his family, that's, you know . . . . He's a good kid anyway.

In conclusion, when you leave this place and this blessing, this *mitzvah*, I can assure you that you will come down. And I can further tell you, although you may forget it, that that is as much of the teaching as this is. And the down and up is all part of the dance. And the game is not to get high but the game is to be. And to be includes highs and lows, until you are no more attached to your high than you are to your low. There's bliss, there's depression. There it all is. There's the whole panorama of maya. All the positive states and the negative states; it's all more stuff. Divine stuff. The leela. And in it all, here we are. Here we are. And the meaning of honoring Siva is to give space to all these forces. To recognize them, to allow their being. To not try to shove them under the rug. There is a terrible habit we have of getting holy too fast. Intellectually, we know where holy is, and we figure out, "Well, I want to be like Swamiji. So I'll put on those clothes and I'll act like that." You do it from outside in. You can't do this game from outside in. You can play at it, but you're going to keep that inner voice being horrified by your hypocrisy. And then you'll say, "I'm really nowhere," and the statement, "I'm really nowhere" is the recognition of being somewhere. That's it. You see, people come to me and say, "I'm no good," "I'm depressed," or "I hate everybody," and I say to them, "If you hated everybody, you wouldn't tell me you hate everybody."

It's like that story I've told about. Some years back at Millbrook, a girl called in the middle of the night and she had taken some mysterious chemical in Los Angeles and she was freaked out and called up, got me on the line and said, "I've gone crazy and I'm gonna kill myself and I'm insane." And she laughed hysterically to show me she was insane. I said to her, "Well, who dialed the phone? You know, the one digit and then the three digits and the three digits and the four digits?" She said, "I did." I said, "Well, would you put her on the phone, because you're crazy?"

So let me say that once the connection has been made, once we have acknowledged each other's existence, once we know we are here, you can't get away. You can't get away. You may go under really deep and feel, "I've lost it," and then you'll see yourself standing there, "I've lost it." And you'll break up. And then it's done, right? You see, the game is, if you're so afraid of all the Siva forces that you keep pushing them away, they keep clinging. It's very interesting to use the gold chain to pull yourself out of the mud. It's called the sattvic chain — of being good and pure and doing good and pure things. It's good to help you get out of other stuff, but remember, you're holding on to a chain and that chain can bind too. You can get caught in good and evil while you're using good and evil as a method; just remember that behind good and evil, we are. Behind good and evil, we are. Siva and Ram are two more faces of that which is indescribable and unknowable and unseeable, but only be-able.

It's really very, very good to be with all of us. Namaste.

The Three Gunas and the Three Types of People

Swami Satchidananda

Most of the days on this retreat have been overcast, with occasional rain. Yet, because of the wonderful harmony of the retreat and the inwardness of the yogic practices, this has not been a problem. This is certainly true on this last full day of the retreat, which has almost a festive atmosphere, as another 200 people come to join the hundreds already here, to hear Swamiji and Ram Dass and to take part in the full weekend program.

The evening talk is Swamiji's last lecture of the retreat. A fund of extremely useful information on the nature of the mind is given, followed by a final exhortation to get into the practice of Karma Yoga to get the mind quickly trained and purified and to live a balanced and happy life. Engage in wholehearted service to others and be happy and free: this is his final message to the 600 seekers gathered at the Monticello Retreat and to the world at large. The message is simple, clear, all-encompassing, and at the same time, eminently practical; a path for which all who earnestly seek the inner peace and joy are fit no matter what their age, background, taste, capacity or station in life, a path leading to the Highest, yet realistic, modern and universally applicable.

The end of our retreat program is more or less nearing. But, wherever there is an end, there is a beginning too. When something ends, something is also beginning, and that's how the days go on and on. There is a day; there is a night. If night comes, then day must come – a cycle. So let us keep watching it. If we can only learn to watch it, then it is all just fun. But until we get to that stage of witnessing, we still have to keep doing. As I said in the very beginning, we are all used to doing something. That's how we're built. Even Sri Krishna in the Bhagavad Gita says, "In My manifested state, when I come into this frame, with this name and form, then even I must be doing something. I can't be quiet." That is the law of the nature, the *Prakriti Dharma*.

There is a beautiful prayer of offering, of surrendering everything unto God, which explains our proper relationship with this Prakriti Dharma. It is usually repeated at the end of any practice: meditation, japa, puja, chanting, everything. Whatever you do, towards the end you say this prayer:

Kaayena Vaachaa Manasendriyair Vaa
Buddhyaatamanaa Vaa Prakriter Swabhaavaat.
Karomi Yad Yad Sakalam Parasmai
Naraayanaayeti Samarpayaami

It means, "Oh Lord Narayana, the Cosmic One, I offer everything unto
you. I offer all the actions done by the body, the mind, the intellect and
the soul which have been due to the functioning of the qualities of the
nature or 'Prakriter Swabhavat'." Swabhava is the inherent nature of
something; Prakriti is the One Lord in manifestation. All that you see as
manifested has this Swabhava or its own nature, which is constantly tossed by the three qualities of nature, *sattva, rajas* and *tamas*.

Sattva is tranquility; rajas, dynamic activity; and tamas is inertness, in-
activity, dullness or laziness. So whenever you feel dull, lazy, drowsy,
whenever you feel like not doing anything, know that the tamasic quality of the mind is predominant. It's the mind that motivates and uses the
body to do things. So whenever you feel dull, then you know that the
tamas has taken over. But then sometimes you feel, "Oh, I must do this, I
must do that." It's a kind of a mood. Don't we go through these things?
Sometimes you can't sit quiet, you have to do something. You even say,
"Oh, I'm *in the mood* to do things. If I don't finish my things while I'm in
this mood, I'll never do it." All of a sudden the mind gets into a rajasic
tendency. It's just common. At that moment, get things done. "Make hay
while the sun shines." Because when you are dull and lazy, however
much you push, you find it difficult. Even if someone pricks you, you get
annoyed. "I've been doing so much, so much, constantly. I'm not even
appreciated, however much I do." You feel that way. And a sane man
will know that you're in a tamasic state and he won't force you too
much.

But sometimes we get into a kind of in-between, a very balanced state.
You feel like doing, but not overdoing. You are neither dull nor too excited. A kind of sane, tranquil state. Then you say, "Ah, I feel like just sitting and meditating." Not that you feel like sleeping. "No, I just feel like
sitting and meditating or just listening to some nice music." It just
happens, without even your wanting. That is the proof that the mind is
being tossed by these three gunas. Sometimes when there is wind, the
flame flickers; when there's no wind, it is steady. It is not just the motives
of the mind alone. Our mind is part of the Cosmic Mind, part of the
Prakriti, or nature. So when the waves — the sattva, rajas and tamas waves
— come, it gets caught in that.

But we can develop the strength of the mind. We can make an ordinary flickering lamp into a hurricane lamp. If there's no shelter, if it's not well protected, you have to always keep it indoors; you can't even open the windows. The minute you open the windows, it seems to be going out. But if you shelter it with a nice chimney, you can take it even into the mid-ocean. That's what you call hurricane lanterns. But within the hurricane lamp, the flame is the same. It's the same flame, but well sheltered. Then it can face even the hurricane. The mind is like that. You can build up the strength of the mind. Then it can face all situations.

But whatever it be, all these movements, as I said before, are caused by the Prakriter Swabhava, the nature of the Prakriti, because everything is made out of these three gunas. If there are no changes in the gunas, everything is tranquil. That is what you call the end of the cycle. In that *pralaya*, or equilibrium, they all stand still. So in a way we need rajas and tamas also. It is the rajas and tamas that create the entire show. As such, our bodies and minds are all part of the Prakriti – the nature. That's why everything can be divided into these three categories. If you read the seventeenth chapter of the Bhagavad Gita, you will see everything divided by their gunas.

Even charity is divided into these three. Like the other day, Rabbi Shlomo Carlebach told about the "holy miser." He was not really a miser but he looked like a miser. Why? Because he didn't do anything to advertise himself. He hid everything; he did everything secretly. He didn't want any praise for what he had done. That kind of charity is sattvic charity, we say. The rajasic charity is when you give something with nice good purpose, like giving to a church or hospital, but you want recognition: "Mr. So-and-So built it." During the consecration ceremony people should come and take a photograph of you and the building and put it in the headlines. That is charity, but it is for name and fame, a rajasic type of charity. Another type is to be lavish and buy a lot of bottles and packs and invite hundreds of friends, "Come on, drink as much as you want." Charity, huh? that's tamasic. It doesn't really help people to grow. By building a church at least you create a devotional feeling in the other men's minds, so it elevates the other people. But this type of charity is tamasic.

Meditation can be tamasic, rajasic or sattvic also. If you meditate all by yourself without others even knowing that you are a Yogi, a meditator, people will think you are just an ordinary man.

You go quietly when there is nobody around and just sit and meditate. You don't expose that you are a devotee, a *sadhak* (seeker). That is sattvic. Sri Ramakrishna used to say, if you are really a sattvic meditator, you will do it when everybody is asleep. You may even make others believe that you are going to sleep. You will lie down, putting your mosquito curtains around, then when the lights are off, you get up quietly and meditate. If anybody turns on the light you can immediately lie down. Let people not think that you are really meditating. Very sattvic and quiet. But the rajasic meditation you could easily guess, hm? (*Swamiji imitates a person appearing to meditate very intensely, sitting very stiff.*) You are a little dull but when you see somebody coming, you sit up more and more stiff, hm? When the people go away . . . you sag down again. You see somebody coming again, you straighten up. It's all for show. You *do* meditate, but you want others to say, "Oh, how long he is sitting." When the ankle aches, if there is nobody there to see, you will move a little; otherwise, no. "It doesn't matter." Getting the pride hurt is worse than getting the ankle hurt. The tamasic type of meditation is where you just sit and immediately go to sleep. You don't even worry about what people think.

Now I am going to tell you something interesting. People do japa with the aid of a *mala* (beads on a string), and it is to have sattvic meditation that you are asked to do your malas quietly. You don't need to expose to ople that you're repeating the mala. And that's why you're asked to keep the mala in a small bag and then put your hand inside and keep repeating. Have you seen such bags? It is a nice L-shaped bag, opening on the side. The mouth of the bag is tied at the wrist. Then you put your hand into that. The mala is inside and when you repeat, the mala rolls within the bag itself. The idea is to hide the mala and hide that you are repeating anything. That is for sattvic japa, not to expose. But you know how it took shape? They make nice beautiful velvet bags, with all nice glittering things on the bag itself and then they expose it. The *mala* is not shown, but the bag is shown, him? It creates more curiosity: "Oh, what kind of mala are you having inside?" Then they will open it and show. "Oh, it's a . . . crystal . . . mala!" Put it in the bag again. The entire purpose is lost then. The human tendency is that way. It wants to show. That is rajasic.

In the same way you can categorize everything into the three gunas, even food. When I first came to the West I saw a couple who took me into the country to spend a weekend. I saw them preparing so much food. I said, "What, just for three people you make this much?" "Oh, no, Swamiji, we are making for the whole week." They make for the whole week, take it home, put it in the refrigerator, take a little bit every day, warm it up and eat it. The Bhagavad Gita says that is very tamasic food — heat it up, cool it, heat it, cool it. It loses everything. The kinds of foods we get here, even the very ingredients are all bleached and I don't know what all. And then in the cooking and cooling and heating we lose even the little bit. It only fills the stomach then. So the Gita says, if you cook, cook for the time. Eat it, finish it. Don't keep it and make it stale and then eat it afterwards. So any stale, old, left-over food is tamasic. And if cooked too long, it's tamasic. This will really create a lot of problems in many of us, hm?

I'm not talking about the bread and things like that. Bread you can bake. I'm talking about anything that has too much moisture in it. Vegetables, for example, or cooked rice. And rajasic food is overly spicy food, a lot of salt and spices and red pepper. So what we call the yogic food is plain, simple, neither too hot nor too stale. And if we want to develop the sattvic tendency, we have to eat sattvic food.

Excitement, or rajas, is a form of disturbance of the mind. So the idea is to keep the mind always tranquil or in your term, always high. Not the other "high." When you go high, that high, you have to come down. From that high, you'll crash down later on. The real high is the medium. The balanced height. So excitement is a kind of disturbance. Depression is another form of disturbance. Balancing is what you call tranquility, or sattva. That is what you call samadhi. Don't think that samadhi means to sit and forget the body and mind and everything and sit like a rock for months. Then even a rock could do better. What is the difference between the rock and yourself? Real samadhi is to keep the mind *samatwam*. Samatwam means equanimity. "*Samatwam Yoga uchyate*: Equanimity is Yoga." Samadhi is that samatwam. Keep the mind well balanced under all conditions.

That's why I always give the example of a wonderful surfer. The one who surfs well is one who can serve well. If we learn to surf, we can learn to serve. Whatever be the waves, the surfer still maintains the balance there. He enjoys that. No more "freaking out," no more frustrations. He doesn't have the fear, "Oh, look at that! A big wave is coming. My goodness, I have to run back." A man who knows surfing will even be waiting for that wave. "Ahh, here it is coming. Let me go in." See? The same wave frightens one and not the other. He is waiting for it. Why? He knows how to balance. So one who knows this balance can be anywhere and everywhere.

Certainly we can't run from anything. Where can we run, from what? People say, "I'm running away from my home; I am renouncing my home." Okay, you have renounced the home. But you got attached to your institute or ashram or community, hm? Wherever you go, you still have to be on the same earth, inhale the same air, drink the same water. You cannot get out of the Prakriti. So instead of running here and there,

stay where you are. Learn to balance. That is the aim in all these practices. No religion asks you to run away or change your occupation. This
morning Ram Dass said clearly that the real Yoga is not just running
away, going into a corner, sitting and closing your eyes, meditating
always. People think that. Or they say, "Well, I don't know, I don't
seem to be fit for anything, I will just do Karma Yoga." You are the
worst person to do Karma Yoga then, because Karma Yoga is the most
difficult one. Just doing things is not Karma Yoga; that is karma. Yes. To
make the karma into Karma Yoga, you should have a wonderful attitude.
A well-balanced mind. Otherwise, don't call it Karma Yoga. That's just
calling poison as if it were nectar. It's in the mental attitude. You should
have a yogic attitude in your karma, then it is Karma Yoga. That is the
most difficult one, and because it is difficult, it will elevate you quickly.
You don't learn this much in any other practice. Everything will teach
you in Karma Yoga. In this sense, a saintly poet once said that the essence
of the Vedas is Karma Yoga. The Vedas say, "Only Karma Yoga will
save you." It's easy to go and close your eyes and say, "Oh, I'm
meditating." But how long can you meditate? You still have to come out
into the world. You have to face the world. You can't be just hiding
yourself, locking yourself indoors always.

This reminds me of a seeker, who went into a Himalayan cave and
locked himself in for several years. He had a couple of devotees, who
would just bring some food, leave it there and go away. He never even
saw anybody. Food was just brought to him and he ate and spent the time
there in meditation. I tried myself for some time. So after several years, he
felt so peaceful, so calm. Ah! Everything was beautiful. He thought that
he had got that samadhi, that equanimity. Nothing could disturb him
now. So he slowly came out of the cave and walked into the village.
Immediately people gathered around him. "Oh, the *mouni* (silent)
Swami! The cave Swami has come!" Everybody was talking about him.
They were saying, "He never talks, never sees anybody! He's just there
inside the cave always." He had created a kind of awe.

It's just like if you close your palm, everybody will be wondering.
Suppose I just keep my hand closed and talk to you, you won't even be
listening to me. Every minute you'll be thinking. "He seems to be having
something in the hand." It's just a closed fist; I don't need to have
anything. In the same way: Keep mouna. It's a good way to make people
think you are really high. It avoids all kinds of troubles. The minute you
open your mouth, you expose yourself, either your ignorance, or how
bad you are. So, if you just keep your mouth shut . . . "Ooooh, "Ooooh,
the mouni Swami, he doesn't talk, he must know something . . ." It's

easy to keep mouna or to just talk and talk and talk. But it's very difficult to limit. To measure your talk is very difficult.

So when he came out, they came and they fell at his feet. He thought, "Oh, they're all looking for me!" And they said, "Oh, Swami, we are so happy to have your *darshan* (presence) after so many years! Please, please tell us, what have you been experiencing all these years? What have you achieved? Did you get some *siddhi* (power) or something?" Then he sat and smiled at them. "Yes."

"Could you please tell us?"

"Well, above everything else, I would like to say that when I went into the cave, I was a very ferocious, angry man. Terrible. Nobody could face me even for a minute. I used to shout and yell at them. Anger was my devilish quality. But in all these years, I completely conquered anger. I never got angry, not even once. That was the biggest siddhi I achieved, to get the mastery over that anger."

"Oh, so nice to hear that. But you say that you were terribly angry before. How is it, all of a sudden, it all went away? In all these years, didn't you burst into anger once, at least?"

"No, not even once, not at all."

"It's really nice to hear that, Swamiji, but it's really a little hard to believe. Could you just think a little and see if at least for one minute, when the devotees brought your food they might not have brought it with enough salt or something. You would have gotten annoyed. Something like that, even once?"

"You fool! How many times do I have to say?? I've been telling you again and again. Do you mean to say that I'm a liar???"

"No, no, Swami. We understand you very well. . . . Do you want to go back to your cave now . . . . ?"

That's it. See? It's easy to say, "I don't have any anger," when there's nobody in front of you to show your anger to. It's easy to say, "Oh, I have renounced everything. I don't even touch money," when you don't even have a dollar bill to call your own. There's no money, so how can you touch? When there is no food to eat, you say, "I'm fasting," or "I have renounced everything." What did you have before? "Well, I didn't have anything." Then, what is it that you renounced? To renounce, you must have had something. So when will you know that you're balanced? When you are in the midst of ups and downs. Otherwise, you will seem to be balanced, but you need to be kept away from the normal life. You will be of no use to anybody. You can't even come out and face life.

It's something like somebody wants to learn swimming. He says, "Oh, the water is cold and I'm mortally afraid of water; I can't go in the water.

But I would like to learn swimming."

I say, "How can you learn swimming without going in the water?"

"Well, teach me here on the land. Because if I don't know how to swim, how can I get into the water?"

Seems to be a kind of puzzle, hm? Without knowing how to swim you can't go into the water. And without water you can't learn how to swim. That's a mystery.

The answer is, select a section where you'll be in the water, and at the same time you'll be safe. Get into shallow water. Tie some rubber tube or something around you, some flotation. The water will go into the nose, mouth, everywhere. It doesn't matter. That's the way you learn. The world also is like that. Go into it. But don't go too deep. Let there be a trainer by your side. Let him hold one end of the rope. Go in. If you are going in too far, he will pull you out. He'll take care of you until you learn. Once you show your capability, he'll say, "Okay, now you go, swim wherever you want. You don't need me any more." That is the relationship, you see, between a seeker and a teacher. He's only there to push you into the water a little, keeping the other end of the rope in the hand. He will watch. If you are going a little too deep, he will pull you out. He'll teach you how to swim, what to do. Then, once he's satisfied, "Okay, now you can go."

So we have to learn and that is what you call Karma Yoga. If you are in the world, you have to do something. Even if you say, "I'm going to sit quietly and meditate," you have to eat something. Even if you say you're not eating anything, you have to inhale the air. Where do you get the air? From the nature. So you are getting something; aren't you going to return something? When you get something, you have to return. Otherwise you are only getting and not giving. We constantly get something from the nature. So we have to return. Otherwise, we'll be exploiting the nature, or God's gifts, if you want to put it that way.

According to the Gita, there are three types of people and dealings. A Yogi is a *yagnyashista*. That means he always gives more than he gets. The second type is an ordinary businessman. He will give exactly what he gets — fair business. If you give a fair businessman ten dollars, he will give you ten dollars; not exactly the same, but ten dollars' worth of articles. Nothing less or more — fifty-fifty, an equal transaction. Then there is the third type. He will give you one dollar's worth, when you give him ten dollars. So, he steals nine dollars from you. Because he's not returning all that he got from you, he's called a thief. So when you don't give at least in return for what you get, you are a kind of thief.

Think how much we are getting from the nature: the very air that we breathe, the sunlight, a space to sit, to walk, to move. And food and water to drink. We're not charged anything for all those things. And we get nice things to see: beautiful flowers, beautiful views. You see, the nature doesn't charge you. Every time you say "beautiful," do you get a bill? No. So you get nice things to satisfy your senses from the nature. What do you give in return? You might at least give as much as what you get. Then you are a fair businessman. If you don't give that much, you are a thief. That's how the Bhagavad Gita puts it. But a Yogi should give even more. You might wonder how. I inhale five hundred cc's of air. And I can return only some carbon dioxide. I don't even retain the quality, I kill it. So should I just breathe the air and give the same air back? Even if I do, I am only a fair businessman. How can I be a Yogi? That is why I say you don't need to return the same thing. Like a businessman, when he gets money, he gives articles in return. In the same way, when you get nourishment from the nature, you return it through your energy, your actions. We are constantly fed enough intelligence, physical strength, everything, by the nature, and we are to return it, a little more than what we get. How can I return the intelligence to nature, the strength to nature? Well, everything is nature. You may get the air here, and you make your return in the form of your energy to your fellow beings, to the people who need it, to the things that need it: an exchange of articles.

That is what you call service. A Karma Yogi should give a little more than what he gets. And that is what we learn in ashrams. The bare minimum of our needs are taken care of, but what we give back is much more. So we learn to be Yogis. And again, the entire ashram — it gets from different sources, contributions and so on. When they get monetary contributions, the ashram need not return money to others, but they can return it in some other way. They can return it through their service. And they are sending prayerful thoughts, praying for the benefit of others. By sending good thoughts, you share the benefit of your own prayer with others. That is also Karma Yoga. So ashrams are only places where you can easily learn to perform your actions as Karma Yoga. That doesn't mean you should do it only at the ashram. You learn there. Then wherever you go, whatever you do becomes Karma Yoga.

And that is what we expect to happen through these retreats. For ten days we have been doing all kinds of things. When you go home, you'll be doing more or less the same. The other day I saw people scrubbing, cleaning, washing, cutting the lawn, doing everything. We do that every day in our homes, or even if you're employed as a gardener, you do it there. But when you're employed, if you are getting $50 a week, your conscience should tell you that you are doing at least $75 work for him. You should know, "Yes, I'm only getting $50, but I have to give more." Don't just look at the time and say: "I only have to work eight hours."

Even for those eight hours, are you really working? Maybe you can cheat him, but you can't cheat the Cosmic Law. There is one big divine computer. It computes everything. It is in here. (*Swamiji points to his heart.*) That is what you call the Judgment Day, but you don't need to wait until the last day. Sometimes the judgment comes immediately, daily or weekly or monthly. All of a sudden something may go wrong in your house. You may have to shell out $500, just for nothing. All of a sudden you may hurt your ankle. You have to go to your doctor. He will just feel the pulse here, and he will feel the purse also. That's all. Gone. All of the money you cheated from the employer gone to somebody. God knows how to adjust. Don't think that you can just cheat and get away with it. The man may not know, but God knows. *That* accountant is really well-trained. Yes, he's a beautiful C.P.A. He's certified. His system never fails. He counts not only your money, but your service, your actions, your thoughts, your attitude. "Well, he pays me, but I don't really want to do the work. Okay, let me finish it somehow and go." You may be doing even more than $50 worth, but if you are not doing it with a good heart and if he gives the pay with good heart, you'll be in the minus column.

This reminds me of an incident that happened in Ceylon once. In Ceylon, there is a beautiful temple of Lord Muruga or Subramanya, a very holy place. There, no one knows what is in the *sanctum sanctorum*. It is never opened. It is always covered with seven screens, not even just one or two. And only one priest can go in and even that is a kind of small family thing. Every year they change the priest and those people should not reveal the thing that is inside to anybody. If they say it, they die. Even today it is there like that. We used to go there and because nobody knows what is inside, they have more devotion to that. "Oh, it must be really something." Because when everything is exposed we say, "Is that all? The carved head in that other temple is a little taller than this and more beautiful." You begin to compare. Because you don't know what is there, the awe is even more, the devotion is more and the devotees really get a lot of benefit that way. It is something like your proverb: Familiarity breeds contempt. If God is going to appear every minute, whenever you want, you may say, "Oh, I'm sorry, I just called you by mistake; be there, I have some work to do. I'll finish it and call you again." Familiarity. It's a human tendency. And that is the reason why God doesn't want to appear before you every minute. He is there in you, but He knows if

He comes out, you will dispose of him soon. So He becomes a scarce commodity. And that's why this temple is kept like that, for the past several hundreds of years. Only the front screen is visible to people.

Originally it was just a plain screen but people are not satisfied in just going and seeing a plain screen, so they started painting nice pictures of the Gods. A beautiful Subramanya — with six heads and His consorts, Valli and Devayani, on either side and His beautiful peacock vehicle. And once a year somebody would give a new one. One year, a friend of mine, a big businessman, was there when I went and he showed me, "Swamiji, this is what I offered the Lord this year."

"Oh, it is beautiful, it's beautiful." I looked and saw at the bottom, the full length, in triple lines, his full name, his address, his business address, telephone, where to contact and the things that he deals in. I said, "Why all this?"

"Well, I just . . . you know." He couldn't say anything.

And I said, "Okay, fine. Come with me; I'll talk to you. Take a piece of paper and pencil." Then I asked him to make a calculation. "Imagine all these three big lines. If you want to put an ad at an important junction in the city, how much would the city government charge you for the advertisement? The city charges for billboards, no? Normally, how much? Say, in the public square in Colombo, if you want to write all this on a big board, how much would it be?

"Oh, that would be at least 1,000 rupees a month."

"Okay. How many people do you think would see that on a given day?"

"On an average, at least a hundred or two hundred people would see it."

"Now, how much did you pay for the screen?"

"Two hundred and fifty rupees."

"Okay, how many people do you think will come to God's place to worship Him?"

"Oh, several thousands, several thousands."

"And will they all see the lines?"

"Yes, sure."

"Do you pay any advertisement charges for this?"

"No."

"You think you can get away with that? Already Lord Muruga has opened a page in His ledger — 'Mr. So and So: 250 rupees towards the screen. His contribution is 250 to Me.' And in His account, every day He would also be writing the advertising costs — 'so many rupees he owes

Me.' After a month, if He calculates how much you have to pay back . . . how much? Why don't you calculate it?"

"Oh, no, Swami, you are just teasing me. If it's really an advertisement and if I had to pay according to what I pay in Colombo, certainly it will be several thousands."

"And do you think you can get away with it? You think He is a fool? You are going to be a debtor, no doubt."

Don't think that you can just get away with things. You have to pay for everything. The account is well adjusted. We used to have a proverb in South India. Suppose somebody goes and takes a loan from another person and is somehow delayed in paying it back. If the person says: "You don't seem to be able to give me the money back. Should I erase it as a bad debt?"

"Oh, no, no, no. Please, please, I will somehow pay you, before I die. Please, if I don't do it, then I'll be born as a dog to watch your doorstep until I pay you back by my service. If I don't pay the money, I'll have to be your watch-dog."

That is how the Cosmic Law acts. And that is the reason why I say that even the people at the Institutes and any ashrams who receive contributions shouldn't think that they can just get away with that. You don't need to return the money as the money, but you have to pray for the donor. If you don't do it, whatever practice you do and whatever spiritual benefit you get, a proper portion of your benefit will go to the donor automatically because you are able to sit and meditate because of his money. You bought the apple to eat because of his money. The apple gave you strength to sit and meditate. So the amount of energy that you got through the apple should go back to him, if not more. So if you are a seeker and if he donates some money to you, thinking that you are a good meditator or seeker who will sit and pray, and if you don't do that or you just do a little bit, all the little bit will go to him; you won't have anything left over for you. And again, if you don't spend the contribution in the proper way, you'll become a debtor because he gives to you for a certain purpose to be used in the proper way. You have to give an account for every cent that you receive. He won't ask you. Not even the government will ask you, because you are tax-exempted. But God will ask you. So let us not just think that even though things come easily I can just sit and enjoy. That's the karma theory.

So now you see how many complications are there in Karma Yoga. One has to take care of everything. That way the mind is quickly trained. It's a vigorous work. The mind can come to the tranquil level, the sattwic level, very quickly; all other practices are more slow. So that's the reason why we say: "Treat everything as Karma Yoga; see that you always give a little more." And that is what you call Yoga. This way you'll be having a continuous retreat even when you go back home. We don't need to think, "Oh, there's no bell ringing, nobody to wake me up; I don't need to go and meditate; I just have to go and do my work." It doesn't matter even if you don't do meditation. If it is too difficult, it doesn't matter, but meditate on this point when you go to work: "Oh, let me do it as an offering to Him." That's why I say Yoga is not just a few selected practices, what you call meditating or asanas or pranayama or chanting. It's all good. If you have time, do that. If you don't have time, it doesn't matter. Don't think that if you don't sit and meditate, if you don't chant, if you don't do puja, or if you don't stand on your head, you'll be unfit for a yogic life. It is the attitude of mind. If you keep this attitude, you won't do things that will disturb your mind. You will keep your balance amidst all the ups and downs. Automatically, everything will come under control.

That's all I want to tell you. If you follow this, you will reach the goal — you will be always joyful and peaceful. Thank you. Om Shanthi.

Questions and Answers on Parents and Children

Swami Satchidananda

My mother feels hurt and rejected because of my devotion to Yoga. She calls me ungrateful. I usually feel peaceful and positive, but when I go to my parents' home, I feel sucked into negativity.

Well, many, many children are in this boat. Yes. I really feel sorry for them because I hear a lot of stories about this. Even the parents call me and complain, "What is this Yoga? I don't understand what it is." And then I say, "Why don't you at least come and see what it is? You say you don't understand it. You don't know what it is. Without even knowing what it is, you ask your child not to do it. At least to pass a judgment, you should know what it is. Do you see your child doing anything wrong? Drinking, smoking, running around? In the name of Yoga, are they not becoming better children?"

"Yes, but I still don't know what it is all about."

Hmm. Well, the only way to know is just come and see what is happening. So, if they don't want to do it, if they don't want to understand, and at the same time if they are adamant in not allowing you to go, then know that your responsibility as a child is over. They are no longer your benefactors. They are either blind — a kind of blind affection — or selfish. They are not thinking of your welfare. You can just ignore that. You don't need to hurt them. But just ignore. Don't even go there. But prove yourself to be a good Yogi. Let others talk to them about you and one day . . . one day they will come. They will call you. They will understand the Yoga through you. Until then, have patience. You don't have to go there and get into negativity.

I'm not trying to separate the children from the parents, but when the parents are against the children's growth, they are not parents anymore. Stay away from them. Renounce them. But don't dislike them. You know the benefit, but they still do not know. Just wait until they know. Any many times it happens. If you just leave it alone, gradually they come. And they understand. That's the only way. Don't think that you are not fulfilling your responsibility as a child. Your first responsibility is to put yourself in the right spot. Be a child of God first.

Many, many great men, they left their home, family, everything, because that was not conducive for them to grow spiritually. That's why they left the home and went away. Not that they hated the parents. No. Later, when they got settled, they went back to the same home and they were received well.

When I'm at home I feel very drawn to this Yoga. It seems like the only sensible way to live. But as soon as I place myself in a yogic environment and start the practices, I feel, "Oh, no; I don't like it, I want to go home." What can I do for this?

Go home. When you're tired of that, come back again. Then it will be a little tastier. Then when you get dissatisfied, go home again, get bitten. Come back. One day you will say, "Every time I go, I get bitten, so I'll stay."

It takes time to understand and enjoy the taste. Other things give you some kind of taste quickly. But this takes time to get rooted and bring the fruit. If you plant spinach, within two days, or ten days, you can pluck some leaves. But if you want to plant a banyan seed, you won't see any leaves for five years. It takes a long time to grow. But it lives long when it grows. Everything is like that.

For instance, "I don't want to learn typewriting in the proper way, using the proper fingers. It is all nonsense and botheration. I can just do this." (*Swamiji imitates typing with two fingers.*) I start typing right away, typing my letters, but the fellow next to me doesn't do that; he takes patience to learn. He just types a, a, a, b, b, b, c, c, c, for weeks and weeks. I think, "Oh, at this rate, when is he going to type a letter? I have already finished a letter." But you see, he's like a tiger. When he started, he was backing up a little. I thought, "Oh, he is just backing up." But then, when I saw him bouncing forward, "Oh, now I know why he backed up!" (*laughter*) so it takes time. Don't expect a result immediately. Yoga fruit is a better fruit, a long-lasting fruit. So it will take time to mature.

So one problem is, if you are in a haste, if you don't see the result quickly, then you feel like stopping. And another is, you have to pay a big price for it. For other things, you can pay easily, small prices. But here you have to pay a big price. As Nirmalanandaji reminded you the other day, "The price is your ego. It hurts a lot." It's not that easy. It is easy to say, "Get rid of the ego." But even the people who come to get rid of the ego, they do some nice things and they wait for the appreciation. On one day someone will type ten letters and bring them, "These are all the letters I typed today; see, we have answered them all."

"Oh, beautiful, great, you are wonderful, glad to see that."

Then everything is okay. But if we just sign it and say, "Take it away," then, "So much work, and not even a word of appreciation."

And you make some nice vegetable one day. "Oh! Beautiful, great." I should say that. Otherwise, "Whatever I do, he doesn't seem to appreciate me."

Appreciation. We wait for appreciation for everything. Even among the students, when they do something, "Oh, I keep on doing it, but he doesn't seem to appreciate it." Even a little thing: "When I was away, I sent a card, and he especially called and said, 'Thank you for your wonderful letter, wonderful card.' He appreciated so much when I was away. Now that I am closer to him, he doesn't even look at me."

That's the natural tendency. Ask yourself, "Why do I want it? Did I do it for his appreciation? Or as a service, as my duty? Does a candle expect my appreciation? 'Oh, you give a nice light!' Does a scented stick ask for my appreciation? Does a flower ask for appreciation?" (*He indicates the flowers around him, on stage.*) They are sitting here all these days. I seldom even look at them. They don't grumble at me. "What, man, we're sitting on either side of you, don't you even see us and appreciate us?" No. Instead they feel, "My business is to be here, that's all. If you like to see, see. I don't even demand it."

That's the attitude a seeker should have. But it comes slowly. It won't come in a day — because you miss that appreciation. But every time you miss something, sit and analyze, "What is it that I miss? Is it necessary that I should get the appreciation? Is that what I want?" If you question yourself, all your feelings, every time, then you'll get the answer. So instead of immediately putting the blame on somebody, the seeker should question all his feelings, or all her feelings, whatever they be. "I'm excited today. Why? Oh, he says I'm fine. Huh? So if I am excited now, then I will expect the same thing every time. Hmm? That's not right." The seeker must be very careful. These are all subtle things, very small. But that will go a long way in your growth, in your control.

So I would tell this young person, "It doesn't matter, whatever it may be, come and go, come and go, come and go. Because the very fact that you are attracted to this, will slowly bring you again and again and one day you'll be permanent." It's something like, you want to learn swimming. Just get into the water. You may feel, "Oh! Get out! Run away!" Then, later, go a little more deep, one gulp of water, run away. And slowly, slowly, you get rid of the fear. And then one day when you start swimming, ah! you enjoy it. Then your mother will have a terrible time to pull you out of the water. For how many hours you are there, "Coming, Mama; coming, Mama," hm? That's why, until you get used to that, be patient.

In the outside world I am constantly upset because I see people around me acting more and more senseless and animal-like every day. At the same time I do not feel ready to live a complete yogic life-style. There are many things I don't want to give up. I feel stuck in the middle.

Well, at least that's a good beginning. And from the middle, look at both sides. Which will really help you? Outside, don't think that you are going to train others, to teach others. If they're animal-like, that's all right. You must have been animal-like before. Nobody's a born saint. You go outside and see the babies crawling. You say, "What babies, crawling! I don't like that!" What were you doing when you were a baby? In some sense *we* are babies. We may have grown up a little. They still have their own tendencies. So we have no right to condemn them. Pity them, and if you have the capacity, help them. Otherwise let them crawl. Let them grow. You don't need to condemn anybody. Everybody will be a saint in time. We should have tolerance. So if they're senseless and animal-like, you need not lose *your* sense. Be sensible in working with them. And if you can't, if you get irritated, then stay away until you have the strength.

I came to the retreat looking for answers to personal problems that need to be resolved. I am feeling peaceful here. But I know that when I get back home the problems will still be there. So far no answers seem to be coming. Is it wrong to look for answers? Should I just keep meditating and put my faith in that?

Keep meditating. You'll get answers. Don't be in a hurry. Now at least you are finding some peace. Find out where the peace comes from. You may say that it's coming from the environment here. In a way, it's true, but the environment is helping you realize your own peace. If only you come to know that, you can find the same peace wherever you go.

At the same time, don't go out to train anybody, to teach them. Take care of yourself. This reminds me of a very useful Yoga *sutra* (aphorism) in Patanjali. If you want to maintain your peace of mind, it's very, very helpful. If you have a paper and pencil, you can even note this point.

Patanjali gives four types of attitudes. Friendliness, compassion, joy, and just ignoring. These are the four different attitudes for the four types of people. What are the four types of people? Happy people, contented;

the miserable people, always unhappy; the virtuous people; and the vicious people. You can probably group all of the people within these four categories: either happy or unhappy, or virtuous or vicious. So whenever you see happy type of people, show friendliness. When you see unhappy people, show compassion. When you see virtuous people, show your joy. And when you see vicious people, ignore them. Don't try to go and teach them, unless they come and ask for your advice. They are not ready to take your advice. If you still feel like saying something, gently say a word. Keep an eye on their feeling, how they are receiving what you are saying. If you know that they are not receiving well, stop saying.

Once on a rainy day, a nice little sparrow was sitting in a comfortable nest. He saw a monkey sitting on a branch getting drenched, totally wet. The little sparrow looked at him and said, "Oh, God. You are a big animal. You have four legs, or at least two hands and two legs. I have only a beak and two little legs. See, I worked hard and made a nice comfortable home. I am not getting wet. I am happy inside the home. I saw you jumping around here and there, playing, but you never thought of the rainy season. If you had thought of it early and made a nice small home like me, you would have been happy. You need not be sitting here and getting wet."

"You, you little creature. You come to advise me, huh? Because you are cozy and comfortable in the rain, huh? So, you are mocking at me. Let me teach *you!*"

He jumped down and tore away the nest. "Come on now. You also get wet. Then you won't come to advise me."

That is what happens. So you don't need to go and give your advice to such people. Stay away from them. Ignore them. Let them learn by their own mistakes. You are not there to teach.

If you maintain these four kinds of attitudes with these four types of people, you maintain your peace. If you see happy people, be friends with them; unhappy, show your compassion — do what you can. With virtuous people, show your happiness, joy. "Oh, that's beautiful, wonderful." Appreciate them. If you see vicious people, always the wise men agree ... (*here Swamiji quotes a saying in Sanskrit and then translates*), "Wherever you see horns, stay away at least $2\frac{1}{2}$ yards. Don't go any nearer because they will strike you. For a horse, stay away at least 5 yards. They may bite or kick you. If you see an elephant, at least 500 yards. And the mischievous troublemakers, if you come across them, before they even see you, run away. Don't even be seen by them." That is a good method. Beautiful advice. It's really helpful.

Sometimes we have courage. "Oh, I can go and help them," you say.

You go there and get absorbed. How many times people say, "I can go and help them." Hmm? Within a week, you also. (*Swamiji imitates smoking pot.*) Yes. They go help them: In providing what they want, and to get more. So let us stay away. We can take care of the world later on. First take care of yourself. If you are not ready, nobody is going to blame you that you didn't take care of it. It's not your responsibility.

Was Mahatma Gandhi using Yoga in politics?

Gandhi followed Yoga, but his main theme was a part of *yama*, the first part of Yoga. He took just two parts of yama, *ahimsa* and *satyam*, nonviolence and truth; these are what he was trying to develop. Even until his death he was trying. He wanted that to be incorporated into the political field also. That's why he asked the Hindus not to fight back. Many of the Hindus were not ready to understand it. So they killed him. It's sort of like teaching truth to unfit students. If you tell them something, and they are not ready, they will kill you. It happens everywhere, every time. I was also condemned because I advocated *brahmacharya* and said that until they are married they should be single. It's just natural. Thank God they spared me. But I did it in a natural way. I did not force anybody. In Gandhi's case, he forced. "If you don't do it," he said, "I will kill myself by fasting." He fasted. When he said, "Unless you stop this trouble, I'm fasting unto death," what does it mean? "If you don't follow me, I'm going to kill myself." Why should I go to that extreme? I'm not forcing anybody. When they come and ask me I tell them, but not without their asking. So in a way Gandhi failed, in forcing Yoga into the political field. As an Indian I say this, for even in India many feel the same way. He was a great man, no doubt, but he was trying to force his truth onto unqualified students. We were not ready. And at the same time it is not possible to use total ahimsa in the political field.

Gandhi's own book was the Bhagavad Gita. He even translated the Bhagavad Gita. A follower of the Gita, he said, "Don't kill the vicious people." I myself could not understand his teachings. He believed it, he is a saint, he can say that and keep quiet. But if he forces that into politics, it brings trouble. So ahimsa doesn't mean not to kill. Killing is a necessity if it comes to that. If an individual refuses, it's all right, but as a group it's very difficult. It takes time. You can't change the whole world overnight. But even though he failed in the political field, personally he gained a lot; that's why the whole world respected him. Truthfulness and nonviolence were his watchwords, and at the same time devotion, Bhakti Yoga. Ram Nam! He trusted God in the name of Ram wholeheartedly, without any condition whatsoever. That's why, even when the bullet passed through him, he said, "Ram! If that is your will, take me." He didn't even want his assassin to be hanged. As a person, he was a great saint. But in the political field, in a way he failed. Even while he was advocating ahimsa, we had our military development. We were building arms. It's not possible to put that into the entire world. Yoga cannot just be made into something political, but individually one can grow. Even individually, for defense sake — you have to defend yourself. If you defend yourself and while defending, if you cause some *himsa* (harm) to somebody, it's still treated as ahimsa. It's a part of nature. The eyelids defend the eyes. The minute something flies in front of them, they defend. So all these vows should be understood properly.

Tenth Day

Staying Together

Brother David Steindl-Rast, O.S.B.

The last guest speaker of the retreat — an old and very dear friend of Swamiji's — is the one who in his own person represents best the dominant spiritual tradition of the West: the Christian tradition. Brother David Steindl-Rast is a Benedictine monk, who has long been concerned with the other major spiritual traditions, and their relation to Christianity, and who has personally involved himself in the practices of one of them: Zen Buddhism. But he had done this not in any sense as a dilution or departure from his own tradition, but always from a deep rootedness in it. He has found that deeper understanding of other faiths is complementary to a deeper understanding of one's own, so that one can see the common ground of all and at the same time respect the differences of each.

Just as Rabbi Gelberman has been helpful in opening up people to the compatibility of the Jewish tradition and Yoga (a source of concern both to those who feel that Yoga might conflict with Judaism and to those who are alienated from their own Jewish background), so Brother David speaks to those who are concerned about the compatibility of Yoga and Christianity. Already much has been said about this, particularly by Swami Nirmalananda, but in his case it was from the perspective of one who had adopted the Hindu form of religion as his own. In the case of Brother David, we see a man of profound Christian conviction — who lives a Christian life — yet sees the unity between Christianity and that universal essence of all religions which we call Yoga.

As East and West are predominantly characterized by the Hindu (and Buddhist) faiths on the one hand, and the Christian on the other, it is fitting that the retreat should close with Brother David's talk. And in closing, Brother David picks up and completes the theme that Swamiji used to open the retreat: coming together and staying together.

In the course of his talk, Brother David discusses the mantram and shows how this is not an exclusively Eastern practice but is to be found in the Christian tradition as well; and he talks also on another subject much discussed during the retreat: the question of householder and monastic life. With his typical lucidity and precision, Brother David shows that the two are not in any way in opposition, that neither represents a more "natural" or more "spiritual" path; that in fact they are complementary ways to the same goal.

Brother David is not a storyteller, but a man with a very clear and exact mind: what one might call a jnani. He requires close attention to what he says, and he repays it. He is able to analyze a problem so as to clear away all confusion, leaving the listener free of all conceptual obstacles — obstacles that often lie unconsciously in the mind.

At the close of his relatively short comments, Brother David also answers questions from

278

the retreatants. The audience, which had listened intently to Brother David's comments, responds to the offer by asking many of those questions which come so readily to mind to persons from a Christian background in their search for a more universal spiritual understanding.

Thank you, Swamiji, and all of you, for inviting me. It's a great joy to be with you. Just to see all these happy faces and shiny eyes, on this beautiful morning, is a great joy. To come, after you have been here for ten days, and then to say something . . . that's like rain on the ocean. Steven picked me up early this morning, and on the way told me about the way things have been going here, and I asked him what he thought might be questions in your minds, so that I can address myself more concretely to what you want to hear at this point of the retreat. He came up with very much the same questions that always arise at the end of a retreat. It's basically: where do we go from here? We don't want to go anywhere. This is such a wonderful place, why do we have to leave? We have been together now for ten days, and it seems like eternity, and now, why do we have to part? And what shall we do then, when we are all alone out there? It's kind of a re-entry panic after you have been out in space for ten days. What's going to happen when we get back into the atmosphere of our daily lives? Well, the point is, stay together, stay together. If you have really come together, in the full sense of the word – which implies not just together with others who speak your language and with whom you feel comfortable, but together with yourself for once, which is so rare – really together with yourself, and therefore, together with God, together with that ground of our being from which we are so easily uprooted and alienated – if you've really come together during these ten days, then stay together. So the question is not so much what are we supposed to do when we are no longer together, but the question is, really, how are we going to stay together?

I would just like to suggest a way of reflecting on our own experience, because sometimes when we reflect, it helps us. We ought not to be disturbed by reflection while we experience; we are just to be experiencing. But then, we have some periods where we can reflect on our experience, and our trouble is that the two often get mixed up with one another. We can't really experience as deeply and as fully as we would like, because reflection constantly gets in our way, and we are constantly distracted from really being there. And then, at other times, when we want to reflect, experience creeps in as a sort of distraction, and doesn't allow us to reflect as clearly and with as much detachment as we should. So this, right now, is a period of reflection on our experiencing, and I would just like to draw out some of the aspects of the experience that you have had during these ten days.

When you are really together with yourself, it is because you accept yourself. The key word here is self-acceptance. So to the extent that you would be able to retain this self-acceptance, you'll be able to stay together with yourself. And you have been together with one another here and enjoyed that and rejoiced in it — as one can clearly see just by the vibrations that one gets when one comes into the place — through selflessness, through selfless service. Selflessness goes very well together with self-acceptance. Somehow you first have to accept yourself and then you become selfless, but you can also go the other way round — just serve in selflessness, and as you serve, you will begin to be able to accept yourself. The two go hand in hand. And there's just one more thing, and that's really the most important, and that's self-forgetfulness. Not to be preoccupied with accepting yourself, not being pre-occupied even with selfless service. Preoccupied in the sense that you think about it, that you constantly have to make an effort toward it. Self-forgetfulness is to go beyond all these efforts to the point where you make the greatest effort, which is to make no effort at all. Then you are no longer preoccupied, "Oh, I must accept myself," "Oh, I must serve selflessly." Instead, you just forget yourself, and that puts you together with God, because before you forget yourself, how could you be together with everything, with the ground of everything — with God?

And now, just recalling your own experience and reminding you of what you yourself know, I'd like to remind you that this togetherness which is really what we're looking for, which is what makes us so happy, is perfectly compatible with being alone, and in fact implies a greater aloneness than our normal way of living, our more superficial way of living. When we are truly together, we are truly alone.

Now, to a certain extent, we experience this as loneliness, but that's not what it's meant to be. To the extent that we experience our aloneness as loneliness, it isn't yet fully purified. We may have to go through periods of loneliness, just as we may have to go through periods of childhood diseases. If you haven't had them, you may not be as well off in later life, or maybe more in danger and not very strong. And so loneliness is not good in itself, but it may be very helpful to you. It is just something to get through, something to be purified. So when you really are together, you're even more alone than in your loneliness, but not in a bad sense. You are solitary.

There's a great difference between being solitary and being lonely.

Loneliness is an aloneness that is cut off from others, and you experience painfully how you are cut off from others. Solitude is an even greater and deeper aloneness, but an aloneness that unites you with all others, an aloneness that is supported by others, that is perfectly compatible with togetherness. And therefore, if we focus on the aloneness in togetherness, we must say that self-acceptance implies accepting our aloneness, accepting it and so redeeming it. Loneliness is overcome by this acceptance of our aloneness. Aloneness in togetherness with others means redeeming the loneliness of others, and we do that by giving them all the support they need in togetherness. But, the other side of this, the other half of this, is that we leave them alone. If we think we are supporting others by togetherness and yet we don't know when to leave them alone, we are not really supporting them – we are infringing on their aloneness. If we just leave them alone, and don't sufficiently pay attention to the need for supporting others, then we just plainly leave them in the lurch, and leave them lonely, and fail very much. So, the two have to come together. You have to develop a very fine sensitivity as to when to leave others alone, and leave them really alone by supporting them in their aloneness.

It is in this sense that we really have to become the mothers of our friends, we have to become the mothers of everybody. We have to enter into the motherliness of God. And of course in our Western tradition, where we speak so often and so insistently about God as our Father, we overlook the fact that He is every bit as much our Mother. We are a little warped in this way, and have great difficulties with this. But it's very important to think of this "Motherliness" that we want to have toward one another. A mother that doesn't support her children isn't a mother. That's the whole idea of motherhood. Even physiologically, a fertilized egg is on the way out, to be discarded by the body, until the womb takes it on. We say it implants itself in the womb. But that's not a very good expression. The womb takes it on. This is a very different thing. By itself, it can't implant itself in the womb, if the endocrine system of the body does not allow this to happen. The body must take it on. So, from the very first moment, life is taken on. If we had not been taken on and supported, we would never have come to birth, any one of us here. So the mother takes on and supports that life. But a mother gives birth, and unless we give birth to one another, we don't become mothers either. We kill life. And every mother knows, I'm sure, how difficult it is to give birth over and over again. Some mothers think it is enough if they give birth to the child once, and then they smother it; smother love, rather than mother love. Children know what that feels like. How difficult it must be for a mother to give birth over and over again, because it's much more difficult to give birth to a teenager than to a tiny baby. And yet, this is absolutely necessary, to constantly let go, let alone. And it is in this sense that we must be mothers towards one another. Only then will we really be able to enter into that Aloneness, which is Aloneness with a capital A, or all capital letters, which spells in a way All One-ness, Aloneness; Alone, All One.

You're all one with yourself. You're all one with all others, because you know how to support them and let them be, and you are one with all, with the universe, with what goes beyond the universe. You are united with God, you're truly together in that sense too, because you're not clinging to anything, and because you are not refusing your relatedness to anything. You're supporting and you're letting be. And that takes tremendous courage. That's very difficult — to be alone and together in this sense. And you may have noticed that the two spiritual paths, the basic spiritual paths, are also closely connected with this aloneness, and this togetherness. It is either the path of the householder, in which the togetherness is clearly emphasized, or it is the path of the sannyasi, the monk, in which the aloneness is clearly emphasized. But if we know from our own experience that togetherness and aloneness are intimately united, really inseparable from one another, then we also see that these two paths are really complementary, and are really leading to the same goal. It isn't as if one were a kind of privileged path, and you try to do that but if it doesn't work out for you, then, well, do the best you can, and choose the other one. Or as if the other one, the path of togetherness, were really the normal path, but if you happen to be some sort of freak or misfit, well then, make the best of it and choose the path to aloneness. It's neither the one nor the other. Because both paths lead, and are designed to lead, to the fullness of life in which we are together. And in married life, it isn't, as the overtones of advertising would have us believe, that the ideal marriage is a pairing of two halves, with each one as just half a creature, and if they fit nicely together, well then you get the ideal couple. But the ideal marriage is a long process in which each one helps the other to become a whole. You see? And in this respect, it has the same goal exactly as the monastic life, namely to make the person whole. And the question is only, "Which is *my* path?"

It's not that one is better or that one is higher or anything of the sort, but we have to start from where we are. That's our trouble in spiritual life, that we always want to start where we are not. But there is no other place to start but where we are. So we ask ourselves, "What is my path?" And it may take a long time until we clearly see which of the two paths will crystalize. But once we see it clearly, then we can commit ourselves.

And we commit ourselves, by one or the other path, to one and the same goal — and that is to become a whole person, to help one another either in the community of single people who live singly for the sake of God, or in the very close togetherness of a married life and of a family — again to support one another, so that each one can become a whole. And it is easier in monastic life to overlook the need to support one another, and loneliness creeps in very easily. It is a kind of professional hazard. And it is easier in married life to overlook the need for solitude and to smother one another, to make one another smaller, to deprive one another of wholeness. That is one of the professional hazards of married life. So as long as we keep our eyes on the professional hazards and keep our eyes on the goal, we will have a much clearer idea as to where we are going, on both paths. In monastic life, it is going to true togetherness by the path of aloneness; in married life, it's a way of going to true aloneness by the path of togetherness.

Now all this sounds nice, but how are you going to do it when you get back to the city? How are you going to stay together when the temptation to be lonely is so great, when the support by others is suddenly withdrawn. I think that this is where, among other things, the mantram comes in. I speak primarily from the experience of the Jesus prayer, which is a Christian mantram. I think that more people who have discovered the spiritual life through the Hindu tradition have revealed a grasp and understanding of the Jesus prayer than people who have come out of the Biblical tradition. It is a very, very old form of prayer, nevertheless. It's probably one of the oldest forms of Christian prayer, going back to the first century supposedly, but at least to the third or fourth century. It is simply a repetition of the name of Jesus in a prayerful way, very much like a mantram. I think that the emphasis is slightly different, in that there's not so much emphasis on the sound and the vibrations that you set up. It's a little more intellectual, because the Biblical tradition is a little more intellectual than the Hindu tradition, for better or worse. But in both cases it isn't primarily an intellectual thing, or an emotional thing; it is a matter of the heart, and that is why the Jesus prayer is also called the Prayer of the Heart. You can't recite a mantram with your head, you can't recite the Jesus prayer with your head. The whole idea is that you bring the mind down to your heart, or as deep as you can. And your heart is that center of your person where you are all one, where you are together. See, if you want to make a statement about some action that you did with your whole person, you say, "I made this decision from my heart of hearts." Or, if you have a conviction that is rooted where you are really together, you say, "In my heart of hearts I am convinced of this." So your heart is a symbol, is an expression, of that togetherness, and the mantram is a prayer of the heart, the Jesus prayer is a prayer of the heart. And every time you recite your mantram, every time you recite the Jesus prayer, you enter again into that heart, into that center in which you are together with yourself, with all others, with God. To come back again and again to this heart — that's why we recite the mantram, that's why every second, with every breath, we pull ourselves together so that we can go out from there and serve.

Now, in our monastery, we have a tradition; it's a particular expression of a broader tradition, and it's closely connected with this prayer of the heart. It's a very practical way of living. I thought I'd share this with you. We call it "the little steps," because all these high-sounding things have to be translated into little steps, and these steps are just three, basically. You can break each one of them down into many others, but basically there are just three. They help us, and they might be helpful to you, when you go back. The first step is not a step at all, but it is to stop before you take a step. This is our biggest problem, that in our enthusiasm or in our downheartedness, or in our forgetfulness — whatever it is — we rush into the next thing, instead of taking a step. And you can't take a step unless you first stop, and gather yourself together. So the first thing is, stop! In your reciting of the mantram, in your reciting of the prayer of the heart, the first benefit you derive from it is, that every time you recite it you stop — not in a static sense, but in this very dynamic sense in which stopping is part of moving, like setting your foot down is part of walking.

The first thing is that you really stop, and the second thing is that you look. It's very much like crossing a street. You stop, look, go. That's really what it amounts to. First you stop; then you look, and looking is a very inadequate term here because what it means is total openness. It's not just a looking, it's a listening, it's an openness of all our senses, but goes beyond the senses; it's an opening of our heart. We really open ourselves, we really let the light fall on everything that is in the present moment; we bring everything in, and then we survey the whole thing. And this may sound like a very clumsy process, because it really has to include our whole past, and all our hopes and aspirations for the future. They all have to come together in this present moment. So it includes all the mistakes that we have made in the past, from which we should have learned, and all the good advice that has been given to us in the past, and all the good things that we've done in the past, and that have laid the foundation of where we are now, and that have given us an impetus towards where we are going, all the hopes and outlooks for the future, and the clear-cut planning for the future. But of course all this is present in a very general way, unless we're dealing with a major decision in our life, where we have to analyze and take maybe a day or days to work this out. But normally this stopping should take no longer than a fraction of a second, and this looking should take no longer than a fraction of a second.

And then the third thing. Now that you look, you may see the next little step ahead of you, just enough to see where to step. And then you go. But you really go, and that is very important. That is something which we also overlook very often. Most of the time when something goes wrong — and that is the time when we stop and check, while we should have stopped much earlier — the first thing we discover is that we didn't stop soon enough. Or we did stop, but we didn't really look. Just those little steps. It is so easy to deceive ourselves in this. We may stop and look. We may even go to people for advice, but we make sure they have their blind spot exactly in the same place as ours. Or we look and we know that there is something over there and we make sure we don't look too closely at the thing, because that is the one thing that gives us trouble. So it is the one thing that eventually causes things to go wrong. So looking means really looking — at everything — and then go.

And how often we fail with that going. Either we don't go at all — we figure we have done all that is necessary or we stop and look and we sit — or we go across, but we go so sluggishly that by the time we come to the middle of the street the light has changed. The cars come zooming by before we ever get anywhere, because we didn't go really. So this "go" part is just as important as the stopping and the looking, and this "go" part is also in the prayer of the heart, in your mantram. Your mantram is something that sends you. And you will never fully understand the word until you do what it sends you to do. The understanding comes with the doing, not with the sitting and mulling it around in your head. The mantram can never be understood in your head, nor the Jesus prayer for that matter. It is a word truly, a word that cannot be translated into any other words or language. And that word will only be understood if we go.

That is really the answer, the second half of the answer, to the question with which we started out. The question was, where do we go from here? Now we have been together and the answer was, stay together! But the other half of the answer is, go! And the two are not incompatible. The thing is that if you really go where the word sends you — that "word" which these ten days were here — then you will go in such a way that you will stay, will never lose this togetherness. That's the way to go, and if you really stay in that togetherness then you will go, you will go beyond yourself, constantly beyond yourself, by self-forgetfulness, by self-acceptance, by selflessness and service.

These were the thoughts I thought I'd share with you. And I would now rather have you bring up questions, either questions that relate to this or any other questions while we are together.

Questions and Answers on Yoga and Christianity

Brother David Steindl-Rast, O.S.B.

What's the Jesus Mantra?

There's an old tradition. I was going to say a monastic tradition, but it isn't really. It's very much a layman's tradition: a very old tradition in the Christian church that goes back to the earliest centuries. It basically consists just in repeating the name of Jesus. And I'm personally convinced — and although one cannot prove it, I think that most scholars are convinced — that this was originally introduced into the Christian tradition by contact with Hinduism, with Hindu monks and with the Hindu practice of mantra. It seems quite obvious there was a great deal of exchange between the near East and India at that time. So it seems that the stimulus came from the East, came from India. All you'd need is just one senior monk who would tell the Christian monks, that's what we do. He can get the idea and from there he can develop it. That's all you'd need. Now that particular monk is not recorded in history by name and date, but we do know that there were monks going back and forth and why shouldn't it happen? All of a sudden it springs up. It crystalized at Mt. Athos. Before that, in the earliest centuries, in the whole Eastern region where monasticism was strongest, the monks would simply repeat the name of Jesus — that was the original form. Then other developments took place in which it was made longer and longer. Maybe, "Jesus"; "Lord Jesus"; "Lord Jesus, have mercy"; "Lord Jesus, have mercy on me"; "Lord Jesus, have mercy on me a sinner." That is the most developed form that I have come across and that's one of the standard forms now found in the Eastern church. It seems a little long to me and I'm not quite clear how you coordinate this with your breath. But people do it. I think they do it with separate breaths, you see. But the simplest form is just the name of Lord Jesus or Lord Jesus, mercy. As you breathe in, you pronounce the name, and as you breathe out you either pronounce nothing or "mercy," "have mercy," or whatever it may be. Mercy is preferable in my mind, because you don't ask for mercy. There are situations in which really you can't ask, and you just say, "mercy."

But it is a breathing-in that takes everything in and names it at that mo-

287

ment. You breathe in and whatever this present situation contains, you open yourself to it and you name it. You know what it's all about, there is no more than that one word. Then you breathe out and you give yourself in service, you respond to the situation, and you breathe in again, you breathe out. Now this has been practiced throughout the centuries, and as I said, Mt. Athos was a center for it because Mt. Athos was a center for Eastern monastic life anyway. This was very much practiced there, and then it was very highly developed also in connection with *mudras*, with particular positions of your hands, and with a particular posture, usually the lotus posture. All these elements may have been developed more or less independently because they are so natural to man, or there may have been more than one connection in which influences came from India. And then some of the greatest writings that date over a period of about a thousand years were collected in the eighteenth century. There had been many many different collections but that final collection was made in the eighteenth century and was published in Venice. It's a huge volume and it's called the *Philokalia*, "The Love of the Beautiful." And it contains texts from all the different Fathers throughout the centuries who have written on this Jesus prayer.

Some of you must be familiar with the prayer from the book *Franny and Zooey*. That's really a whole book about the Jesus prayer and the only problem is that it's such a good book. It's about many things, and some people overlook the most important thing for Salinger and that's the Jesus prayer. So, you might even want to reread it under that aspect. In the book, references are made to the *Philokalia* and also to another little book that's more popular because it's more easily accessible and that's *The Way of a Pilgrim*, the story of a Russian pilgrim. It's a little autobiography and probably also partly fictitious. It was published in Russian about a hundred years ago and is now available in paperback in English. I'm sure many of you have read it. It's a story of a man who wants to pray all of the time — that's the Biblical formulation: We ought to pray at all times — but he doesn't know how to do it. In other words, he wants to keep in contact with God, he wants to keep together at all times. So he finally finds an old monk who teaches him this Jesus prayer and that's where the book begins. He describes how he's being taught and how he goes on and practices it and leaves everything behind and just travels for years and years as a pilgrim throughout Russia. He describes all the beautiful experiences he has as he meets different people and the things that happen to him and how people treat him and how he helps them by doing nothing else but just repeating this one mantram over and over again, the prayer of the heart. He is a man that lives out of the heart and so he is really united with the heart of the world. That's where we all hang together and so he can speak to everybody, heart to heart. That's why he can speak to people from all different walks of life. Russia at that time was divided into different castes who would have nothing to do with each other, but he can speak to everybody because he speaks the language of the heart. It's a very beautiful book, published by the Seabury Press in paperback and those of you who haven't come across it can easily get it.

Are the principles of reincarnation compatible with the Christian doctrine?

The answer is yes. It's very simple, because we are talking about the *principles* of reincarnation. And if I understand them correctly, they are some very basic answers to some very basic questions that human beings have had at all times. Like: Is there justice? Is everything to be worked out? Because we see just such a little stretch of the way in which this justice is worked out, it looks like injustice in some cases. And so we ask ourselves, is there justice? And the answer is, yes. That's the answer that every religious person has given. And reincarnation is just one image under which the answer is given.

And another question is: If a person dies, as most people die, neither being so good that you say this person now becomes one with the Knower, one with Ultimate Reality, nor so bad that you'd have to say that person is just lost, just disintegrated and goes down the drain or something like that, what happens to that person? Most people die in this state. There's a beautiful passage, a beautiful scene, in Ibsen's play *Peer Gynt*. Most of the other plays by Ibsen are more familiar to students, but *Peer Gynt* is probably his most important play, and it's so very different from all the others. It's really a cosmic play. Peer Gynt is Everyman. He goes through all the ups and downs. He leaves his bride Solveg at the moment when she comes to him. She is the absolute perfect love for him. And he's an outcast and he deserves to be an outcast and he knows he deserves to be an outcast. He lives in the mountains and he builds his own house. And just when the house is almost finished, Solveg appears on the scene in her snowshoes, having come all the way through the snow up into the high mountains and says, "I've come to be with you." And that so completely knocks him off his feet, that he just goes out to gather some wood and he never comes back to the house. He spends his whole life everywhere in the world, messing his life up in every possible way and doing some good things, too. And then he comes back home, but not quite home, just close to home, when he's a very old man. He meets Death now, in the woods. Death comes in the form of a buttonmaker.

You see, in Norway at that time, these buttonmakers went from one village to another, and they cast lead into little buttons. And Death is a buttonmaker and says to him, "You are one of those buttons that didn't turn out, and you have to be recast now." Peer Gynt is terribly upset and he tries to prove that he was good enough to go to heaven. But for everything that he did good, he did something wrong, too. And so Death finally says, "You can't go to heaven. You're really not good enough." And he sees that. It doesn't take much persuasion. Then he tries to prove that he's at least bad enough to go to hell, because he much prefers to go to hell than to be recast, you see. Just completely undone. But he can't find proof that he's bad enough to go to hell. He goes to all the different people, and he did a lot of bad things, you see. He sold idols to the heathens, and made a fortune, then somebody comes along and proves that he gave some of that money to the missions. So he isn't good enough to go to heaven, and he isn't bad enough to go to hell. And just at the point when the buttonmaker comes for the last time, to recast him, he hears singing, and that's the famous Solveg's song which everybody knows who has ever seen *Peer Gynt*. He hears her singing, and she's a very old woman, and she's still sitting in front of the house where he left her. And she is singing a cradle song. And he bends his head in her lap and he keeps saying he hopes now that she will be the one that proves that he was really bad enough to go, at least, to hell. And she is the one that proves that he was. He says, "But where was I all this time? Where was I? I am not." And she says, "You were in my heart." She gives birth to him; she becomes his mother at that point.

That comes back to our being mothers to one another and to being together in this sense. Again, one of the principles of reincarnation is the conviction that there is no man who has to be simply recast. We are. But we often are not good enough to go to heaven and so something else has to happen to us. The Christian answer to this is purgatory. And I think that it's very important for me, coming out of the Christian tradition, to bring up purgatory, when you ask about reincarnation, because it's the same answer to the same questions. I do not take the image of purgatory literally, just as I don't take that of reincarnation literally. I don't believe that there is a fire burning somewhere, and that I will be kind of purified through fire, but I do believe that the purification will be as a purification through fire, every bit as much.

So I do not want to be pressed to accept any particular imagery of reincarnation. It is for me a beautiful, poetic, strong, mythical image, with which I can totally identify, just as I totally identify with purgatory, and there's no incompatibility. But the moment that I press purgatory, as some people have done, with a more primitive mentality, I can't accept it any more. And the moment I press reincarnation in any concrete mode, I can't accept it anymore. But I think I accept it more fully by not insisting on the literalness of it.

If I'm a Catholic and I meditate at home and I don't go to church, is it a sin?

First of all, nothing can be a sin if you don't recognize it to be a sin. Secondly, I believe that a person who is serious enough to meditate at home would be serious enough to have given serious consideration to this and would not simply stay at home out of laziness. Now, normally, Christians, for over two thousand years, have gotten together on one particular day of the week to break bread with one another and to celebrate the presence of the risen Lord among them. That's a great thing. That is not something that is easily discarded by anybody who really believes in Christ, because just as a family tradition, that's tremendous, if you think about that. Every Sunday for two thousand years we got together and did the same thing. You might normally want to be in on it. And that is why this community of believers put such an important premium on it. And they say that it is even a grave sin if you don't come. But, as I said, if you're in tune with what is happening there and you do not recognize that this is a sin, it is no sin for you. You may one day recognize that this is really something that you ought to do and then if you didn't do it it would be a sin. You may be encouraged by the fact that so many Christians, who are good Christians and good people by any standards, and deeply spiritual, *do* consider it important to get together and break bread. Then it will encourage you to take a more positive view of it.

This past week we have heard about yogic monastic and householder life. Could you explain a bit about Christian monastic communities. How do they compare with Eastern monasticism?

Well, this is a very big question, and I will restrict myself to one very small aspect which I consider somehow the clue, so that from there you can follow it up. First, we have to say that in the Catholic Church today we have a vast multitude of religious orders and only very few of them are monastic. First, you have to make this distinction. So the vast majority of those hundred and sixty thousand religious that we have just in the United States right now are not primarily, not strictly, monastic. They are people who serve God in their neighbor and that is not possible without that dimension of finding yourself, of being together with

yourself. But the monastic tradition, which comprises a very small frag-
ment of religions, is primarily concerned with being together with
yourself. Now, I've said enough about the two being absolutely inseparable from one another, so that you can see that there's a monastic
element to anyone's life who serves others, and there is a service aspect to
anyone who emphasizes this finding yourself, being together with
yourself.

You're familiar with the fact that this is also central to the Eastern
tradition, getting together with yourself, getting yourself together, finding yourself. In both traditions, it's done by meditation. In the Western
monastic tradition it is done by meditation that has the emphasis on the
outward manifestation of God, while in the Eastern tradition the
emphasis is on the inward manifestation of God. Now, again, the two are
absolutely inseparable from one another. But that's why, in the Western
tradition, the monastery, the way it looks, the way it's built, the schedule,
the things you do, the scriptures, the reading, the study, have such a
strong emphasis — because that is all outward manifestation. The Benedictine tradition, out of which I myself come and which has influenced all
the various monastic trends in the Western Church — it's the oldest in a
way — emphasizes mindfulness. Doing everything with mindfulness,
handling everything with mindfulness. One of the important passages is
that every pot and pan in the monastery should be handled as if it were
the sacred vessel on the altar. Not *as if*, really, in the last analysis, but
because they *are* the sacred vessels of the altar, because the whole monastic
life is conceived as a life of worship, of constant communion with God.
And you communicate with Him through the chalice that stands on the
altar. And this is then extended to your contact with other human beings,
with learning, with environment, with everything. Not that we have
done a particularly good job of it, I must admit, but if we were to sit back
and be satisfied and say we've done a great job of it, we'd be just as much
on the wrong track as if the Eastern tradition were to sit back and say,
we've done a great job in finding the inward manifestation of God. We
have tried. Both traditions have tried very hard. I'm inclined to think,
maybe because the grass is always greener on the other side of the fence,
that the Eastern tradition has done a little better in establishing methods
of really coming to a deep communion with the inward manifestation of
God, than we have done in establishing methods to come to a deep communion with the outward manifestations of God. But give us time, we
are much younger. We have a lot to learn, we have a long way to go.
Besides, as I say, the two overlap. What one has accomplished is accomplished for everybody else. It's a common search; it's a pooling of

resources. That's how I would see it. Admittedly, it's not much of an answer, it's just a point in which direction to find the answer, and I hope it'll be helpful in this respect.

Would you please speak on the Mass and its relation to Yoga, if any?

Well, of course, one could speak about the Mass for hours, but again I will try to just bring out one point or so. And that is that Yoga, as Swami Venkatesananda has told us, "yokes" everything together. Yoga is the understanding that yokes God and man together. It comes from the same word as the English word "yoke" — it unites. And the Mass is in its center, in the center of this yoking together, this uniting together of the human-Divine. Or rather, it is the celebration, the re-enactment, the making present here and now of that yoking that took place throughout history and came to a head at one particular point in history, at the death and resurrection of Christ. That's why it is a re-enactment and a re-celebration, making present again this death and resurrection of Christ. And it is celebrated in the form of a meal, of a breaking of bread. Because that was the image that Jesus used throughout his life to show how all are one with one another and one with God. When you really break bread you are one — you are never as much your self as when you share with others. You're together with your self, you're together with all others. Limitless.

What is sin?

What is sin? This brings up the distinction between what is objectively wrong, and what is sin. Sin is always subjectively wrong. If it isn't subjectively wrong, it can't be sin, no matter how objectively wrong it is. But we have a responsibility to inform ourselves in many different ways of what is right and what is wrong. Our whole life is this informing and to fail in this is already a sin, something which we know we ought to do and we don't do it. You see, life tells us that we ought to open ourselves to life, and if we do, we open ourselves to all the right and wrong, all the do's and don'ts that are implicit in life. So, it isn't very likely that somebody who is really trying to live fully will not recognize some of those major mistakes, like killing and lying. Yet on the other hand, just think about those millions and millions of people that have been killed just in recent years. Did all those who killed them really sin; did they recognize that they were doing something wrong? I am not prepared to say that. It was a terrible disaster. It was a disaster for their own souls too, because nobody can injure anybody else without injuring himself. You may not be aware of that, if you are that blind. But there is a distinction between sin and doing wrong. You can do wrong·without sinning, if you don't recognize it as a sin. That's simply a way of speaking about it. It's a terminological question. If you want to use the term sin in a different sense, well, anybody's free to use words anyway they want. But I think it helps to clarify it in this way.

Could you speak about the problem of evil? We have heard the Hindu play-of-Maya explanation. Why does God permit alienation, evil, self-destruction, less than humanity, or less than divinity to occur?

The answer in Christian theology is that evil and sin are mysteries and that you cannot fathom them and cannot give the answer. Now, that isn't really so far removed from that play-of-maya answer either, because that play is also a mystery. We don't quite understand why. It's just a very beautiful way of saying it. Now I myself like that play-of-Maya idea, and I find it perfectly compatible with Christian tradition, even with Old Testament tradition, because in the Book of Wisdom it says that the Wisdom of God delights in playing all the time on the face of the Earth, and that's what it's all about. We can go very wrong, and we have gone very wrong in the West, by overlooking this idea that in the last analysis everything is play. We have made everything so purpose-oriented that in the end we ask ourselves, "If he's really God, why does He need the world? What purpose could *that* be?" It's not a purpose. He needs nothing if He's really God. So why does He create? Because He plays. You look around and it's very obvious that He plays. Just the way things look. It's very playful. We don't always look that playful, but if you look at the birds and at the flowers and so forth, it's a very playful universe. And so I think the idea that God's divine Wisdom plays in the universe, is perfectly compatible with the Biblical tradition. You still haven't explained the mystery of evil. It remains a mystery. You just can't fathom it. But you have said something that at least makes you capable of living with it, and dealing with it, and avoiding evil and sin; and that's a great help.

We can take the next two questions together.

Did you ever feel an intellectual or emotional conflict in yourself from practicing Zen, Catholicism, and Hinduism? How did you come to study from different traditions rather than staying within one?

Please explain how zazen (the practice of Zen Buddhism) fits in with your spiritual practices? Would you compare it with mantra meditation?

No, I would not compare it with mantra meditation. But, maybe this was an invitation for me to do so. If so, then I will try to compare it. But it's something very different.

First, did I ever feel a conflict? Yes, because I come out of a very traditional Christian background in Austria where I was born. Some 98% are Catholics, so it's about as traditional as any country can be, and it never had a Reformation really, for better or worse. Anybody who comes from Austria is very much stuck in one tradition, and so there is a certain fear, I guess. We are always fearful of giving up our own traditions or of questioning. Of course, if you have an open mind, it isn't fear so much, but, "Well, I wonder, are we really still on the right track?" Or something like that. But I didn't go out and browse around to see if there wasn't something that I could add to my Catholic tradition. I must admit, I don't know whether this would be desirable or not; but at any rate, I didn't do it. I always had the feeling that one tradition is already too big to do justice to in one lifetime, so stick with it and don't browse around. This is one of my favorite quotes of Swamiji: If you want to find water, keep digging. So I knew I could keep digging for the rest of my days.

But through circumstances, I was faced with other traditions, and I had the tremendous privilege of meeting Swamiji and meeting Eido Roshi and meeting other men of very very different spiritual traditions. The moment I met them I could recognize — maybe because I was dedicated to my own tradition — that we were all speaking the same language, that we were all trying to do the same thing, and the more different it got outwardly, the more clearly I could see how much it was the same inwardly. I'm not saying it's all the same. I'm saying it's very very different, just as different as you can possibly make it, and if you haven't quite recognized how different it is, well then, go on, and you will see how different it is. But the more different it is, the more it also becomes one. That's the paradox. And this is how I would like to wind this up, because this paradox is really anchored in the central paradox of the Christian faith.

What is that central paradox? Not the divinity of Christ or the Incarnation or the Resurrection or anything like that. The central mystery of the Christian faith is the mystery of the Trinity. Of the Triune God. And again, to talk about Trinity, it isn't sufficient to talk about that mystery. But the way it looks to someone who stands in the Christian tradition is this: That it is always the one God, whom Christians recognize as Triune, whom everybody seeks. And in seeking Him, you can focus — as the

Biblical traditions: Jews, Christians, Moslems, have done — on his Word. You can focus on the fact that he speaks to us. Now this is tremendous and you never come to an end with that. So you live by the Word of God as it manifests itself around you and within you and in everything that you experience. You are really centering on God speaking to you.

But you can also center on the silence of God out of which this Word comes and into which this Word leads. The silence embodied in the Word of God seems to me where Buddhists and particularly Zen is at: preoccupied with the silence of Ultimate Reality every bit as much as we are preoccupied with the fact that Ultimate Reality speaks to us and we have to respond. It isn't either-or. The Word and the silence are not separable from one another. And that is precisely the insight where Hinduism and Yoga come in: the yoking together of the Word and the silence. You say, "It isn't one over against the other, but I listen to the Word so deeply, I give myself to the Word so totally, that the Word will lead me into that silence out of which it comes." That is the gesture that Yoga makes in all its various forms. That's the Hindu gesture. Of course, that's not a dead-end road where finally you are stuck now in the silence and there is emptiness, nothing else. When you are really deeply silent, the silence comes to Word; it's like a deep lake that overflows, and flows into the Word. And the Word through understanding returns into the silence.

That's why the notion of the Trinity is such a dynamic notion in Christianity. The early Fathers, Greek Fathers, called it the "round dance" of the Trinity. Within God there is room for a round dance. This play of Maya has its roots even there: Where the Father, what Christians call Father, the abyss of God, expresses Himself totally in this one eternal Word, which is the Son, whom we have come to know in Jesus. Others have come to know Him in other ways. Many people have come to know, but it is always the one Word because there is only one Word and this then finds its manifestation in different ways in different times. For Christians this one Christ is the central event and we would betray our tradition if we didn't acknowledge this. That's what it was for me. That's what it is for most Christians although that doesn't exclude other possibilities for other people.

God speaks through a rainbow or through any experience or through some other human being. And we can understand this Word of God only because we have the Spirit of God. This is again New Testament. St. Paul says, "No one can understand what's in the mind of a man except the Spirit of that same man." I alone know what's in me. And so no one can understand what's in the mind of God except the Spirit of God. And then he goes on and says, "And we have received that Spirit so that we can understand." And that Spirit is what Christians call the Holy Spirit. That's the Spirit of God. And we have all received it from the very first moment of our life, and we can open ourselves more and more to it so that, in this Spirit, we will understand what the Word of God in a given situation says to us, and will allow this Word to lead us into that silence from which it comes. In other words, we'll dance with the Trinity; we'll enter into that tremendous dance of God.

Closing Comments by Retreatants

As is traditional at Integral Yoga retreats, on the last day, after the final talk, the retreatants themselves get the opportunity to come up and express their thoughts and feelings. It is shortly before noon as Hari invites every retreatant who wishes to do so to come up one at a time. He invites them to share their experiences on the retreat, or to sing a song, or to read a poem, or even to offer criticisms and suggestions as to how the retreat could have been run better — this is described as offering a few pickles, the idea being that the sweet always tastes a little sweeter if it is interspersed with something a little sour. Or, if they wish, retreatants may simply express their thanks, and in fact this is what many of the retreatants who speak choose to do.

This time of the retreat never fails to be moving. All during the ten days, each retreatant has been observing silence. This means that all their feelings have remained within, to be transformed through the inner practices or expressed through the chanting — but in any case not to be dissipated in the normal way of just talking. This leads to an intensification and purification of feelings, but it also sometimes leads some retreatants to feel that they are perhaps the only ones who are going through difficult changes — everyone else around them seems (as do they to others) serene and peaceful.

Now, at the time of the retreatants' sharing, everyone recognizes their own experience in the expressions of others. In many way, this is the high point of the retreat.

Woman: I think all of us probably have done a great deal of searching here. I can remember as a child I was always talking to God, but as I got older, I just got all clogged up and stopped. And then when I got to college, I did my homework and I got through and got a couple degrees. I was always taking home all these books. Since I'm an intellectual, I just really went the gamut. I read everything. But it was just words. It was just nothing. And I was really stagnant. I have been very very stagnant for a long time. I even went through psychotherapy, but I don't think I grew in my heart.

This is my first time ever to be with Swamiji and with all of you. It was just through some Integral Yoga classes that I started subscribing to the magazine and I just looked at Swamiji's face and said, "This is what we all want. It's just so beautiful, and it's so real." So I thought, "Well, I just have to get that peace, too." Even my husband was very eager for me to come. He said, "Even though we both can't come, we'll still grow, because you'll bring back something." I don't know how to take it back except maybe slowly I'll start living it. But I just have so much to take back. I remember my husband asking me from another room, "Oh, Satchidananda's going to be there?" And I said "Yes." Can you imagine how I'm going to explain about "Satchidananda"? (*laughter*) Another thing I know, just in looking in all your faces, is that you really do have love and you really do have peace. And I know that this is what we want. I don't think I'm near that at all, but I know for the first time that I'm free. (*applause*)

Girl: I had a terrible time getting used to this place. I hated it for quite a few days. But I knew I had to stay, because of the confrontation. I was basically very upset with it because it made me see that I was ashamed of myself, and to see how inadequate I felt in certain ways. So I knew I had to stay. And I stayed. I tended to be on the periphery of things but in some ways it had to affect me. And I knew that I had to come up here and speak. I knew I had to do it, because it's been probably the major turning point in my life. And I thank you all. And I thank Swamiji. (*great applause*)

Man: There're just a few things I'd like to share with you. Just before I came here I was in California, and I went up for one day to Yogaville West and they said, "That's not a retreat. That's a yogic circus they're going to have there!" All the retreats in the past haven't had the kind of program we've had here. As joyous as they've been, they've been more . . . austere. Of course they were the stepping stones to this kind of a retreat. And another reason retreats seem to get better is because we seem to get better!

But this particular format was absolutely incredible, because it was truly ecumenical. People could come from different walks of life – we saw bhaktis: Jewish bhaktis, Hindu bhaktis, bhakti bhaktis; we saw jnanis, we saw everything, in all different combinations, presenting things in their own way, in their own time – and it was just incredible. That was one thing.

Another thing I want to mention: I just had this realization that in another few years we're going to be out there like Swamiji wants us to be – not sitting away in seclusion someplace, but out there being in some way essences of him and his teachings. Doing whatever we're doing, whether it's rapping, teaching, or making music, we're just going to be.

That's what I learned both from Swamiji and from Ram Dass — just to be, and don't try to look to expectations. Now that I can just accept and be, I can see that we're all going to be and be beautiful and things are going to change. (*applause*) Om Shanthi.

Swamiji: And if you're all going to "bee," there'll bee a lot of honey! (*laughter*) Hm?

Woman: There are two things I want to say. I was at the Annhurst Retreat two years ago and what I felt and learned there helped me survive for two years. And now I am here, and I am overwhelmed by how the whole thing just seems to have spread out and melted into the soil. Thank you.

Girl: Thursday morning I decided to come to this retreat. And Thursday afternoon I was on my way. And right now I am in kind of a bad time in my life. But I want to thank you for not letting me drop, but picking me up. (*she cries*) And I never met you before. I want to tell you that I'm afraid of the effect that you're going to have on my life. (*light laughter*)

Man: Here's just a little something that I'd like to sing, that I feel pretty deeply in my heart. And I feel that you all feel the same way too about this wonderful man here. (*singing*) "Should my heart not be humble, should my eyes fail to see, if I walk and I stumble, stay with me — Swamiji. You're the glow of the morning, that's the prelude to the dawn. If we know you're by our side, we'll go on. We'll be strong." Thank you. (*great applause*)

Woman: I just want to say that all year long I worked with little children. And it's very easy to love little children. But being here with Satchidananda and being here with you has turned me on to the little child within myself and in all of you too. You're all beautiful. Thank you. (*applause*)

Woman: I'm very full. I was trying to get to the retreat all last week. But I couldn't get up here. I had job interviews every day. And I finally made it very late Friday night. I've been very full all weekend. Every joyous thing that happened. And all of you — I've been crying half the weekend, but not from sadness, from joy. And this beautiful lady over here, this mother who's here with her daughter and her son. I have a daughter twenty years old. I've been trying to get her to come to a retreat with me since last year. And I haven't been able to get her here yet. And these three are so blessed and it's my desire that some day my daughter and I can share all of you and Swamiji and all of this beauty and love together. Thank you all. (*great applause*)

Swamiji: Thank you.

Man: Thanks very much to the IYI in New York for making this possible. I didn't think I'd be here. I think they've taught me to not use my mind but to just be. Thank you. Thank you, Swamiji. (*applause*)

Woman: I just wanted to say that this was a real sweet-and-sour retreat. And I'd like to thank Brother David for articulating and understanding the sour. I really felt at times that real loneliness and alienation. But I'd especially like to thank Swamiji for the sweet. I've begun to realize that the guru does live within each one of us.

Woman: I was really hidden a long time. And a couple of years ago a miracle happened. Something took me out of the San Francisco suburbs and took me shopping for a mantram. (*laughter*) I guess I would have gone to the Safeway if they had been on sale.

Swamiji: "Safe" way? (*great laughter*)

Woman: Yes, I went to the 'Satchidananda Safe-Way" — and it's been a wild two years. And now I think of Swamiji not only as the beautiful laundryman but the great tenderizer in the butcher shop. He just takes his cleaver and he just keeps hammering away at my heart. Just trying and trying to tenderize it some more. Thank you, Swamiji, and thank you all.

Boy: I have a secret and I want to share it with everyone. It has something to do with what you do when you leave here. You have some anxieties about the trip coming to an end, so to speak. And it took me nine months to learn this, so I'll pass it on.

Last summer I went to a retreat, and shortly after that I got on a 450 Honda, and for nine months I rode through the U.S. and Mexico and parts of Central America. Before I left I took a little folder that had a picture of Swamiji on it from the IYI. It's free, you know, you don't have to pay anything for it. And when I packed my bags I couldn't leave that out. I had to take it with me.

So I carried it with me on the motorcycle everywhere I went. I hung it up now and then. Sometimes I did and sometimes I didn't. But I looked at it when I noticed that I was carrying it. And it would get to be raining in New Orleans and there was no place to stay and I'd end up in some garage: I'd paste the picture up on the wall. When I climbed a mountain in Guatamala I'd paste it up on a tree. Everywhere I went I was carrying Swamiji with me. And I kept looking at the picture and I kept wondering, who is this man? What does he do? But I said, it's okay, just keep carrying Swamiji. And I'd get out on the bike every day and I'd do my Honda Yoga. (*laughs*) But while I did it all, I kept carrying that picture and I found that I was pasting it up on the wall more and more. So that's the secret. What do you do when you leave here? You carry Swamiji with you. (*applause*)

Woman: A couple of weeks ago I wrote Swamiji a letter to ask him if it would be all right to go to the September Retreat in California, because I'd be eight months pregnant. He wrote back very quickly, and the first thing that fell out of the envelope was the brochure for this retreat. "Why is he sending me this? I wanted to go to the September retreat." I read the letter and he said, "Well, you're only five months pregnant now. Why don't you come to this one?"

Well, I live in California, and it's an awful long way, and a lot of money to come out here. But I've got the time, I've got the money, and Swamiji *did* suggest it. He said it was just a suggestion, but I don't believe it! (*laughter*)

So, here we are, my husband and I. We'd been wandering around for almost a year now, ever since we'd left the Institute, sort of getting emptier and more drained. We thought we were making our life better and better 'cause we were having all these "experiences" of going to Tahiti and all these things, but we came back to California because we weren't finding what we were looking for. We just kept getting worse and worse. So we said, "Well, we can't get much worse." So we came out here to the retreat.

I wrote a letter to Swamiji. I gave it to him when I got here. I just cried in the letter and I said, "You can write me a letter when I get back home". But the next day, "Swamiji wants to see you." And I thought "Oh no . . .!" I was sick; I had a fever; I didn't feel well, and I was just shaking. But both of us went in and Swamiji said, "Oh, changes, so many changes." And I just said, "God, I don't feel like the same person at all." And he said, "You look so dry, you look so dry." And I thought, "Yes, I felt so drained and so dry, as if all the life had gone out of me since I'd left the Institute." I'd actually left everything there. I couldn't really practice. I was meditating, but it was just so dry. Most of the time if was just blugh.

So we talked to Swamiji and asked him what we should do, and he said, "Well, maybe you should move up by Yogaville." The Ashram? And I said, "Oh, no." Because my husband and I had this conflict – he didn't want to live in an ashram and I do. Then I looked at my husband and he said, "Well, why don't we move up by the Ashram?" And I looked. He amazed me. "You want to move up there?" So I guess we're going to go move up there.

Swamiji said that we looked so dry when we came here. Now, I feel like I've just been watered and watered and watered. (*laughter*) I felt like I'm just blooming again. I really do feel that way, like my whole life has been reborn. And I would like to thank you all.

Swamiji: You don't look dry now, hm? This couple is really a very exemplary couple. I should tell you that when they came to Santa Cruz for the first time, they saw me, they heard me, and they immediately joined the Institute. They just opened up their hearts. They had some money, and at that time we were planning to buy a house for Santa Cruz. They said, "Here is the money. Take it and use it." They gave all the money to buy the house there. And then still their karma took them away. They went around here and there. But now they've come back, hm? So they're open-hearted people. Even the bright sun gets clouded once in a while, but the clouds don't remain there. They get dispersed. Only keep up the spirit. The clouds will pass away. Nothing's going to stand in the way.

Actually, she came here very much dried, but she's very much changed within these few days. That's how we can see that there's a hope for everybody. Don't get disturbed because some dense cloud comes in the way. The sun is always behind, hm? Know that for certain. It's only a temporary cloud hiding you from seeing the sun. My master Swami

Sivananda always used to say, "Even this will pass away." *Even this will pass away.* You can call that "this" anything you want, whether it is a white cloud or a dense cloud. It's all fleeting, changing. So just keep watching. Don't get frightened. Even this excitement will pass away, hm? If you want to cling to that excitement – "I must have it always "– then when it goes, you are sad. So clinging to the pleasures, as well as putting a negative attitude to the sufferings, both are bad. Treat them alike. Let them come. They're different types of clouds. But you just be there. Know that the sun is always shining."

Woman: I have a list. It's a very short list, but I tried. Some of the grass needs cutting. The buildings are a little too spread out. The topography is very hard on bare feet. (*laughter interspersed throughout*) You asked for pickles. I think when Swamiji asks for something, we should try to do it. It rained a lot. Everybody has to admit it rained a lot. I didn't get to go swimming. It was boring here and there a little bit, come on, right? Does anybody here dislike getting up early? There are your pickles! (*Swamiji can be heard making sounds of agreement, "Yea . . . hmm"*) Let's see a show of hands of people that think it either rained too much or they didn't swim or they didn't sleep enough or they don't like to get up early . . . your pickles. (*Swamiji: "Good, fine . . ."*) My last pickle is that it has to end. (*applause, and Swamiji can be heard really enjoying it. He says, "Beautiful. I want it. I got it. Hm?" Laughs.*)

Boy: Hello. I haven't worked in a year and I have a very big debt to about 25 million people in Canada who have been paying for my unemployment insurance. But I'll pay it back somehow! I feel I'm like a bull who's sort of stomping the ground before he rushes forward. I'm going to go anytime. It's going to happen. The last job I had I would stand in front of 20 people, immigrants who didn't speak English, and say, "Ah, good morning." I was a teacher. I'm ashamed to say I was a teacher. Swamiji, how does it feel to help people wake up?

Swamiji: It's nice.

Boy: I want to thank you for all you've given me, for all you've given us. Thank you. (*applause and Swamiji can be heard in the background saying "good morning."*)

Girl: What's so overwhelmingly and so passionately and vibrantly real is that Swamiji is surely the incarnation of Love. (*applause*)

Swamiji: Who won't love such faces? Even a wild animal who looks at such faces will melt — why not a Swami? Look at these faces, hm? The beauty, the love; *you* make me love. I can't do anything else. It's so beautiful. You teach me how to love.

Girl: The last time I saw Swamiji was at Hunter College, and I asked him to help me put out my fire, so that's why I'm here. And I'd like to share with you something that happened to me on this retreat. The first retreat I went on was the Easter Retreat and getting out of the car I banged my head. And on this retreat, on the third day, before meditation I banged my head again. And walking to meditation I said, what's going on? I keep getting hit on the head (*laughter*) and I said, I think somebody's knocking at my door. And it felt awfully good. And I want to thank Swamiji for all his blessings and all of you because my heart has melted. Thank you. (*applause*)

Boy: I'm really just the hard-assed kid from Brooklyn: the hippie, the theater freak, the acid-tripper. But then somebody gets up and talks and I'm sitting on the floor watching them and all of a sudden I start crying because their love comes through, you know, it just keeps coming through. I went to my first retreat two months ago, to see why people in white at the Institute were saying things like, "Wow, Wow!" (*laughs*) So I came as a skeptic because that's my nature, and I met Swamiji and said "Wow!" It's just unreal how lucky we are to be in the presence of somebody like this.

You know, I'm from New York City and paranoia is rampant there. Suddenly for 10 days I never thought about losing my camera. I never thought that somebody was going to sock me in the head. It wasn't a conscious decision. I just never thought of it. It was just gone. All of you have that trust too, because you don't feel that tension from anybody. You all have the tears, and you all have the love, and you all have the smiles, and you all have the doubts, too, but it doesn't matter; you all have that thing. And that's what freaks me out. At the last retreat I was a retreatant and it was my first retreat. And this time I'm on the staff and I can only say thank you for letting me serve you. (*applause*)

Girl: Hello, when I came here I was very confused. I had a lot of trouble trusting people and everything and now that I've been here I can't explain what it is but all that is changed somehow, and I feel a lot better. Thank you. (*applause*)

Boy: I fully expected this retreat to be the greatest experience in my life — and I wasn't let down. It's the greatest experience in my life. You're beautiful. You've been told a million times. Thanks from the bottom of my heart. (*applause*)

Woman: When I first came here and I saw people bowing to Swamiji and to their brothers and sisters, I was really astounded. I thought you only do that to God when you're in church! So it kind of came together!

I left my husband not long ago and decided that men were uchk! But I really appreciate the way that the men here have just let the barriers down and let the love from me as a sister just come out. It's almost always that way with my sisters because women are just kind of flowing, but here it was the same with the brothers too.

And one more thing: it really helped to hear from the people in whites. I don't even know if you call yourselves disciples or what you are, but to hear your stories and to find out that you're really human and you have the same hang-ups and problems and joys that I do, made me start feeling like one of you. Thank you. (*applause*)

Woman: Last Thursday I got "detached" from my Indian bedspread and I really felt very badly about it, but then I realized that it was exactly what needed to happen to me. I'm so attached to all my possessions, I just own so much, and eat so much food — got to have it, have it. So thank you, whoever took it. It was like the kriya cleansing. (*laughter*) (You can hear Swamiji laughing a lot.)

Also, I've been smiling all week, and I never smiled this much at all. And just thank you so much, everybody who has been smiling back at me. In the city I'm just so scared of all those people, and I never smile at anybody, and especially those people on the subway that, you know, (*high-pitched laughter*) . . . and when I see somebody like that, I'm just going to keep smiling at them and smiling at them until they just have to break down . . . (*applause*)

Girl: I have a friend who ran around being chased by the FBI for about nine months before he decided to accept the word of God and face up to induction into the Army. And now he's in Fort Sill, Oklahoma. I visited him there right before I came to this retreat and I kept asking him questions like; "How can you stand it? How can you take what they're giving you? And HOW can you keep this schedule up all the time?" And I'd ask him questions like; "What time do you have to be here and what time do you have to be there?" And he'd just look at me and answer and laugh, and just shake his head. And I really didn't understand at all what he was trying to say until I came here and realized that he knew what Karma Yoga is all about. He accepted perfectly. It is not what you do but how you do it. And through the grace of Swamiji I can see that now. Thank you. (*applause*)

Woman: Most of the first few days I had a terrible time, really terrible. The only ones I could communicate with were the chipmunks. That's really true. And the reason that it was such a bad time was because I have a lot of trouble with words like God and guru and holy. Then I have that terrible ego trip, where I sit on the side and say, "I'm not holy," and I cry. I'm sure many of you have gone through it. And a lot of things happened like people started reaching out very much by smiles and looks and a hand and a hug. I got such a tremendous feeling of family here that I will carry it back with me. It means very much to me. And then when Shlomo came and he sang about holy beggers, then even the word holy was all right. (*laughs*) Then I could handle it. It's just gotten better and better. Yesterday, when Ram Dass was starting to sing that song "Listen, listen, listen, to my heart's song, I will never forget you, I will never forsake you" — I couldn't sing. I just sat there. You know, I'm a singer, I love to sing and chant all the time. But I couldn't sing at first. So I just looked at all of you. I just looked at so many faces that I loved. I felt so much love in the faces that all of a sudden my mouth opened up and there it came and I was swaying back and forth. And it was just tremendous for me. And the message that I'm going to carry back for myself about holiness and about God, is just to let my heart be open as much as possible and to look into the faces of people and to find God and guru and holiness in everybody and everything I see. Thank you very much. (*great applause*)

Swamiji: And that transformation came into you because in the very beginning you recognized the chipmunks. Hm? (*laughter*) Then you recognized the monks! (*more laughter*)

Young man: OM, brothers and sisters and holy fathers. I come from India. The only person who worries too much about me when I am away from home is my mother. She always thinks, "How will my son be in that foreign land? Will he be taken care of well by his friends, will he be loved and fed?" So today I can truly write to my mother, "Dear Mother, don't worry about your son, he's surrounded by the holiest of the holy brothers and sisters and the most divine Father." (*applause*)

This is right from the bottom of my heart. I don't even know how I'm going to write to her. My father has chanted all his life. He sings holy songs of Krishna. Every morning and evening when I was a little boy I used to go with him to the temple and sing the songs with him, but then I went to college and I became "intelligent," and I said, "What are these kirtans and all this?" That didn't fit with my thinking. You know in college they don't teach about God, particularly in India. So with that intelligent mind I came here, went to college again. When my father finds out that his son is becoming a little kirtan singer again, he's just going to flip out! (*lots of laughter and applause*)

I was in India just three months ago. I visited several ashrams, and I learned about Yoga, but believe me, the gathering of the retreat and the love and the warmth and the joy and the purity we have here is as holy as the holiest of the ashrams of the Himalayas. And we were blessed by Swamiji to put us in that divine situation. One thing I noticed when I was visiting all the ashrams was about Americans. In all those ashrams there are more foreigners than Indians, and out of all the foreigners, there are more Americans than people from any other country. And one thing I saw in them is that they're very *intense*. They will do anything they are told by the masters who are running the ashrams. They'll sit and chant; they'll eat any food they are given; they'll never complain about anything, they'll just do their thing, so intensely, without evaluating and analyzing. It was just amazing, and as an Indian, I was saying, a lot of times from my ego, "Hey, how can you do this, how can you do that?" but not Americans. I'm now seeing the same thing here. One quality you Americans have is the intensity. When you play, you play with intensity. When you play baseball, you don't play anything less than the world series. (*laughter*) When you go out in the space you don't go out any place less than the moon. So when you become devotees you don't know anything less than God. (*great applause*)

And I can see this in all these faces here – that we want nothing but God; you know, that's what we want. You say, "If you have it, give us, Swamiji." And Swamiji keeps saying, "Yes, you come to my feet and you'll get it. You become a devotee and you'll get it." And he really means it. Now we have all this energy, and we all want that real getting closer to God. But what about the other people? What about the people who wanted to come to the retreat but just couldn't make it for a number of reasons? I think one of the things we can do when we go back is to bring five more people — each one of us — to the next retreat, so we will keep multiplying like that. Then the whole world could be a heaven one day. Thank you. (*applause*)

Woman: I would like to say that I came here because I needed the association of all you fine people, and it was through the mercy of God and the grace of the guru that I found myself when I'd fallen away from my spiritual practice. You find yourself doing that when you're involved in the business world. I really needed this life and my spirit has been lifted. I feel that I can go back and go forward instead of backward, to serve selflessly instead of being a slave to my ego, and it's just really overwhelming. (*applause*)

The next person to come up and share her feelings is Sister Peggy. She is one of the small staff of four Catholic sisters who manage the Monticello camp site, which has been rented for the occasion of this Yoga retreat. These sisters, who cooperated very beautifully with the retreat staff, have more or less remained in the background during the past ten days — so much so that most retreatants have been unaware of them.

Sister Peggy: I hope I'll be able to express to you the feelings that we have and that we have been trying to explain to each other these past few days. We work here, four of us, and it unfortunately becomes a business. We become overactive. I want you to know that the presence of the Yoga staff and of yourselves has given us new eyes to love our place and to love each other. I was thinking last night that it will be so sad to come to this hall next week, when it's empty, but it won't be empty. I want you to know that you've left us a beautiful legacy. And we really have that in our hearts. The gentleness of all of you has saved us even despite ourselves. We were trying to keep at it feverishly, and we weren't able to. And we're so grateful, so extremely grateful for that. Just now we received some very very tragic news. Sister Christine, who is the administrator here, has just lost her mother a few moments ago. The call just came. And I want you to know that their love relationship was a magnificent one. But please know that in the Divine Providence you have really prepared her for this most traumatic experience of her life.

You have gentled her and given her a gift of peace, that's going to allow her to accept this as Grace. Thank you so much. (*applause*)

Man: The thing that has saved me is that I've been able to laugh a lot. I need to laugh a lot, 'cause I'm very scared. (*laughter*) I was scared before I came. And sometimes I'll be scared again. But those are temporary states, and in between I've been able to be myself more than in any other stretch that I can think of. And that's very important. Before I came I was afraid of submitting to ten days of austerity or I don't know what. But the great gift that Swamiji gives me is that when a delusion is its heaviest and when the mask is firmly in place, Swamiji's love cuts through all of that. When I'm guarding myself, his love cuts through all of that. Swamiji's given that gift to me many times ... but he still sneaks it up on me when I'm not looking. And the gift that *you* all have given to me, that I'll treasure always, is to be so many and to be so different outwardly, but to have shown me over and over again the humanity and the divinity that is within us all. Thank you. (*applause*)

The last person to share her feelings is Shanthi, Swamiji's personal secretary.

Shanthi: Knowing that you're all about to go out into the world I just want to share with you some words that Swamiji gave me at one of the several times that I was thinking of leaving him. I am telling you these words because they are the words that guru and God are telling us at every moment if we can only hear them. Swamiji asked me, "Well, you're going out. What is the one thing that you always know that you should remember? What one thing is there?" And I said, "I know, Swamiji, that I love you." And he said, "Well, even if you forget that, you should remember that I love you." Thank you.

Concluding Comments

Swami Satchidananda

This is the end of the retreat. After the closing comments by the retreatants, there is a final meal together, prepared and served by the retreat staff, and then everyone will be leaving to go back to their homes. Before adjourning to the meal, however, Swamiji takes the opportunity to make some concluding comments, as a final word to all those who will be taking back this experience into their regular lives.

You have really made me speechless! We are all beginning to feel instead of to think and talk. We have been hearing people saying how they feel. But truly you can never put your feelings into words. It's impossible. Words have their limitations. You can't even bring out one hundredth of what you feel. And now if you're all going to feel this much just by being with a few of us, imagine how *we* must feel by being with so many of you loving, loving people.

This itself is a proof that we are all born with that divine love, divine purity. We have that element in us. There's no need to go and ask anybody in order to feel that. God made man in His own image and likeness. What other proof do you want? And that is the very reason why we feel that beauty, that tranquility, that flowing love. Not just because of one or two individuals, but because we're all really expressing our true nature here. Somehow, temporarily, all the elements that were hiding our true nature were left outside. They have already had to wait outside for ten days. I'm sure by this time they would have got tired and gone away. So when you go back, you won't be seeing them anymore. That is what the retreat is meant for. Just to bring out our true nature, and to realize and live in that.

The Hindu scriptures say that whoever goes to take a bath in the Ganges, the holy river, goes with all his sins, but the minute he steps into the water, the sins stay on the shore, because they can't go into the river. If they do, they'll get completely dissolved. They know that and just stay out. So he takes a bath. And as long as he's in the water he's pure, beautiful, but unfortunately he can't stay that way long. The minute he walks out, they come to him again.

311

And that's what happens when we go into solitude or into prayer or into meditation for a few minutes or hours. When we stop, they are waiting to catch us again. But in the retreat, because we have been here long enough to assure ourselves about our own beauty, or own truth, we are getting rooted in this knowledge. So when you go back home you will still go with this awareness and they won't come to attack you any more. Some of them have even gone away because they got tired of waiting for you. They thought that you were not going to come any more, so they have gone to see some other people in whom they can live, hm? That is the benefit of this secluded atmosphere. When you get rooted in this knowledge, you will go out and be able to handle things very easily without getting affected by them.

So that's why this is not the end of the retreat. This is the beginning of a new life. You're going to carry this truth, the beauty, the love that you have experienced, with you when you go. Who made it? It's not just one or two individuals or the Swamis and the teachers or the staff members. We were only watchmen to remind you and to see that no one came and disturbed your peace. We were just your friends. So you were enjoying your own beauty. You created the atmosphere. When the opportunity was given, the dormant, beautiful tendencies in you came to the surface. So that's what you call satsang, the company, the group environment.

So now, just to remind you of what you should be doing when you go back — more or less as a conclusion — remember that you are born physically and mentally pure. You are born with all the divine qualities like that of a baby. When we were born, how beautiful our faces were! Without any kind of make-up. Everybody loved our faces. Why? Because of the beauty within. The child has that tranquility. It never gets caught in these ups and downs, the dualities. To the child, nothing is big, and nothing is small. Give a golden doll — it will play with it. Take it away and give it a clay doll, it will play with that. It doesn't feel any difference. It doesn't know who is an enemy and who is a friend; who is rich, who is poor; who is black, who is white; who belongs to what country or what religion. And that is the secret of why it's so beautiful — because the mind is so tranquil.

As we grow we seem to be getting involved in these intellectual gymnasiums, hm? In a way, when I even heard some of the questions asked of Brother David, I felt, "What is this? Why should we go into all these intellectual things?" If you have faith, go ahead. But nobody can force that faith into you. It cannot be proved. How do you know that so and so is your mother? You just feel it. You don't ask your mind. "Is she mother?"

You ask your heart; it tells you. It's all in you. Truly speaking, everything is divine.

Every morning, the Indian village housewife gets up and comes to clean the front yard. Then she goes back to the cow shed in the back yard, and she just picks up some cow dung, rolls it into a nice ball, brings it, and puts that right in front of the entrance of the house. She draws a nice diagram, a kind of mandala, to make it a little more beautiful, and then she puts this cow-dung ball right in the middle. Then she puts a little sandlewood paste, ash, burns a little camphor in front of it, falls prostrated, and says, "God Ganapathi, You are the remover of all interferences, all disturbances, all troubles. Please protect me, protect my house, my children, my family for the whole day." And then she walks in to do all her work. She knows that she herself went to the back yard and brought a little cow dung. Until she went there and brought it and put it here, it was just cow dung. She will never do the same thing, prostration, with a lump of cow dung that is still in the yard. You may call it a blind faith or foolishness or whatever it be. She doesn't worry about what you think. To her that ball of cow dung which she picked and planted there is Ganesh, the elephant-headed God who is going to protect her and her house for the whole day. What does it mean? What makes that separate ball of cow dung Ganesh and the big heaps of cow dung just ordinary dirt? Faith. If you believe it's so, it is so. If you don't believe it, even if the Lord Ganesh comes and sits in front of you, you'll say, "Hey, what is this, who are you, get out! I'm a little frightened of you!"

Your religion, your God, your Guru, your teachers, your parents, your friends . . . they're all with you because you trust. You believe it to be so. You believe somebody is your friend, so he is your friend. The minute somebody comes and tells you something against him, and you believe it, the next second he is no longer your friend. Is it not so? So who makes the friend and foe? Your mind. Who makes the God and Devil? Your mind. It's all from within. That's why we don't need to worry about God. God is there. We are not creating God. We cannot create Him or eliminate Him. He is there. But we are trying to understand with our own minds. If you have that faith, you see. If you don't have it, you see something different. That's the reason you don't need to go and disturb anybody's faith. If you don't believe in something, it doesn't matter. You don't believe it. But at least you believe in something else. Take that as your approach. Why should everybody believe the same thing?

I often give this example: If I believe in my own pudding which I enjoy so much, does it mean that I must force that belief into you and say that you must all eat pudding, otherwise you will go to hell? If you come and say, "No, no, I like bread and butter," and a third man comes and says, "No, I must have only Macrobiotic," a fourth man will say, "You're all fools, the only proper food is spaghetti!" No, we all have the same hunger, but we satisfy it with so many different kinds of foods. It is the same in the spiritual field also.

Another point I would like to tell you before you go back home. Many people tell me, "My job is not really yogic; I have to serve meat or do this or that." I say, if you can't get any other job, it doesn't matter; do the one you have until you get a better one. And when you do it, don't hate that. Love it, because somebody is going to eat that. If you inject your hatred into that, he will have stomach trouble. Do your job and at the same time pray to God, "God, I don't know. This is what You gave me. I'm just doing it as part of my service, not for my own sake but because I have to get some money to support myself and my family. If you think I should not be doing this, find a good job for me. I am also on the lookout ... but until I get a good job, I can't be starving, I have to do something."

There is the story of Vyadan in the Hindu scriptures. He was a butcher who was also a great Karma Yogi. Yes, even a butcher could be a Karma Yogi. He even initiated a seeker who had spent years and years in the forest. The seeker went to him and said, "I was asked to come to you for initiation. But I see that you are a butcher! How is that possible?"

"Well, that is my *swadharma,* my duty. It just happens that way. I have to be here but I'm not doing it for my own joy. It is my duty, and whenever I cut an animal I see the dedication of that animal and I pray, "Oh animal, you gave your life to feed these men. Let me also give my life to feed everybody like you do."

So, we should think that way also. Every action could be made holy. Whatever be your job, think that way. Don't curse the job; don't curse the boss, but be thankful. At least he is helping you to get your food and pay the rent. You must be thankful to him. That will build up a good understanding between the boss and you. And if you are the boss, treat the others as your colleagues helping you, not as servants.

Ultimately, all these jobs are needed for the welfare of the humanity in one way or another. So treat that as your Karma Yoga. Then come back to your house, rest, relax, and treat your family as God given. God brought some people to be under your care. Take good care of them. And if you happen to be a man of solitude who is staying away from any personal responsibilities to dedicate himself for the whole community as a monk, perform *that* duty.

And when you leave the retreat, take care of your food also. It can still be Yogic. Don't think that you will ever die without all those proteins! I'm surviving all these years without all that. An elephant is stronger than any animal and it is a strict vegetarian. With all their vitality, monkeys are vegetarians. Almost all the animals are vegetarians: horses, cows, goats. . . . All the wild animals are carnivores. That's why I say, "Live the life of the retreat." Try to go to bed early so that you can be up early. Even at home you can go to bed at 10 o'clock if you want, or at the latest, 10:30. Don't stay up too long seeing all these "Kung Fu" (*lots of laughter*) or Perry Mason! You've seen enough. If you really don't feel like sleeping, repeat any chant or mantram.

That's another important point, as Brother David reminded us. Mantra repetition is there in every religion. So repeat your mantram until you feel sleepy. Just sleep with mantram and you'll wake up with mantram. Even if you are awakened all of a sudden in the middle of the night for some reason, get up with that mantram. So let the mantram be part and parcel in your life. When you drive you can repeat the mantram. Constant mental repetition is very beneficial.

And then, just sleep like a baby. Don't worry about tomorrow. We don't know whether there is a tomorrow or not until we wake up again, is it not? Who knows if we are going to wake up or not? You yourself don't know. You are at the mercy of the Mother Goddess. You're just putting your head on the lap of the Mother. Feel that way when you put your head on the pillow. Treat that pillow as the soft lap of the Mother: "Mama, I'm just lying on your lap. Put me to sleep. If you think I am fit and useful, wake me up. Otherwise take me, because what am I doing here? Your work. If you think I am fit to do some more work tomorrow, hire me; otherwise fire me." That's Yoga.

If you are constantly that relaxed — physically and mentally — you express your divinity. People will see that you are God. I am sure that at least for some time people are going to say that to you: "Hi, what is happening with you? Is that what the retreat taught you?" Certainly, they're all going to ask you. Everybody will see the change in you.

I'm really eager to tell you that you should keep up this life and maintain this as you have been doing. That's all I want to tell you. And God bless you for all these beautiful, beautiful days. If our roads cross, we may meet each other physically; otherwise spiritually we are never separate. We are one. God bless you.

Glossary

ahimsa — non-injury.

ajnana — lack of Self-knowledge.

apana — descending energy within the body.

Aquarian Age (Eng.) — Age of peace and expanded consciousness which many believe to be coming.

Arjuna — Sri Krishna's disciple in the Bhagavad Gita.

asana — firm, steady posture for meditation; also Yoga postures done for health.

ashram — spiritual community.

Ashtavakra — ancient Indian sage of the Epic period.

Ashtavakra Gita — lit. "Song of Ashtavakra"; his spiritual teachings.

astral plane — subtle plane.

Atma(n) — true Self.

(Sri) Aurobindo (1872–1950) — Indian Yogi and sage of Pondichery, S. India, who wrote widely and who conceived Auroville, a spiritual city near Pondichery.

Avatar — God manifest in a human form.

Bar Mitzvah (Hebrew) — Jewish ceremony celebrating a boy's entry into manhood.

bastrika — bellows breathing technique which cleanses the blood, alerts the mind and awakens the dormant energy within.

Be Here Now — by Ram Dass, Lama Foundation, 1971; practical book on modern yogic life.

Benares — city in India where many Hindus go to die, believing they will be liberated.

Bhagavad Gita — lit. "Song of God"; section of the Mahabharata epic which gives Sri Krishna's instructions to Arjuna on all aspects of Yoga.

Bhagavan — the Lord in the personal aspect.

bhakta — devotee

Bhakti Sutras — attributed to Narada; authoritative text of Bhakti Yoga. Translation available by Swami Prabhavananda, Vedanta Press, Hollywood.

Bhakti Yoga — yogic path of devotion.

bija — lit. "seed"; refers to powerful, universal mantrams normally given in mantra initiation from a qualified guru.

Bodh Gaya — place of Buddha's enlightenment in Northern India.

Brahma — creative aspect of God.

brahmachari — one who practices brahmacharya.

brahmacharya — lit. 'Wandering in Brahman'; sense control, especially sexual continence.

Brahman – Absolute God or the pure static Consciousness.

(chakras) – subtle psychic centers along the spinal column which awaken during deep meditation.

chid – knowledge or consciousness.

darshan – lit. "vision"; experience of seeing a divine form or presence.

dasa – servant.

devatas – divine forms; aspects of the one Supreme Divine Consciousness.

dharma – righteousness; duty; the Cosmic Plan.

Durga – divine aspect as Mother; consort of Lord Siva.

Ganga (Ganges in English) – holy river in Northern India.

Gopala – Sri Krishna as a baby or small child.

gopi(s) – milkmaid devotees of Sri Krishna (as the Cowherd Boy); represents how all souls are the lovers of the One Supreme Lord.

gunas – qualities of nature.

guru – lit. "remover of the darkness"; spiritual guide.

Guru Poornima Day – full moon day of July, set aside for honoring the spiritual teacher.

(Sri) Hanuman – greatest devotee of Sri Rama; said to have had the form of a monkey. His story is told in the Ramayana epic.

Hari – name and mantram of the Lord, especially as Lord Vishnu, the preserving aspect.

Hari OM – a universal mantram.

Hatha Yoga – system of physical postures, breathing techniques, relaxation and cleansing practices for good health as well as a preparation for meditation.

Himalayas – holy mountains in Northern India.

householder (Eng.) – married person.

I Ching – philosophical and oracular book of China.

ida – the subtle nerve channel along the left side of the spinal column.

initiation – usually means receiving a meditation technique (such as a mantram) from a guru along with a portion of his energy which awakens that mantram within. Can also refer to the ceremony with which one enters Sannyas (the monkhood or renunciate life).

Ishta Devata – one's chosen deity which one worships and meditates upon.

Jaganath Puri – a famous Krishna temple in Puri, India.

Jai! – "victory".

japa – repetition (of a mantram).

jiva – individual soul.

Jnana Yoga – yogic path of self-analysis and awareness.

jivanmukta – liberation while living.

jnani – one who knows the Self.

Kabir or Kabirdas (1440–1518) – Indian poet-saint who preached brotherhood between Indian Moslems and Hindus.

Kali — Lord as Mother; consort of Lord Siva.

kamya — with desire for selfish result.

karma — action and reaction; destiny.

Karma Yoga — yogic path of selfless action, dedicating the results of one's actions to God or humanity.

kevalya — emancipation; liberation.

King Janaka (Raja Janaka) — a king during Epic period; known as the ideal Karma Yogi, he ruled a kingdom yet was rooted in Self-knowledge.

kirtan — chanting the names of God; mantra chanting.

(Sri) Krishna — avatar of Lord Vishnu, the preserving aspect of the Supreme; giver of the *Bhagavad Gita.*

(Sri) Krishna Chaitanya (1485–1533) — great Bhakti saint and devotee of Sri Krishna. Sometimes thought to be another avatar of Vishnu.

kriya — lit. "action"; sometimes refers to certain Hatha Yoga cleansing techniques; can also refer to the preliminary stage of Raja Yoga as expounded by Patanjali.

kundalini — lit. "serpent power"; the Divine Power dormant within each person.

Lakshmi — Divine Mother; consort of Narayana (Vishnu).

Lama Anagarika Govinda (1898–) — German-born, Tibetan Buddhist lama and scholar.

leela — lit. "play"; the entire creation as the Play of the Lord.

(Sri) Ma Anandamayi (1896–) — great Indian woman saint; guru of Swami Nirmalananda.

Mahabharata — one of the two great Hindu epics; tells the story of a war between two parts of the same family, representing the struggle between the good and evil forces in the mind of a seeker. Also tells of the avatar Sri Krishna.

Maharaj Ji — teenage Indian teacher who has many devotees in the U.S. Founder of Divine Light Mission.

Maharaji — Indian saint and guru of Ram Dass.

Maharishi (Mahesh Yogi) — proponent of Transcendental Meditation and founder of the International Meditation Society.

Maha Vakyas — four great Vedantic formulas: "Prajnanam Brahman" — Pure Consciousness is Brahman; "Aham Brahmasmi" — I am Brahman; "Tat Twam Asi" — Thou art That; and "Ayam Atma Brahma" — This Atman is Brahman.

mala — rosary used for counting number of mantrams repeated.

mantram — sound symbol of the Divine.

maya — illusory world of names and forms.

(Saint) Mirabai (1547–1614) great poet-saint and devotee of Lord Krishna.

moorthi – image; embodiment; statue.

mouna – silence.

(Swami) Muktananda – Indian Siddha guru with an ashram at Ganeshpuri, S. India,

mukti – liberation.

Mundaka Upanishad – one of the twelve principal Upanishads according to Shankara.

Muruga – Hindu deity; son of Lord Siva.

nama-rupa prapanjam – the name-form world.

Namaste – "Salutations to you." A respectful Indian greeting.

Narada – supposed to be the son of Goddess Saraswati and a great devotee of Lord Narayana who wanders throughout the universe chanting God's names and playing the veena (an Indian stringed instrument).

Narayana – Vishu; the preserving aspect of God.

Nayanar(s) – the name of sixty-three Siva devotees famous for sticking to one vow throughout their lives.

Neti, neti – "Not this, not this." Vedantic formula to remove false identification with names and forms.

nirvana – lit. "nakedness"; liberation.

nisang – unspiritual company.

nishkamya – without desire for selfish result.

niyama(s) – observances in Raja Yoga: purity, contentment, austerity, study and self-surrender.

OM – Sound symbol of the Absolute.

Oy Gevalt! Oy Vey! (Yiddish) – Ejaculations; something like, "Oh my!"

Padma Sambhava – founder of Tibetan Buddhism.

padmasana – lotus posture; thought to be the most ideal pose for pranayama and meditation.

(Sri) Panduranga – an incarnation of Lord Vishnu, the preserving aspect of God.

Parabrahman – Supreme Brahman or Absolute God or Consciousness.

Paramahamsa Ramakrishna (1836–1886) – great Indian saint; guru of Swami Vivekananda.

Paramahansa Yogananda (1893–1952) – Indian Yogi and guru; founder of the Self Realization Fellowship.

Paramatma(n) – Supreme Atma or true Self.

Parvathi – Divine Mother; consort of Lord Siva.

Patanjali (possibly 2nd Cent. AD) – compiler of the *Yoga Sutras,* the authoritative text of Raja Yoga.

pingala – subtle nerve channel along the right side of the spinal cord.

Prakriti – nature.

prana – life force, vitality.

pranayama – control over the life force; often refers to certain breathing practices designed to help one gain such control.

puja – worship.

Puranas – auxiliary scriptures of Hinduism written to popularize the Vedic truths through legends about the divine Incarnations, saints and devotees.

Purusha – the true Self.

raja – king.

Raja Yoga – the yogic path of mind control through ethical perfection, steady pose, control of prana, senses and thoughts and ultimate absorption in pure Consciousness.

rajas – restlessness, activity.

(Sri) Ram or Rama – an incarnation of Lord Vishnu, the preserving aspect of God; told of in the Ramayana. Also a powerful purificatory mantram.

(Sri) Ramakrishna Paramahamsa – see Paramahamsa Ramakrishna.

Ramana Maharshi (1879–1950) – great Indian Jnana Yogi.

Ramayana – Hindu epic telling the story of Sri Rama, avatar of Lord Vishnu.

Ravana – demon king whom Rama vanquished in Ramayana story; represents our lower nature.

rishis – ancient Indian sages who formulated and practiced Yoga.

sadhana – spiritual discipline.

sahaja – natural; continuous.

Saivite – worshiper or Lord Siva.

samsara – illusory round of births and deaths.

samskara – mental impression.

Sanatana Dharma – Eternal Truth; the names Indians give to their religion, known to others as Hinduism.

sanctum sanctorum (Latin) – inner temple shrine where Deity resides.

sanga – company, group.

Sannyas – monastic order organized by Shankaracharya in the 8th century AD.

Sannyasi(n) – monk (feminine – sannyasini).

Sanskrit – ancient scriptural language of India.

sant – saint.

Santji – shortened form of respect and endearment in addressing an Indian saint.

Saraswati – Goddess of learning; represents sattvic aspect of Divine Mother.

Sat – Truth.

Satchidananda – Truth – Knowledge – Bliss Absolute.

satsang – spiritual company.

Satya Yuga – Age of Truth where all are righteous.

sattva – Purity, tranquility.

seevan (Tamil) – individual soul (same as Sanskrit "jiva").

Self-Realization Fellowship – Yoga organization founded by Paramahansa Yogananda.

shalom (Hebrew) – hello, goodbye, and peace.

shakti – power; divine energy; feminine principle or aspect of God.

(Sri) Shankara or Shankaracharya (686–718 AD) – Indian jnani and bhakta who established the order of Sannyas; great reformer of the Hinduism of his day; thought to be avatar of Lord Siva.

shanthi – peace.

Shrimad Bhagavatam: classic Hindu scripture.

siddha: one who possesses siddhis.

siddhis: occult powers obtained through yogic practices.

Sita — Rama's wife: incarnation of Lord Krishna.

Siva — destructive and regenerative aspect of God; also Supreme Lord; auspiciousness.

Siva Lingam — egg-shaped symbol of Lord Siva.

Sivan (Tamil) — Siva.

(Swami) Sivananda (1887–1963) — great Indian Yogi; Swami Satchidananda's guru.

Sivaratri — festival honoring Lord Siva.

Sivoham — "I am Siva"; Vedantic formula used in Jnana Yoga.

Sixty-three Nayanar Saints, by Swami Sivananda, Divine Life Press; stories of South Indian Siva devottees.

sloka — verse.

Soham — "I am He" (meaning Brahman or God); Vedantic formula in Jnana Yoga.

Sri — title of respect and reverence; also used as we use "Mr."

sushumna — central subtle nerve channel through the spinal column through which the kundalini rises in deep meditation.

Swami — a monk, used as title in front of a monk's name.
(For individual Swamis mentioned in text, please see their name; e.g. for Swami Vivekananda, see Vivekananda.)

Swamiji — respectful and endearing form in addressing a Swami.

tamas — inertia, dullness, sloth.

Tamil — South Indian language; Swami Satchidananda's native tongue.

Tantra Shatras — scriptures concerning ritual worship of Vishnu, Siva and Shakti.

Tantra Yoga — Yoga of ritual worship of Vishnu, Siva or Shakti.

tapas or tapasya — austerity or penance; accepting sufferings which come to oneself, while not inflicting sufferings on others.

Tat Twam Asi — "Thou art That" (meaning Brahman, the Absolute God); Vedantic formula in Jnana Yoga.

Tukaram (1568–1650) — Indian poet-saint and great devotee of Vishnu.

Tulsidas (1511-1637) — Indian poet-saint who composed a highly devotional version of the Ramayana.

untouchables — outcastes; below even the lowest Hindu caste. They do the most menial tasks and until recently were not even allowed to worship in the temples.

Upanishads — the last section of the Vedas, describing the Absolute Brahman and the path to Self-realization; the Vedanta.

Vedanta — lit. "end of the Vedas"; the Upanishads, where the truth about Brahman is described.

Vedas – Hindu scriptural revelations; the oldest world scriptures.

Vibhishana – Ravana's (q.v.) virtuous brother who took refuge at Sri Rama's feet and was accepted although he came from the enemy's camp.

Vishnu – the preserving aspect of God; avatars are held to be incarnations of this aspect.

(Swami) Vivekananda (1863–1902) – dynamic Yogi and one of the first to bring Yoga to the Western world.

yantra – visual symbol of the Divine.

yamas – restraint or control; first step in Raja Yoga: truthfulness, non-injury, non-stealing, continence and non-hoarding.

Yagnavalkya – Indian sage of the Epic period.

Yidalach (Yiddish) – Jews.

Yoga – union of the individual self with the Universal Self; communion.

Yoga Sutras – authoritative Raja Yoga text compiled by Patanjali.

Yogananda – see Paramahansa Yogananda.